Prostate Cancer: Symptoms, Diagnosis & Treatment - 2nd Volume

Prostate Cancer: Symptoms, Diagnosis & Treatment - 2nd Volume

Topic Editors

**Ana Faustino
Paula Oliveira
Lúcio Lara Santos**

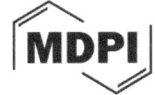

Basel • Beijing • Wuhan • Barcelona • Belgrade • Novi Sad • Cluj • Manchester

Topic Editors

Ana Faustino
University of Évora
Évora
Portugal

Paula Oliveira
University of Trás-os-Montes
and Alto Douro (UTAD)
Vila Real
Portugal

Lúcio Lara Santos
Portuguese Institute of
Oncology
Porto
Portugal

Editorial Office
MDPI AG
Grosspeteranlage 5
4052 Basel, Switzerland

This is a reprint of the Topic, published open access by the journals *Current Oncology* (1718-7729), *Diagnostics* (ISSN 2075-4418) and *Uro* (ISSN 2673-4397), freely accessible at: https://www.mdpi.com/topics/prostate_Cancer2.

For citation purposes, cite each article independently as indicated on the article page online and as indicated below:

Lastname, A.A.; Lastname, B.B. Article Title. *Journal Name* **Year**, *Volume Number*, Page Range.

ISBN 978-3-7258-2783-1 (Hbk)
ISBN 978-3-7258-2784-8 (PDF)
https://doi.org/10.3390/books978-3-7258-2784-8

© 2024 by the authors. Articles in this book are Open Access and distributed under the Creative Commons Attribution (CC BY) license. The book as a whole is distributed by MDPI under the terms and conditions of the Creative Commons Attribution-NonCommercial-NoDerivs (CC BY-NC-ND) license (https://creativecommons.org/licenses/by-nc-nd/4.0/).

Contents

Alessandro Cicchetti, Marianna Noale, Paola Dordoni, Barbara Noris Chiorda, Letizia De Luca, Lara Bellardita, et al.
Patient-Factors Influencing the 2-Year Trajectory of Mental and Physical Health in Prostate Cancer Patients
Reprinted from: *Curr. Oncol.* **2022**, *29*, 8244–8260, https://doi.org/10.3390/curroncol29110651 . . 1

Guangyu Sun, Zhengxin Liang, Yuchen Jiang, Shenfei Ma, Shuaiqi Chen and Ranlu Liu
Clinical Analysis of Perioperative Outcomes on Neoadjuvant Hormone Therapy before Laparoscopic and Robot-Assisted Surgery for Localized High-Risk Prostate Cancer in a Chinese Cohort
Reprinted from: *Curr. Oncol.* **2022**, *29*, 8668–8676, https://doi.org/10.3390/curroncol29110683 . . 18

Mehmet Asim Bilen, Akinyemi Akintayo, Yuan Liu, Olayinka Abiodun-Ojo, Omer Kucuk, Bradley C. Carthon, et al.
Prognostic Evaluation of Metastatic Castration Resistant Prostate Cancer and Neuroendocrine Prostate Cancer with [^{68}Ga]Ga DOTATATE PET-CT
Reprinted from: *Cancers* **2022**, *14*, 6039, https://doi.org/10.3390/cancers14246039 27

Dongho Shin, Seunggyun Ha, Joo Hyun O, Seung ah Rhew, Chang Eil Yoon, Hyeok Jae Kwon, et al.
A Single Dose of Novel PSMA-Targeting Radiopharmaceutical Agent [^{177}Lu]Ludotadipep for Patients with Metastatic Castration-Resistant Prostate Cancer: Phase I Clinical Trial
Reprinted from: *Cancers* **2022**, *14*, 6225, https://doi.org/10.3390/cancers14246225 37

Islam Kourampi, Ioannis-Panagiotis Tsetzan, Panagiota Kappi and Nityanand Jain
PARP Inhibitors in the Management of BRCA-Positive Prostate Cancer: An Overview
Reprinted from: *Uro* **2023**, *3*, 40–47, https://doi.org/10.3390/uro3010006 48

Elisa Bellei, Stefania Caramaschi, Giovanna A. Giannico, Emanuela Monari, Eugenio Martorana, Luca Reggiani Bonetti and Stefania Bergamini
Research of Prostate Cancer Urinary Diagnostic Biomarkers by Proteomics: The Noteworthy Influence of Inflammation
Reprinted from: *Diagnostics* **2023**, *13*, 1318, https://doi.org/10.3390/diagnostics13071318 56

Laura García-Zoghby, Cristina Lucas-Lucas, Mariano Amo-Salas, Ángel María Soriano-Castrejón and Ana María García-Vicente
Head-to-Head Comparison of [^{18}F]F-choline and Imaging of Prostate-Specific Membrane Antigen, Using [^{18}F]DCFPyL PET/CT, in Patients with Biochemical Recurrence of Prostate Cancer
Reprinted from: *Curr. Oncol.* **2023**, *30*, 6271–6288, https://doi.org/10.3390/curroncol30070464 . 70

Vinayak G. Wagaskar, Osama Zaytoun, Swati Bhardwaj and Ash Tewari
'Stealth' Prostate Tumors
Reprinted from: *Cancers* **2023**, *15*, 3487, https://doi.org/10.3390/cancers15133487 88

Chung-Hsin Chen, Chung-You Tsai and Yeong-Shiau Pu
Primary Total Prostate Cryoablation for Localized High-Risk Prostate Cancer: 10-Year Outcomes and Nomograms
Reprinted from: *Cancers* **2023**, *15*, 3873, https://doi.org/10.3390/cancers15153873 99

Leandro Lima da Silva, Amanda Mara Teles, Joana M. O. Santos, Marcelo Souza de Andrade, Rui Medeiros, Ana I. Faustino-Rocha, et al.
Malignancy Associated with Low-Risk HPV6 and HPV11: A Systematic Review and Implications for Cancer Prevention
Reprinted from: *Cancers* 2023, *15*, 4068, https://doi.org/10.3390/cancers15164068 112

Hendrik Ballhausen, Minglun Li, Elia Lombardo, Guillaume Landry and Claus Belka
Planning CT Identifies Patients at Risk of High Prostate Intrafraction Motion
Reprinted from: *Cancers* 2023, *15*, 4103, https://doi.org/10.3390/cancers15164103 125

Jucileide Mota, Alice Marques Moreira Lima, Jhessica I. S. Gomes,
Marcelo Souza de Andrade, Haissa O. Brito, Melaine M. A. Lawall Silva, et al.
Klotho in Cancer: Potential Diagnostic and Prognostic Applications
Reprinted from: *Diagnostics* 2023, *13*, 3357, https://doi.org/10.3390/diagnostics13213357 142

Matthieu Vermeille, Kira-Lee Koster, David Benzaquen, Ambroise Champion, Daniel Taussky, Kevin Kaulanjan and Martin Früh
A Literature Review of Racial Disparities in Prostate Cancer Research
Reprinted from: *Curr. Oncol.* 2023, *30*, 9886–9894, https://doi.org/10.3390/curroncol30110718 . 157

Moisés Rodríguez Socarrás, Juan Gómez Rivas, Javier Reinoso Elbers, Fabio Espósito, Luis Llanes Gonzalez, Diego M. Carrion Monsalve, et al.
Robot-Assisted Radical Prostatectomy by Lateral Approach: Technique, Reproducibility and Outcomes
Reprinted from: *Cancers* 2023, *15*, 5442, https://doi.org/10.3390/cancers15225442 166

René Fernández, Cristian Soza-Ried, Andrei Iagaru, Andrew Stephens, Andre Müller, Hanno Schieferstein, et al.
Imaging GRPr Expression in Metastatic Castration-Resistant Prostate Cancer with [^{68}Ga]Ga-RM2—A Head-to-Head Pilot Comparison with [^{68}Ga]Ga-PSMA-11
Reprinted from: *Cancers* 2024, *16*, 173, https://doi.org/10.3390/cancers16010173 175

Emmanuella Oyogoa, Maya Sonpatki, Brian T. Brinkerhoff, Nicole Andeen, Haley Meyer, Christopher Ryan and Alexandra O. Sokolova
Mixed Adenosquamous Cell Carcinoma of the Prostate with Paired Sequencing on the Primary and Liver Metastasis
Reprinted from: *Curr. Oncol.* 2024, *31*, 2393–2399, https://doi.org/10.3390/curroncol31050178 . 188

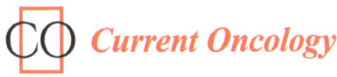

Article

Patient-Factors Influencing the 2-Year Trajectory of Mental and Physical Health in Prostate Cancer Patients

Alessandro Cicchetti [1], Marianna Noale [2,*], Paola Dordoni [1], Barbara Noris Chiorda [1], Letizia De Luca [1], Lara Bellardita [1], Rodolfo Montironi [3], Filippo Bertoni [4], Pierfrancesco Bassi [5], Riccardo Schiavina [6], Mauro Gacci [7], Sergio Serni [7], Francesco Sessa [7], Marco Maruzzo [8], Stefania Maggi [2], Riccardo Valdagni [1,9,10,†] on behalf of The Pros-IT CNR Study Group

[1] Prostate Cancer Program, Fondazione IRCCS Istituto Nazionale dei Tumori, 20133 Milan, Italy
[2] Aging Branch, Neuroscience Institute, National Research Council, 35128 Padua, Italy
[3] Molecular Medicine and Cell Therapy Foundation c/o, Polytechnic University of the Marche Region, 60121 Ancona, Italy
[4] Prostate Group, Italian Association for Radiation Oncology (AIRO), 20124 Milan, Italy
[5] Department of Urology, Policlinico Gemelli, Catholic University of Rome, 00168 Rome, Italy
[6] Division of Urology, IRCCS Azienda Ospedaliero-Universitaria di Bologna, 40138 Bologna, Italy
[7] Department of Urologic Robotic Surgery and Renal Transplantation, Careggi Hospital, University of Florence, 50134 Florence, Italy
[8] Medical Oncology Unit 1, Veneto Institute of Oncology IOV-IRCCS, 35128 Padua, Italy
[9] Department of Oncology and Hemato-Oncology, Università degli Studi di Milano, 20122 Milan, Italy
[10] Unit of Radiation Oncology, Fondazione IRCCS Istituto Nazionale dei Tumori, 20133 Milan, Italy
* Correspondence: marianna.noale@in.cnr.it; Tel.: +39-0498218899
† The Pros-IT CNR study group members are listed at the end of the article.

Abstract: This study aimed to examine the physical and mental Quality of Life (QoL) trajectories in prostate cancer (PCa) patients participating in the Pros-IT CNR study. QoL was assessed using the Physical (PCS) and Mental Component Score (MCS) of Short-Form Health Survey upon diagnosis and two years later. Growth mixture models were applied on 1158 patients and 3 trajectories over time were identified for MCS: 75% of patients had constantly high scores, 13% had permanently low scores and 12% starting with low scores had a recovery; the predictors that differentiated the trajectories were age, comorbidities, a family history of PCa, and the bowel, urinary and sexual functional scores at diagnosis. In the physical domain, 2 trajectories were defined: 85% of patients had constantly high scores, while 15% started with low scores and had a further slight decrease. Two years after diagnosis, the psychological and physical status was moderately compromised in more than 10% of PCa patients. For mental health, the trajectory analysis suggested that following the compromised patients at diagnosis until treatment could allow identification of those more vulnerable, for which a level 2 intervention with support from a non-oncology team supervised by a clinical psychologist could be of help.

Keywords: prostate cancer; health related quality of life; SF-12; growth mixture model

1. Introduction

Prostate cancer (PCa) is one of the leading cancers diagnosed in adult males worldwide, with an estimated incidence of 1,436,000 new cases and an age-standardized incidence rate of 49.9 per 100,000 person-years [1]. Even if the stage of cancer detection with an early diagnosis is important for most cancer survival, for PCa, considering the extremely high one- and five-year survival rates, the stage of detection could be less important [2]. Cutting-edge diagnostic tools and treatments have improved numerous patients' quality of life (QoL). However, it is well established that PCa patients may show early signs of psychological distress (e.g., anxiety, depression) in addition to physical problems [3,4]. PCa diagnosis represents a stressful life event that, together with treatment, can significantly impact the patient's psycho-emotional status and QoL. Although medium to long-term physical and mental QoL trajectories seem to differ and to be relatively stable in many patients [4], depression, anxiety, signs of post-traumatic stress disorder, pain, sexual problems, difficulty in urinating, along with other disturbances or symptoms, have frequently been reported during the initial and later stages of the disease [5]. Indeed, for non-metastatic PCa patients, anxiety and depression appear to be at their highest levels during the pre-treatment phase. Men reported significantly less anxiety, better mental health and feeling of depression following the initial phase of the treatment [6,7], with treatment decision-making having an impact on patients QoL [8]. As the psychological well-being of PCa patients is critically important, and adjustment to the disease is positively related to QoL levels [9–11], more knowledge about the possible trajectories and evolution of both physical and psychological states in patients facing PCa is needed. However, when evaluating longitudinal data, the heterogeneity in QoL trajectories among patients within a population may be masked by analyses based on mean effects; the growth mixture models (GMM) approach could be interesting since it assesses the existence of different trajectories within a population when grouping variables are not known a priori [12,13]. For this reason, the current work described the physical and mental QoL trajectories in Italian male adults diagnosed with non-metastatic PCa to determine who could benefit from personalised care support tools enabling the best possible clinical and personal outcomes [14]. Patients participating in the Pros-IT CNR study and monitored over two years after diagnosis were considered and data examined using the GMMs approach; socio-demographic and clinical variables were analysed with treatment patterns as potential predictors of the trajectories.

2. Materials and Methods

2.1. Participants

The design of the Pros-IT CNR project has been described in detail elsewhere [15]. It is a longitudinal, observational study aiming to monitor QoL in a sample of Italian patients diagnosed with biopsy-verified prostate cancer, beginning in September 2014. Ninety-seven Urology, Radiation Oncology and Medical Oncology facilities in Italy were involved in the project, and 1705 treatment-naïve patients were enrolled. A baseline assessment at the time of diagnosis and evaluations 6, 12, 24, 36, 48, and 60 months later were foreseen by protocol [16]. The data collected during the baseline assessment included demographic and anamnestic information, the initially formulated diagnosis, the cancer stage, the risk factors, comorbidities, and health-related QoL scores. Data regarding the cancer treatments and patients' QoL scores were collected at each follow-up examination.

The Ethics Committee of the coordinating centre (Sant'Anna Hospital, Como, Italy; register number 45/2014) and all the hospitals or health care facilities involved in the project approved the study protocol. The study was carried out according to the Declaration of Helsinki principles, and all of the participants signed informed consent forms.

2.2. Outcome Variables

The patients' general QoL was assessed using the Italian version of the Short-Form Health Survey (SF-12 Standard v1 scale) [17], which is composed of two summary measures: the Physical Component Score (PCS) and the Mental Component Score (MCS). The SF-12 is a widely recognised, reliable, and valid measure of health-related QoL commonly used in multicenter trials. Indeed, Gandek et al. showed that "for large group comparisons and longitudinal monitoring, the differences in measurement reliability of the SF-12 and SF-36 are less important". In fact, in a study such as this one, which focuses on "measuring overall physical and mental health outcomes rather than an eight-scale profile, the SF-12 may be advantageous" [18]. The score on each domain and the total score of each patient were computed using the algorithms suggested by Apolone et al. [17]. The possible range of scores on each section is between 0 and 100, with 100 indicating the best self-perceived health.

2.3. Predictor Variables

The patients' socio-demographic variables at diagnosis, their clinical variables, including comorbidities, the Gleason score, the clinical T-score, the prostate-specific antigen (PSA) level at diagnosis, as well as their PCa treatments, and their urinary, bowel, and sexual QoL at the time of diagnosis were considered as predictors.

The PCa treatments carried out up to the 24-month follow-up assessment were classified as follows:

1. Active surveillance (AS). The patients who did not remain in the group up to the 24-month follow-up were excluded;
2. Nerve-sparing radical prostatectomy (NSRP);
3. Non-nerve sparing exclusive radical prostatectomy (NNSRP);
4. Exclusive radiotherapy (RT);
5. Radiotherapy plus androgen deprivation therapy (RT plus ADT, not considering patients on ADT after radiotherapy for cancer recurrence).

Patients treated with adjuvant radiotherapy, adjuvant ADT after prostatectomy, or brachytherapy were not included in our analyses. The same applied to the patients who dropped out of active surveillance (Figure 1).

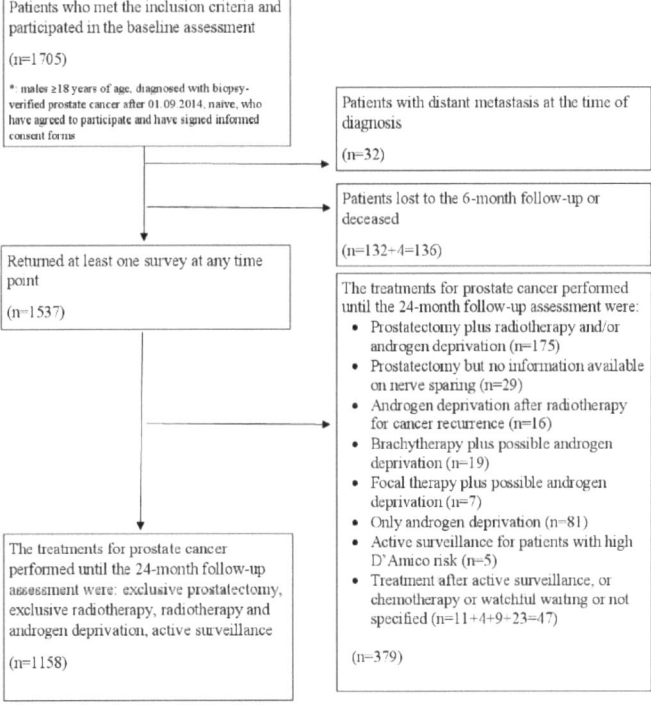

Figure 1. Flow Diagram of the Pros-IT patients.

The University of California Los Angeles-Prostate Cancer Index (Italian UCLA-PCI) [19,20] was used to evaluate urinary (UF), bowel (BF) and sexual (SF) function.

2.4. External Comparison

The MCS-12 and PCS-12 score distributions of the participants in the Pros-IT CNR project were graphically and statistically compared with those of an extensive survey conducted at the beginning of 2000 by the Italian Institute of Statistics (ISTAT) of the general Italian population and the oncologic group that also used the SF-12 questionnaire. The survey was carried out on a sample of 140,000 citizens; for the comparisons, we selected (i) the group of cancer patients ($n = 598$) and (ii) the group of male citizens within the same age range as the patients enrolled in Pros-IT ($n = 14{,}291$).

Raw data from that investigation were not available; statistical information regarding the distribution of the PCS and the MCS values were retrieved from the literature [17]. Mean values and the standard deviation were used to generate the data distribution.

2.5. Statistical Analysis

The data of the participants who underwent one or more of the follow-up assessments were analysed; missing values were not imputed. Summary statistics are expressed as means ± standard deviation (SD) or median and (Quartile 1 (Q1), Quartile 3 (Q3)) for quantitative variables and frequency percentages for categorical variables.

GMMs were applied to identify trajectories within the Pros-IT CNR population. When individuals are expected to experience different changes over time both in terms of strength and direction, a simple mean based trajectory could mask differences; modelling techniques considering heterogeneity in change over time could be preferred [21], and GMMs are statistical techniques that have been used to describe group differences in changes over time, estimating an average growth curve for each identified class, calculating intercept, slope and growth parameter variance by maximizing the log-likelihood function [12]. For each individual, the probability of belonging to each identified class is estimated on the bases of observed data, and participants are assigned to the group with the higher posterior probability, considering also the possible contribution of covariates [22]. SAS Proc Traj was used to identify the subgroups of participants with similar QoL trajectories [23,24], and the following steps were considered:

- the optimal number of groups was identified by fitting several models ranging from single to 5-group models;
- the shape of the trajectories was identified considering polynomials of varying degrees for each group, starting with a cubic specification, and then dropping non-significant polynomial terms;
- The model fit statistics (Bayesian Information Criterion (BIC)), the value of group membership probability and the average posterior probability (entropy) were considered to identify the best model:
  - the magnitude of the difference in the BIC ($2\Delta BIC > 10$) was used to choose between less or more complex models.
  - the analysis aimed to identify groups including at least 5% of the population;
  - the average posterior probability of membership was ascertained for each group; values greater than 0.7 indicate adequate internal reliability.

Chi-square or Kruskal-Wallis tests were then applied to evaluate unadjusted differences between the trajectory groups identified. Multinomial logistic regression models were used to evaluate the variables associated with the trajectory groups. Age at diagnosis, education, marital status, living arrangements, family history of prostate cancer, comorbidities, diabetes, body mass index (BMI), the PSA at diagnosis, the Gleason score, the clinical T-Stage, UF, BF, and SF at diagnosis (highest quartile vs lower quartile according to the distribution in the sample), and the PCa treatments were considered independent variables. Models were also adjusted for the time between the end of PCa treatment and the last follow-up assessment the patient underwent.

Additional GMM and logistic models were defined stratifying age according to its median value (<70 vs. ≥70 years).

A *t*-test was performed to compare the MCS-12 and PCS-12 scores with the ISTAT population.

All the statistical analyses were performed using SAS software version 9.4 (SAS Institute, Cary, NC, USA).

3. Results

Patients (n = 1705) were enrolled in the Pros-IT CNR study, and their characteristics at diagnosis have been described in detail elsewhere [16]. Data regarding the PCa treatments the patients underwent, excluding participants with distant metastasis at diagnosis (n = 32), were available for 1158 patients and included NSRP (n = 311), NNSRP (n = 187), RT (n = 334), RT plus ADT (n = 252) and AS (n = 74) (Figure 1).

Patients undergoing other treatments (n = 379 patients) were not considered in the present report. One thousand thirty-three participants (89%) underwent the 12-month follow-up assessment, and 804 (69%) underwent the 24-month one. Table 1 presents the characteristics at diagnosis of the patients included in the analyses; patients treated with RT and RT plus ADT were older, had more comorbidities and had higher-risk disease features in comparison with those treated with NSRP, NNSRP or AS.

Regarding the following analysis, we differentiated between:

- a statistically significant difference (p < 0.05);
- a minimal clinically important difference (MCID) in the mental or physical domain, i.e., how much of a difference in scores would result in some change in clinical management that is to be considered clinically meaningful [25]. Empirical findings from distribution based methods studies showed a tendency to converge to the $\frac{1}{2}$ SD criteria as a meaningful moderate difference [26,27]. In the following analysis, we considered the conservative estimate approach by Sloan and colleagues for a minimum clinical important difference (MCID = 1 SD) from the patient's perspectives [28,29]. This large effect size considers differences that overcome the limitations due to any subjective (the patient) and objective (the questionnaire) bias or error.

Table 1. Characteristics at the time of diagnosis of the Pros-IT population considered.

	Overall (n = 1158)	Nerve-Sparing Exclusive Prostatectomy (n = 311)	Non-Nerve-Sparing Exclusive Prostatectomy (n = 187)	Exclusive Radiotherapy (n = 334)	Radiotherapy and Androgen Deprivation (n = 252)	Active Surveillance (n = 74)	*p*-Value §
Age at diagnosis, years, mean ± SD	68.8 ± 7.4	63.2 ± 6.8	66.9 ± 6.1	72.8 ± 5.2	72.5 ± 5.9	66.9 ± 6.5	<0.0001
Education > lower secondary school, n (%)	562 (49.2)	178 (57.6)	100 (53.8)	144 (43.6)	97 (39.8)	43 (58.1)	<0.0001
BMI ≥ 30 kg/m², n (%)	177 (15.6)	34 (11.1)	29 (15.5)	56 (17.1)	50 (21.0)	8 (10.8)	0.0179
Current smoker, n (%)	166 (14.6)	48 (15.8)	35 (18.9)	43 (13.2)	29 (11.7)	11 (15.3)	0.2554
Diabetes mellitus, n (%)	172 (14.9)	23 (7.4)	28 (15.0)	57 (17.2)	59 (23.4)	5 (6.8)	<0.0001
3 + moderate/severe comorbidities *, n (%)	174 (15.0)	32 (10.3)	22 (11.8)	59 (17.7)	50 (19.9)	11 (14.9)	0.0089
Family history of prostate cancer, n (%)	187 (16.3)	71 (23.1)	32 (17.5)	39 (11.7)	37 (15.0)	8 (10.8)	0.0015
T staging at diagnosis, n (%)							
T1	557 (50.2)	200 (65.6)	97 (55.4)	131 (41.6)	63 (25.9)	66 (93.0)	<0.0001
T2	445 (40.1)	102 (33.4)	72 (41.2)	150 (47.6)	116 (47.8)	5 (7.0)	
T3 or T4	107 (9.7)	3 (1.0)	6 (3.4)	34 (10.8)	64 (26.3)	0 (0.0)	

Table 1. Cont.

	Overall (n = 1158)	Nerve-Sparing Exclusive Prostatectomy (n = 311)	Non-Nerve-Sparing Exclusive Prostatectomy (n = 187)	Exclusive Radiotherapy (n = 334)	Radiotherapy and Androgen Deprivation (n = 252)	Active Surveillance (n = 74)	p-Value §
Gleason score at diagnosis, n (%)							
≤6	535 (46.6)	186 (60.0)	76 (40.9)	155 (47.1)	48 (19.1)	70 (98.6)	
3 + 4	279 (24.3)	78 (25.2)	49 (26.3)	86 (26.1)	65 (25.9)	1 (1.4)	<0.0001
4 + 3	157 (13.7)	27 (8.7)	36 (19.4)	47 (14.3)	46 (18.3)	1 (1.4)	
≥8	177 (15.4)	19 (6.1)	25 (13.4)	41 (12.5)	92 (36.7)	0 (0.0)	
PSA at diagnosis, ng/mL, median (Q1, Q3)	7 (5.1, 10)	6.3 (5, 8.7)	6.9 (5.1, 10)	7 (5.1, 9.9)	8.9 (6.3, 14.3)	6.2 (4.9, 7.7)	<0.0001
D'Amico risk class, n (%)							
Low	303 (26.7)	120 (39.1)	43 (23.6)	70 (21.4)	10 (4.0)	60 (85.7)	
Intermediate	494 (43.5)	152 (49.5)	97 (53.3)	146 (44.7)	89 (35.7)	10 (14.3)	<0.0001
High	338 (29.8)	35 (11.4)	42 (23.1)	111 (33.9)	150 (60.3)	0 (0.0)	
UCLA PCI UF, mean ± SD	93.7 ± 15.1	96.5 ± 10.7	94.2 ± 15.0	91.9 ± 17.1	92.4 ± 16.5	93.8 ± 15.0	0.0006
UCLA PCI UB, mean ± SD	89.1 ± 22.7	92.8 ± 20.0	92.3 ± 19.5	86.2 ± 24.5	84.7 ± 25.8	92.5 ± 17.0	<0.0001
UCLA PCI BF, mean ± SD	93.6 ± 13.4	96.1 ± 9.3	94.3 ± 12.9	91.7 ± 15.4	91.8 ± 15.0	94.5 ± 12.6	0.0004
UCLA PCI BB, mean ± SD	93.7 ± 17.6	92.3 ± 12.9	94.6 ± 16.0	92.9 ± 18.4	90.4 ± 22.7	95.9 ± 14.4	0.0100
UCLA PCI SF, mean ± SD	50.2 ± 31.7	66.6 ± 27.0	56.4 ± 29.2	37.9 ± 30.3	37.9 ± 29.2	61.1 ± 30.2	<0.0001
UCLA PCI SB, mean ± SD	63.9 ± 34.8	71.8 ± 32.2	61.7 ± 35.1	58.7 ± 36.5	58.8 ± 34.8	75.7 ± 27.2	<0.0001
SF-12 PCS, mean ± SD	51.9 ± 7.2	53.7 ± 5.7	52.6 ± 6.7	50.8 ± 7.8	50.2 ± 8.3	52.7 ± 6.1	<0.0001
SF-12 MCS, mean ± SD	49.5 ± 9.7	49.3 ± 9.4	47.9 ± 10.0	50.2 ± 9.7	49.2 ± 9.9	50.9 ± 9.2	0.0300

SD: Standard Deviation; BMI: Body Mass Index; Q1: Quartile 1; Q3: Quartile 3. SF-12: Short-Form Health Survey; PCS: Physical Component Subscale; MCS: Mental Component Subscale. UCLA: University of California Los Angeles-Prostate Cancer Index; UF: Urinary Function; UB: Urinary Bother; BF: Bowel Function; BB: Bowel Bother; SF: Sexual Function; SB: Sexual Bother. Scores ranges from 0 to 100, with higher scores representing better quality of life in relation to functions or symptoms. * Based on Cumulative Illness Rating Scale (CIRS); § p-value from Chi-square or Fisher exact tests for categorical variables, generalised linear model after testing for homoschedasticity (Levene test) or Kruskal-Wallis test for continuous variables.

3.1. MCS Analysis

3.1.1. MCS at Diagnosis

At diagnosis, the mean MCS baseline value for the whole population was 49.3 with a SD of 9.4, which is the MCID for the mental status (Table S1).

While the average value in the patients undergoing AS (50.9 ± 9.2) was significantly higher than that of those undergoing NNSRP (47.9 ± 10), it was not clinically relevant. This finding will be examined at greater length in the discussion. Since no significant differences were found between AS vs. NSRP, RT or RT plus ADT (49.3 ± 9.4, 50.2 ± 9.7, 49.2 ± 9.9, respectively), the patients had similar mental statuses at the onset before they underwent different cancer treatments. In terms of age, if we consider the median age of our population as a threshold, the mean MCS value in the patients < 70 years old was 49.0 ± 9.6 vs. 49.9 ± 9.8 in those aged ≥70 years ($p = 0.0282$).

3.1.2. MCS over Time

The mean MCS values rose during the first 6 months after diagnosis; they also rose during the following 6 months and then fell between the next 12-month and the 24-month follow-up assessments (Figure 2).

Three trajectories for the MCS scores over the 24-month period analysed were identified (Figure 2; Table S2). We report in this section the baseline intercept mean coefficient (BIM), i.e., the baseline mean score according to the trajectory group, the trajectory score at 2-years of follow-up (2yrFU), the posterior group membership probability (GrMemb), i.e., the likelihood for all the patients within the group to be described by that trajectory

- The "reference group" (Trajectory Group 3 (75% of the patients with GrMemb = 0.97)): the patients in this group showed constantly high scores throughout the 24-month follow-up period. BIM was 53.9, 2yrFU was 51.4.

- The "recovering group" (Trajectory Group 2 (12% of the patients with GrMemb = 0.87)): this group of patients started with low scores at diagnosis, then presented higher values at the 6-month follow-up, which they maintained until the end of the assessment. The difference between the baseline mean value for trajectory 2 members (34.3) and the total population mean value (49.3) exceeded the MCID. The mental health improvement exceeded the MCID in the first six-month follow-up, and then trajectory 2 members had normal range of values for the following follow-up time (Figure 2, black line).
- The "permanently low score group" (Trajectory Group 1 (13% of the patients with GrMemb = 0.92)): this group of patients started with low scores. The scores first fell to an even lower level and then surged upwards. BIM was 39.2, the nadir was 34.2, and the 2yrFU was 44.1. The difference with the total population mean value at the baseline exceeded the MCID. In contrast with the group 2 trajectory, the more considerable discrepancy was recorded at 6 months (34.2), where the average value for the population was 51.0.

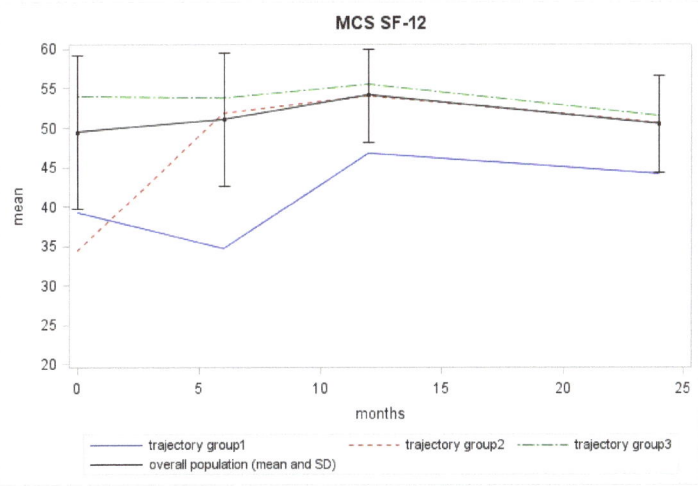

Figure 2. The mean MCS scores across the timeline of the 4 evaluations for the Pros-IT participants.

The predictors that significantly differentiated the MCS trajectories, evaluated using multinomial logistic regression analysis and considering Trajectory Group 3 (constantly high group) as a reference, were: age at diagnosis, comorbidities, a family history of prostate cancer, and the UF, BF, and SF scores at diagnosis (Table 2).

With respect to the constantly high group (Trajectory Group 3), patients in the "recovering group" (Trajectory Group 2) were younger at diagnosis and had higher levels of comorbidity. At diagnosis, high comorbidity levels were also significantly associated with Trajectory Group 1 membership ("permanently low score group"). A family history of prostate cancer was also significantly related to both Trajectory 2 and 1 memberships. The UF, BF and SF scores at diagnosis in the lower quartile (i.e., worst self-perceived functions) were associated with Trajectory 3 ("reference group") with respect to Trajectory 2 ("recovering group") membership. The lower quartile of UF and BF score was also associated with Trajectory 3 with respect to Trajectory 1 ("permanently low score group") membership.

A sub-analysis of the three MCS trajectories of the patients older and younger than 70 is included in the Supplementary Materials.

Table 2. Predictors of the trajectory class membership for the Mental Composite Score (MCS).

MCS SF-12	Trajectory 2 vs. 3		Trajectory 1 vs. 3	
	OR (95% CI)	p-Value	OR (95% CI)	p-Value
Age at diagnosis (years)	0.94 (0.91, 0.97)	0.0003	0.98 (0.95, 1.01)	0.2278
Education > lower secondary school	1.13 (0.76, 1.68)	0.5417	1.34 (0.89, 2.00)	0.1605
Marital status, married vs widowed, divorced or never married	1.39 (0.51, 3.80)	0.5257	1.12 (0.44–2.82)	0.8157
Living arrangement, with other vs alone	1.68 (0.52–5.46)	0.3908	1.84 (0.64–5.28)	0.2563
BMI ≥ 30 kg/m^2	0.82 (0.68, 1.19)	0.1784	1.04 (0.79, 1.38)	0.9759
Diabetes mellitus	0.88 (0.61, 1.10)	0.5628	1.00 (0.61, 1.70)	0.9580
Family history of prostate cancer	1.87 (1.17, 2.99)	0.0092	1.70 (1.03, 2.82)	0.0392
3 + moderate/severe comorbidities *	1.90 (1.16, 3.11)	0.0112	1.86 (1.15, 3.02)	0.0114
Current smoker	0.84 (0.48, 1.46)	0.5327	1.27 (0.74, 2.17)	0.3865
D'Amico risk class, high vs. intermediate/low	1.58 (1.00, 2.49)	0.0501	0.95 (0.59, 1.51)	0.8207
Prostate cancer treatments				
NNSRP vs. NSRP	1.23 (0.70, 2.14)	0.4757	1.13 (0.55, 2.32)	0.7350
RT vs. NSRP	0.69 (0.37, 1.27)	0.2331	1.58 (0.82, 3.02)	0.1716
RT plus ADT vs. NSRP	0.62 (0.30, 1.28)	0.1927	1.83 (0.88, 3.84)	0.1082
AS vs. NSRP	0.86 (0.35, 2.10)	0.7435	1.84 (0.78, 4.35)	0.1648
Distance between the end of treatment and follow-up assessment, days	1.01 (0.97, 1.05)	0.5037	1.05 (0.92, 1.10)	0.7563
UF at diagnosis §, highest quartile vs. lower ^{1}	0.55 (0.35, 0.85)	0.0075	0.52 (0.34, 0.79)	0.0024
BF at diagnosis §, highest quartile vs. lower ^{2}	0.43 (0.29, 0.65)	<0.0001	0.36 (0.24, 0.54)	<0.0001
SF at diagnosis §, highest quartile vs. lower ^{3}	0.48 (0.29, 0.80)	0.0051	0.77 (0.45, 1.32)	0.3369

NSRP: Nerve-Sparing Exclusive Radical Prostatectomy; NNSRP: Non Nerve-Sparing Exclusive Radical Prostatectomy; RT: exclusive Radiotherapy; RT plus ADT: Radiotherapy and Androgen Deprivation Therapy; AS: Active Surveillance; UF: Urinary Function; BF: Bowel Function; SF: Sexual Function; * Based on Cumulative Illness Rating Scale (CIRS); § Based on University of California Los Angeles—Prostate Cancer Index (UCLA-PCI). ^{1} UF = 100 vs. <100; ^{2} BF = 100 vs. <100; ^{3} SF $\geq$ 80 vs. <80.

3.2. PCS Analysis

3.2.1. PCS at Diagnosis

At diagnosis, the mean PCS value was 51.9 with a SD of 7.2 (Table 1). The mean score at diagnosis in the patients undergoing AS (52.7 ± 6.1) was significantly higher than that in the patients undergoing RT or RT plus ADT (50.8 ± 7.8 and 50.2 ± 8.3, respectively; Table 1). There were no significant differences between NNSRP and NSRP (53.7 ± 5.7, 52.6 ± 6.7, respectively).

3.2.2. PCS over Time

Mean PCS values in the overall population were substantially flat over the 24 months analysed (Figure 3).

Two trajectories for the PCS scores in the Pros-IT participants were identified (Figure 3; Table S3):

- The "reference group" (Trajectory Group 2 (85% of the patients with GrMemb = 0.98)): this group of patients showed constantly high scores throughout the 24-month follow-up, with a BIM of 53.2, a 2yrFU of 52.6;
- The "decreasing group" (Trajectory Group 1 (15% of the patients with GrMemb = 0.92)): this group of patients started with low physical scores at diagnosis (BIM = 42.9). The scores fell to an even lower level at the 6-month follow-up, and they continued to decrease until the 24-month follow-up assessment (2yrFU = 37.7). The difference between the baseline mean value for this trajectory group and the overall mean exceeded the MCID. The decline with time increased the distance in PCS for these patients and the trajectory Group 2.

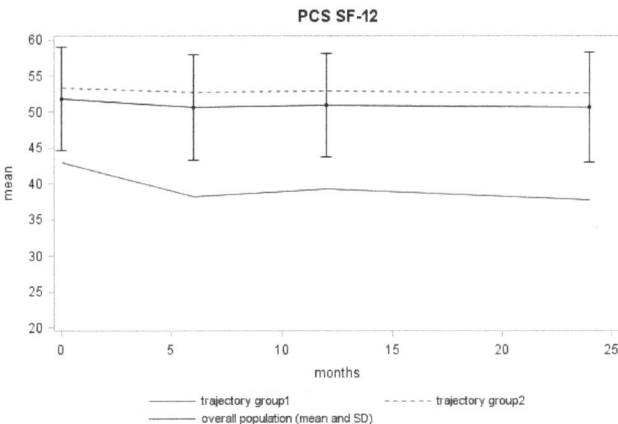

Figure 3. The PCS SF-12 scores across the timeline of the 4 evaluations for the Pros-IT participants.

The patient characteristics significantly associated with the PCS trajectories are outlined in Table 3.

Table 3. Predictors of the trajectory class membership for the Physical Composite Score (PCS).

	Class 2 vs. 1	
PCS SF-12	OR (95% CI)	*p*-Value
Age at diagnosis (years)	1.02 (0.97, 1.07)	0.4128
Education > lower secondary school	0.99 (0.60, 1.65)	0.9752
Marital status, married vs widowed, divorced or never married	1.02 (0.32, 3.30)	0.9691
Living arrangement, with other vs alone	1.23 (0.33, 4.64)	0.7632
BMI $\geq$ 30 kg/m^2	0.97 (0.67, 1.40)	0.8644
Diabetes mellitus, *n* (%)	1.99 (1.11, 3.59)	0.0214
Family history of prostate cancer	1.02 (0.52, 2.03)	0.9466
3 + moderate/severe comorbidities *	1.23 (0.67, 2.26)	0.5144
Current smoker, *n* (%)	1.35 (0.65, 2.82)	0.4193
D'Amico risk class, high	0.70 (0.40, 1.23)	0.2142
Prostate cancer treatments		
NNSRP vs. NSRP	1.05 (0.35, 3.15)	0.9327
ER vs. NSRP	3.01 (1.24, 7.30)	0.0150
RT plus ADT vs. NSRP	3.56 (1.18, 10.7)	0.0246
AS vs. NSRP	1.19 (0.24, 5.96)	0.8342
Distance between the end of treatment and follow-up assessment, days	1.06 (0.98, 1.13)	0.6156
UF at diagnosis §, highest quartile vs. lower [1]	0.55 (0.33, 0.94)	0.0284
BF at diagnosis §, highest quartile vs. lower [2]	0.47 (0.28, 0.78)	0.0032
SF at diagnosis §, highest quartile vs. lower [3]	0.47 (0.21, 1.07)	0.0727

NSRP: Nerve-Sparing Exclusive Radical Prostatectomy; NNSRP: Non Nerve-Sparing Exclusive Radical Prostatectomy; RT: exclusive Radiotherapy; RT plus ADT: Radiotherapy and Androgen Deprivation Therapy; AS: Active Surveillance; UF: Urinary Function; BF: Bowel Function; SF: Sexual Function. * Based on Cumulative Illness Rating Scale (CIRS); § Based on University of California Los Angeles—Prostate Cancer Index (UCLA-PCI). [1] UF = 100 vs. <100; [2] BF = 100 vs. <100; [3] SF $\geq$ 80 vs. <80.

The "decreasing group" was associated with high levels of diabetes. Moreover, lower quartile scores at diagnosis for UF and BF were significantly associated with the "decreasing group" membership. A borderline significant protective effect was also found for SF. This finding suggests that patients included in the Trajectory 2 Group had a compromised health condition. RT and RT plus ADT prostate cancer treatments, as opposed to NSRP, were significantly associated with the "decreasing group" trajectory membership.

A sub-analysis of the PCS trajectories younger and older than 70 is included in the Supplementary Materials.

3.3. Health Status Comparison with the Italian Population Collected by the ISTAT

The current study compared the PCS and MCS distributions in the Pros-IT study participants with those reported by the ISTAT. Particularly, the PCS and MCS in the men in the same age groups as those in the Pros-IT participants and in the group (male and female) with cancer were analysed. We generated the ISTAT distribution from the mean and standard deviation values included in the report and considered an asymmetrical normal distribution (toward the left tail). The distributions shown are thus not exact and have only a graphical meaning. Tables in Supplementary Materials (Tables S4 and S6) and the *p*-value coming from the *t*-test of the distributions have statistical meaning. Finally, we compared the impact of comorbidities on the PCS and MCS in the two studies.

3.3.1. Age Groups in the Men (Tables S4 and S5)

The ISTAT investigation presented the MCS and PCS in 6 age range divided by gender. We compared the Pros-IT distributions (855 patients) with the values obtained from the ISTAT male participants (14,291 citizens). Figure 4a,c show the distributions and analysis for MCS and PCS, respectively.

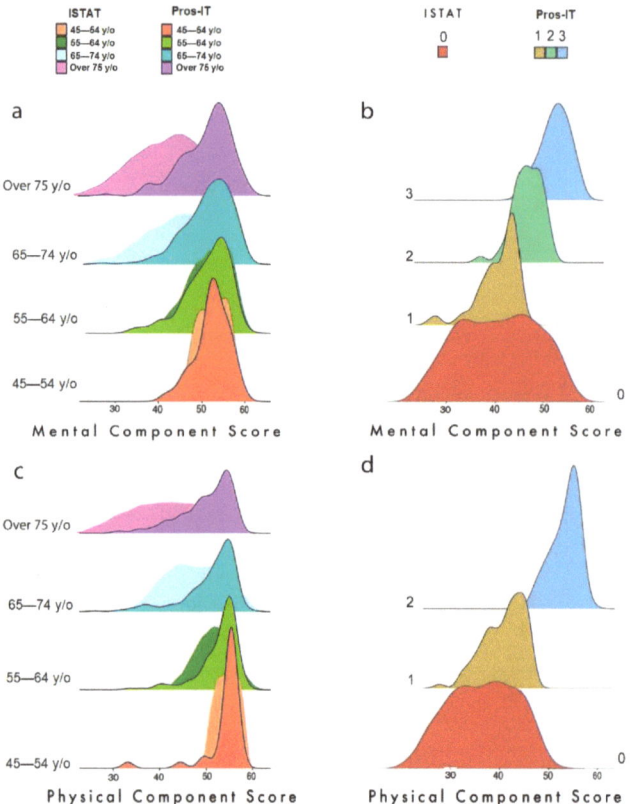

Figure 4. (**a**) Distribution of MCS scores of the Pros-IT and ISTAT populations according to age groups; (**b**) Distribution of MCS scores in trajectories for Pros-IT participants and of the ISTAT cancer patients; (**c**) Distribution of PCS scores of the Pros-IT and ISTAT populations according to age groups; (**d**) Distribution of PCS scores in trajectories for Pros-IT participants and of the ISTAT cancer patients.

A *t*-test was used to compare the distributions according to the statistical values reported in Table S4. A significant difference (*p*-value < 0.001) was found for both domains in the 65–74 and 75+ year ranges. For PCS, a significant *p*-value was also found in the 55–64 year-old group.

In both plots Figure 4c,d the ochre distribution depicts the 1st trajectory group; the powder blue one represents the 2nd trajectory group and the green one represents the 3rd trajectory group (defined only with regard to the MCS analysis); the red one represents the scores of the ISTAT population.

3.3.2. Cancer Pathology (Tables S6 and S7)

The ISTAT analysis showed the distribution of the mental and physical scales in individuals with several diseases, including cancer pathology. These data were used to compare the global health condition of the prostate cancer patient in Italy (represented by Pros-IT cohort, 684 patients) instead of the state of cancer patients (any cancer, characterised by the ISTAT subgroup of 598 citizens) (Figure 4b,d show the distributions and analysis for MCS and PCS).

To facilitate the comparison, we examined the average distribution overtime for the Pros-IT participants (the average distribution of the MCS/PCS at the five time-points) of the trajectory groups defined by our analysis, i.e., 3 groups for MCS and 2 for PCS.

We can infer from the comparison of the statistics in Table S6 that the mental condition of the Pros-IT patients was superior (*p*-value < 0.001 for the *t*-test comparing the distributions) to that of cancer patients in 87% of the cases. Only patients in Trajectory Group 1 (13% of the Pros-IT population) had a comparable mental state. As far as the PCS was concerned, the Pros-IT prostate cancer patients showed a significantly better average score for both trajectories (*p*-value < 0.001).

3.3.3. Impact of Other Diseases on the MCS and PCS (Tables S8 and S9)

Apolone and colleagues showed (reported here in Table S9) the relationship between PCS/MCS classes and the average number of comorbidities. The same table designed for the Pros-IT study (Table S8) confirmed a similar inverse correlation with comorbidities for PCS and MCS. Our findings indicated that the Pros-IT participants in the highest deciles had a mean of less than one comorbidity, while those in the first deciles had a mean of two or more diseases. This was true for both the PCS and MCS.

4. Discussion

The current study investigates the physical and mental QoL trajectories in Italian male adults diagnosed with PCa, who have been monitored for more than two years. In general, participants had a good QoL status, although some findings require further consideration.

For the mental domain, a large percentage of patients (trajectory 3) showed good mental health throughout the 24-month follow-up period. At the time of diagnosis, a limited number of patients (trajectory 1 and 2) experienced a clinically meaningful difference from the average value for the Pros-IT cohort. The evolution of these patients showed two different patterns with time. Twelve per cent of patients started with low mental health at the time of diagnosis but recovered 6 months after the event, suggesting that discomfort was likely generated by the cancer event and the uncertainties on the care path for these patients. Indeed, it can be hypothesised that after the patient has come to terms with the diagnosis [30] and has reached an agreement with health care professionals about treatment [10], he perceives less stress and, as a result, shows lower anxiety and better coping strategies (i.e., the constantly changing cognitive and behavioural efforts to manage specific external and/or internal demands) [6,31–33]. Most acute prevalences of depression, anxiety and psychological distress seem to occur before and after the conclusion of treatment, with possible negative impacts on QoL [7].

Another small percentage of patients (13%) showed low mental health at baseline, but they also did not manifest an improvement over time. In fact, in the core phases of the treatment, they experienced a further decrease in their mental health. Unlike patients in trajectory 2, they could have a limited array of resources to cope with the disease. It is worth noting that half of these patients (around 1/20 patients) were also included in the PCS trajectory 1. Thus, a discrepancy with the average population at two years could be explained by the impact of physical health on mental conditions.

As far as the participants' mental health was concerned, our results showed no clinical differences between the various treatments groups at the time of enrolment. Some predictors of mental health trajectories (younger men with 2 or less moderate/severe co-morbidities, no familiarity with PCa, and good mental health at the time of enrolment) were more likely to maintain stable mental health throughout the follow-up period. As previous studies have highlighted, age at diagnosis [34] and comorbidities [35] are critical predicting factors conditioning the path of mental health.

Regarding physical health, the patients with lower scores embarked on their path with a compromised health condition reflected by diabetes mellitus and worse urinary and bowel function. A significant *p*-value was also found for RT and RT plus ADT as opposed to NSRP in Trajectories 1 and 2. It is worth noting that the two trajectories started out with an important difference in the baseline value. Patients treated with surgery had a better health condition (see Table 1 for further details) and were able to face the treatment modality. On the contrary, patients who underwent RT and RT plus ADT worsened with time, but it is not clear if this could be associated with the divergent ways with which the more physically impaired group faced the treatment. The best clinical approach has to be selected for these patients to limit the discrepancy after treatment.

Several studies analysed the longitudinal evolution of physical and mental condition in PCa patients, averaging the scores according to the received treatment. Punnen et al. [36] reported similar trend; in particular, mental health remained stable over time with little difference across treatments while the adjusted physical function had a decline at 2 years, but no differences were highlighted between surgical and non-surgical treatments. Hoofman et al. performed a similar analysis dividing by PCa with favorable and unfavorable risk disease [37]; none of the treatment groups reported a clinically meaningful decline in physical function, emotional well-being, or energy and fatigue scores. In line with our scores, they confirmed that baseline physical functions were highest for men who underwent prostatectomy and lowest for those who underwent radiotherapy. Again, in the Protect study, no significant differences among the treatment groups in the physical and mental health sub-scores of the SF-12 scale were found [38]. Similar results at 2 years were reported by a multicentric Spanish trial using the SF-36 scale [39].

Considering factors associated with worse trajectories, a systematic review conducted by Vissers et al. found that cancer patients with diabetes had lower physical functioning and vitality [40]. Another study further demonstrated that cancer patients with diabetes had significantly lower levels of physical function and mental health over time compared to those without diabetes [41], and this result was partially confirmed in PCa patients [42], in accordance with our results. Reeve and colleagues evaluated longitudinally the impact of comorbidities evaluated with the Index of Coexistent Diseases on QoL, and they found a significant impact on physical component but no effect on the mental status [43], in contrast with our findings which was supported, instead, by Chambers et al. [4].

4.1. Comparison with ISTAT Study

Finally, we compared our findings with those of the ISTAT's survey focusing on the health state of the Italian population. For patients under 65, there was considerable overlap between the MCS distributions in the ISTAT (in the patients without cancer) and Pros-IT population. As far as the physical domain was concerned, the overlap in distribution was restricted to the group of patients under 55; for the other groups, the physical health condition of the current Italian prostate cancer patient was better than that of the average population 20 years ago. Concerning cancer (all types) patients investigated by the ISTAT study, the patients in Trajectory 1 showed better physical and mental scores. Given its favourable prognosis, the low impact of treatments' side effects (compared to others), the lack of chemotherapy, and a longer life expectancy, non-metastatic PCa patients seems to have a more negligible effect on mental and physical health than other malignancies [17]. This distance is much more evident if we compare patients with the absence of any other comorbidities. Indeed, both the analysed cohorts have highlighted how the presence of two or more comorbidities can reduce the mental and physical score by 20 to 30 points (see also Table in Supplementary Materials). Although the ISTAT analysis is out of date, recent studies [38,44,45] proved that physical and mental components of health in low-intermediate risk PCa are very similar to those reported by the general population.

4.2. Study Limitations

The current study has some limitations. First, since the participating centres were involved voluntarily, a selection bias cannot be excluded. Second, just as for all observational studies, it may be susceptible to confounders. Third, the information on patients experiencing supportive care during follow-up was not included in the data collection. Moreover, data on patients' income and social networks, that might have affected QoL, were not considered and thus not available for analysis. Fifth, there was considerable variability in the times between the diagnosis and the onset of each treatment type; the models were anyway adjusted considering the temporal distance between the end of treatment and the follow-up assessment. Furthermore, different combinations of RT and ADT in terms of starting time and duration is another unmeasured confounding factor for our study. Finally, even if SF-12 has been proved to be responsive to positive change in patients with improved general health and performed well in distinguishing between patients who had improvement in general health and those with worsened general health, caution should be used to evaluate positive change in SF-12 since they could be too responsive to detect "noise" and not clinically significant differences [46]; however, in our analyses on SF-12 changes over time, we did not consider only statistically significant differences, but also MCID, which represent the differences that should be considered as clinically meaningful.

5. Conclusions

The study indicates that the vast majority of PCa patients, excluding those with distant metastasis at diagnosis and those treated with chemotherapy or ADT, appear to find a good psychological state once they have come to terms with the diagnosis and have begun their course of treatment. No clinical differences in mental and physical health were found in the various treatments groups at the time of enrolment. Age, diabetes, number of comorbidities, family history of PCa and bowel/urinary dysfunctions were the patient/clinical factors most influencing the probability of deviating from the high mental and physical health. The trajectory analysis in the two years after the cancer diagnosis highlighted the importance of assessing mental health, coping strategies and psychological and interpersonal resources at PCa diagnosis to identify patients who may benefit from personalised support. At diagnosis, patients with impaired mental health (1 over 4) could take advantage of different level of intervention. For patients with transient distress (trajectory 1 in our study), information leaflets or discussions with peers (other PCa patients) and cancer specialist staff could reduce the baseline gap with patients in stable mental condition. For patients with persistent mild distress, the decision making and the treatment itself could not be sufficient to restore a good mental state and level 2 intervention (mild care) with support from a non-oncology team supervised by a clinical psychologist could be of help to reduce differences at two years from diagnosis. The analysis suggested that following these patients between the diagnosis and the treatment could allow for discriminating between those with a good array of resources (trajectory 2) and those more vulnerable (trajectory 1).

Supplementary Materials: The following supporting information can be downloaded at: https://www.mdpi.com/article/10.3390/curroncol29110651/s1, Figure S1: The MCS (m) and PCS (p) scores of the Pros-IT patients with color density distribution; Table S1: Responses to the 12-Item Short Form Survey (SF-12) by the Pros-IT patients at the time of diagnosis (n (%)); Table S2: Characteristics at the time of diagnosis of the Pros-IT patients classified according to the three trajectories identified by the Mental Component Score (MCS) of the Short-Form Health Survey (SF-12); Table S3: Characteristics at the time of diagnosis of the Pros-IT patients classified according to the two trajectories identified by the Physical Component Score (PCS) of the Short-Form Health Survey (SF-12); Table S4: Mean and standard deviation by age group for MCS-12 and PCS-12 in Pros-IT and ISTAT studies; Table S5: Quartiles divided by age groups for PCS and MCS SF-12 distributions in Pros-IT and ISTAT studies; Table S6: Mean and standard deviation among oncologic Italian citizens (ISTAT) and among Pros-IT patients in trajectory groups identified for MCS-12 and PCS-12; Table S7: Quartiles for MCS and PCS SF-12 distributions in each trajectory groups identified for Pros-IT patients and for oncologic Italian citizens (ISTAT); Table S8: The number of comorbidities (mean and standard deviation (SD)) in the Pros-IT population according to the PCS and MCS deciles; Table S9: The number of comorbidities (mean and standard deviation (SD)) in the ISTAT population according to the PCS and MCS deciles.

Author Contributions: Conceptualization, M.N., A.C. and S.M.; formal analysis, M.N. and A.C.; writing—original draft preparation, M.N., A.C., P.D., L.D.L. and S.M.; writing—review and editing, B.N.C., R.S., F.B., S.M., M.G., S.S., F.S., L.B., R.M., P.B., M.M. and R.V.; supervision, S.M. and R.V. All authors have read and agreed to the published version of the manuscript.

Funding: Pros-IT CNR is a non-profit observational study. Takeda Italia S.p.A. provided an unconditional grant to the CNR to cover the costs of the preparatory meetings, the meetings of the advisory committees and the PIs, and the cost of developing a web platform for data entry.

Institutional Review Board Statement: The Ethics Committee of the coordinating centre (Sant'Anna Hospital, Como, Italy; register number 45/2014) and all the hospitals or health care facilities involved in the project approved the study protocol.

Informed Consent Statement: Informed consent was obtained from all subjects involved in the study.

Data Availability Statement: The datasets generated and/or analysed during the current study are not publicly available due to the study protocol, which planned that data would be available only to the collaborating scientists within the study.

Acknowledgments: The authors wish to thank Linda Moretti Inverso for reviewing the English version of this paper. The Pros-IT CNR Group: Anna Rita Alitto (Roma); Enrica Ambrosi (Brescia); Alessandro Antonelli (Brescia); Cynthia Aristei (Perugia); Michele Barbieri (Napoli); Franco Bardari (Asti); Lilia Bardoscia (Reggio Emilia); Salvina Barra (Genova); Sara Bartoncini (Torino); Umberto Basso (Padova); Carlotta Becherini (Firenze); Rita Bellavita (Perugia); Franco Bergamaschi (Reggio Emilia); Stefania Berlingheri (Brescia); Alfredo Berruti (Brescia); Barbara Bigazzi (Firenze); Marco Borghesi (Bologna); Roberto Bortolus (Pordenone); Valentina Borzillo (Napoli); Davide Bosetti (Milano); Giuseppe Bove (Foggia); Pierluigi Bove (Roma); Maurizio Brausi (Modena); Alessio Bruni (Modena); Giorgio Bruno (Ravenna); Eugenio Brunocilla (Bologna); Alberto Buffoli (Brescia); Michela Buglione (Brescia); Consuelo Buttigliero (Torino); Giovanni Cacciamani (Verona); Michela Caldiroli (Varese); Giuseppe Cardo (Bari); Giorgio Carmignani (Genova); Giuseppe Carrieri (Foggia); Emanuele Castelli (Torino); Elisabetta Castrezzati (Brescia); Gianpiero Catalano (Milano); Susanna Cattarino (Roma); Francesco Catucci (Roma); Dario Cavallini Francolini (Pavia); Ofelia Ceccarini (Bergamo); Antonio Celia (Vicenza); Francesco Chiancone (Napoli); Tommaso Chini (Firenze); Claudia Cianci (Pisa); Antonio Cisternino (Foggia); Devis Collura (Torino); Franco Corbella (Pavia); Matteo Corinti (Como); Paolo Corsi (Verona); Fiorenza Cortese (Alessandria); Luigi Corti (Padova); Cosimo De Nunzio (Roma); Olga Cristiano (Avellino); Rolando D'Angelillo (Roma); Luigi Da Pozzo (Bergamo); Daniele D'agostino (Padova); David D'Andrea (Bolzano); Matteo Dandrea (Padova); Michele De Angelis (Arezzo); Ottavio De Cobelli (Milano); Bernardino De Concilio (Vicenza); Antonello De Lisa (Cagliari); Stefano De Luca (Torino); Agostina De Stefani (Bergamo); Chiara Lucrezia Deantoni (Milano); Claudio Degli Esposti (Bologna); Anna Destito (Catanzaro); Beatrice Detti (Firenze); Nadia Di Muzio (Milano); Andrea Di Stasio (Alessandria); Calogero Di Stefano (Ravenna); Danilo Di Trapani (Palermo); Giuseppe Difino (Foggia); Marco Fabiano (Napoli); Giuseppe Facondo (Roma); Sara Falivene (Napoli); Giuseppe Farullo (Roma); Paolo Fedelini (Napoli); Ilaria Ferrari (Varese);

Francesco Ferrau (Messina); Matteo Ferro (Milano); Andrei Fodor (Milano); Francesco Fontana (Novara); Francesco Francesca (Pisa); Giulio Francolini (Firenze); Giovanni Frezza (Bologna); Pietro Gabriele (Torino); Maria Galeandro (Reggio Emilia); Elisabetta Garibaldi (Torino); Pietro Giovanni Gennari (Arezzo); Alessandro Gentilucci (Roma); Alessandro Giacobbe (Torino); Laura Giussani (Varese); Giuseppe Giusti (Cagliari); Paolo Gontero (Torino); Alessia Guarneri (Torino); Cesare Guida (Avellino); Alberto Gurioli (Torino); Dorijan Huqi (Bolzano); Ciro Imbimbo (Napoli); Gianluca Ingrosso (Roma); Cinzia Iotti (Reggio Emilia); Corrado Italia (Bergamo); Pierdaniele La Mattina (Milano); Enza Lamanna (Ravenna); Luciana Lastrucci (Arezzo); Grazia Lazzari (Taranto); Fabiola Liberale (Biella); Giovanni Liguori (Trieste); Roberto Lisi (Roma); Frank Lohr (Modena); Riccardo Lombardo (Roma); Jon Lovisolo (Varese); Giuseppe Mario Ludovico (Bari); Nicola Macchione (Novara); Francesca Maggio (Imperia); Michele Malizia (Bologna); Gianluca Manasse (Perugia); Giovanni Mandoliti (Rovigo); Giovanna Mantini (Roma); Luigi Marafioti (Cosenza); Luisa Marciello (Prato); Alberto Mario Marconi (Varese); Antonietta Martillotta (Cosenza); Salvino Marzano (Prato); Stefano Masciullo (Bergamo); Gloria Maso (Verbania); Adele Massenzo (Cosenza); Ercole Mazzeo (Modena); Luigi Mearini (Perugia); Serena Medoro (Ferrara); Rosa Molè (Catanzaro); Giorgio Monesi (Novara); Emanuele Montanari (Milano); Franco Montefiore (Alessandria); Giampaolo Montesi (Rovigo); Giuseppe Morgia (Catania); Gregorio Moro (Biella); Giorgio Muscas (Cagliari); Daniela Musio (Roma); Paolo Muto (Napoli); Giovanni Muzzonigro (Ancona); Giorgio Napodano (Salerno); Carlo Luigi Augusto Negro (Asti); Mattia Nidini (Mantova); Maria Ntreta (Bologna); Marco Orsatti (Imperia); Carmela Palazzolo (Messina); Isabella Palumbo (Perugia); Alessandro Parisi (Bologna); Paolo Parma (Mantova); Nicola Pavan (Trieste); Martina Pericolini (Roma); Francesco Pinto (Roma); Antonio Pistone (Salerno); Valerio Pizzuti (Grosseto); Angelo Platania (Messina); Caterina Polli (Prato); Giorgio Pomara (Pisa); Elisabetta Ponti (Roma); Antonio Benito Porcaro (Verona); Francesco Porpiglia (Torino); Dario Pugliese (Roma); Armin Pycha (Bolzano); Giuseppe Raguso (Reggio Emilia); Andrea Rampini (Arezzo); Donato Franco Randone (Torino); Valentina Roboldi (Bergamo); Marco Roscigno (Bergamo); Maria Paola Ruggieri (Reggio Emilia); Giuseppe Ruoppo (Reggio Emilia); Roberto Sanseverino (Salerno); Anna Santacaterina (Messina); Michele Santarsieri (Pisa); Riccardo Santoni (Roma); Giorgio Vittorio Scagliotti (Torino); Mauro Scanzi (Brescia); Marcello Scarcia (Bari); Riccardo Schiavina (Bologna); Alessandro Sciarra (Roma); Carmine Sciorio (Lecco); Tindaro Scolaro (La Spezia); Salvatore Scuzzarella (Lecco); Oscar Selvaggio (Foggia); Armando Serao (Alessandria); Sergio Serni (Firenze); Marco Andrea Signor (Udine); Mauro Silvani (Biella); Giovanni Silvano (Taranto); Franco Silvestris (Bari); Claudio Simeone (Brescia); Valeria Simone (Bari); Girolamo Spagnoletti (Foggia); Matteo Giulio Spinelli (Milano); Luigi Squillace (Pavia); Vincenzo Tombolini (Roma); Mariastella Toninelli (Brescia); Luca Triggiani (Brescia); Alberto Trinchieri (Lecco); Luca Eolo Trodella (Roma); Lucio Trodella (Roma); Carlo Trombetta (Trieste); Marcello Tucci (Torino); Daniele Urzì (Catania); Riccardo Valdagni (Milano); Maurizio Valeriani (Roma); Maurizio Vanoli (La Spezia); Elisabetta Vitali (Bergamo); Stefano Zaramella (Novara); Guglielmo Zeccolini (Vicenza); Giampaolo Zini (Ferrara).

Conflicts of Interest: The authors declare no conflict of interest.

References

1. Collaboration GB of DC. Global, Regional, and National Cancer Incidence, Mortality, Years of Life Lost, Years Lived With Disability, and Disability-Adjusted Life-Years for 29 Cancer Groups, 1990 to 2016: A Systematic Analysis for the Global Burden of Disease Study. *JAMA Oncol.* **2018**, *4*, 1553–1568.
2. Hawkes, N. Cancer survival data emphasise importance of early diagnosis. *BMJ* **2019**, *364*, l408. [CrossRef] [PubMed]
3. Korfage, I.J.; Hak, T.; de Koning, H.J.; Essink-Bot, M.-L. Patients' perceptions of the side-effects of prostate cancer treatment—A qualitative interview study. *Soc. Sci. Med.* **2006**, *63*, 911–919. [CrossRef] [PubMed]
4. Chambers, S.K.; Ng, S.K.; Baade, P.; Aitken, J.F.; Hyde, M.K.; Wittert, G.; Frydenberg, M.; Dunn, J. Trajectories of quality of life, life satisfaction, and psychological adjustment after prostate cancer. *Psychooncology* **2017**, *26*, 1576–1585. [CrossRef] [PubMed]
5. De Sousa, A.; Sonavane, S.; Mehta, J. Psychological aspects of prostate cancer: A clinical review. *Prostate Cancer Prostatic Dis.* **2012**, *15*, 120–127. [CrossRef] [PubMed]
6. Korfage, I.J.; Essink-Bot, M.-L.; Janssens, A.C.; Schröder, F.H.; De Koning, H.J. Anxiety and depression after prostate cancer diagnosis and treatment: 5-year follow-up. *Br. J. Cancer* **2006**, *94*, 1093–1098. [CrossRef] [PubMed]
7. Watts, S.; Leydon, G.; Birch, B.; Prescott, P.; Lai, L.; Eardley, S.; Lewith, G. Depression and anxiety in prostate cancer: A sys-tematic review and meta-analysis of prevalence rates. *BMJ Open* **2014**, *4*, e003901. [CrossRef] [PubMed]
8. Cuypers, M.; Lamers, R.E.D.; Cornel, E.B.; van de Poll-Franse, L.V.; de Vries, M.; Kil, P.J.M. The impact of prostate cancer diagnosis and treatment decision-making on health-related quality of life before treatment onset. *Support. Care Cancer* **2017**, *26*, 1297–1304. [CrossRef]

9. Villa, S.; Kendel, F.; Venderbos, L.; Rancati, T.; Bangma, C.; Carroll, P.; Denis, L.; Klotz, L.; Korfage, I.J.; Lane, A.J.; et al. Setting an Agenda for Assessment of Health-related Quality of Life Among Men with Prostate Cancer on Active Surveillance: A Consensus Paper from a European School of Oncology Task Force. *Eur. Urol.* **2017**, *71*, 274–280. [CrossRef]
10. Bellardita, L.; Valdagni, R.; Bergh, R.V.D.; Randsdorp, H.; Repetto, C.; Venderbos, L.D.; Lane, J.A.; Korfage, I.J. How Does Active Surveillance for Prostate Cancer Affect Quality of Life? A Systematic Review. *Eur. Urol.* **2015**, *67*, 637–645. [CrossRef]
11. Watson, E.; Shinkins, B.; Frith, E.; Neal, D.; Hamdy, F.; Walter, F.; Weller, D.; Wilkinson, C.; Faithfull, S.; Wolstenholme, J.; et al. Symptoms, unmet needs, psychological well-being and health status in survivors of prostate cancer: Implications for rede-signing follow-up. *BJU Int.* **2016**, *117*, E10–E19. [CrossRef]
12. Ram, N.; Grimm, K.J. Growth Mixture Modeling: A Method for Identifying Differences in Longitudinal Change Among Un-observed Groups. *Int. J. Behav. Dev.* **2009**, *33*, 565–576. [CrossRef] [PubMed]
13. Kwon, J.-Y.; Sawatzky, R.; Baumbusch, J.; Lauck, S.; Ratner, P.A. Growth mixture models: A case example of the longitudinal analysis of patient-reported outcomes data captured by a clinical registry. *BMC Med. Res. Methodol.* **2021**, *21*, 79. [CrossRef] [PubMed]
14. Bombard, Y.; Baker, G.R.; Orlando, E.; Fancott, C.; Bhatia, P.; Casalino, S.; Onate, K.; Denis, J.-L.; Pomey, M.-P. Engaging patients to improve quality of care: A systematic review. *Implement. Sci.* **2018**, *13*, 98. [CrossRef] [PubMed]
15. Noale, M.; Maggi, S.; Artibani, W.; Bassi, P.F.; Bertoni, F.; Bracarda, S.; Conti, G.N.; Corvò, R.; Gacci, M.; Graziotti, P.; et al. Pros-IT CNR: An Italian prostate cancer monitoring project. *Aging Clin. Exp. Res.* **2017**, *29*, 165–172. [CrossRef]
16. Porreca, A.; Noale, M.; Artibani, W.; Bassi, P.F.; Bertoni, F.; Bracarda, S.; Conti, G.N.; Corvò, R.; Gacci, M.; Graziotti, P.; et al. Disease-specific and general health-related quality of life in newly diagnosed prostate cancer patients: The Pros-IT CNR study. *Health Qual. Life Outcomes* **2018**, *16*, 122. [CrossRef]
17. Apolone, G.; Mosconi, P.Q.L. *Questionario Sullo Stato di Salute SF-12. Versione Italiana*; Guerini e Associati Editori: Milano, Italy, 2005.
18. Gandek, B.; Ware, J.E.; Aaronson, N.K.; Apolone, G.; Bjorner, J.B.; Brazier, J.E.; Bullinger, M.; Kaasa, S.; Leplege, A.; Prieto, L.; et al. Cross-validation of item selection and scoring for the sf-12 health survey in nine countries: Results from the iqola project. International quality of life assessment. *J. Clin. Epidemiol.* **1998**, *51*, 1171–1178. [CrossRef]
19. Hamoen, E.H.; De Rooij, M.; Witjes, J.A.; Barentsz, J.O.; Rovers, M.M. Measuring health-related quality of life in men with prostate cancer: A systematic review of the most used questionnaires and their validity. *Urol. Oncol. Semin. Orig. Investig.* **2015**, *33*, 69.e19–69.e28. [CrossRef]
20. Gacci, M.; Livi, L.; Paiar, F.; Detti, B.; Litwin, M.; Bartoletti, R.; Giubilei, G.; Cai, T.; Mariani, M.; Carini, M. Quality of life after radical treatment of prostate cancer: Validation of the Italian version of the University of California-Los Angeles Prostate Cancer Index. *Urology* **2005**, *66*, 338–343. [CrossRef]
21. Andruff, H.; Carraro, N.; Thompson, A.; Gaudreau, P.; Louvet, B. Latent Class Growth Modelling: A tutorial. *Tutor. Quant. Methods Psychol.* **2009**, *5*, 11–24. [CrossRef]
22. Nguena Nguefack, H.L.; Pagé, M.G.; Katz, J.; Choinière, M.; Vanasse, A.; Dorais, M.; Samb, O.M.; Lacasse, A. Trajectory Modelling Techniques Useful to Epidemiological Research: A Comparative Narrative Review of Approaches. *Clin. Epidemiol.* **2020**, *12*, 1205–1222. [CrossRef]
23. Jones, B.L.; Nagin, D.S.; Roeder, K. A SAS Procedure Based on Mixture Models for Estimating Developmental Trajectories. *Sociol. Methods Res.* **2001**, *29*, 374–393. [CrossRef]
24. Noale, M.; Bruni, A.; Triggiani, L.; Buglione, M.; Bertoni, F.; Frassinelli, L.; Montironi, R.; Corvò, R.; Zagonel, V.; Porreca, A.; et al. Impact of Gastrointestinal Side Effects on Patients' Reported Quality of Life Trajectories after Radiotherapy for Prostate Cancer: Data from the Prospective, Observational Pros-IT CNR Study. *Cancers* **2021**, *13*, 1479. [CrossRef] [PubMed]
25. Jaeschke, R.; Singer, J.; Guyatt, G.H. Measurement of health status: Ascertaining the minimal clinically important difference. *Control. Clin. Trials* **1989**, *10*, 407–415. [CrossRef]
26. Osoba, D. The clinical value and meaning of health related quality-of-life outcomes in oncology. In *Outcomes Assessment in Cancer*; Lipscomb, J., Gotay, C., Snyder, C., Eds.; Cambridge University Press: Cambridge, UK, 2005; pp. 386–405.
27. Norman, G.R.; Sloan, J.A.; Wyrwich, K.W. Interpretation of changes in health-related quality of life: The remarkable universality of half a standard deviation. *Med. Care* **2003**, *41*, 582–592. [CrossRef] [PubMed]
28. Sloan, J.; Symonds, T.; Vargas, D.; Fridley, B. Practical Guidelines for Assessing the Clinical Significance of Health-Related Quality of Life Changes within Clinical Trials. *Ther. Innov. Regul. Sci.* **2003**, *37*, 23–31. [CrossRef]
29. Sloan, J.A. Assessing the Minimally Clinically Significant Difference: Scientific Considerations, Challenges and Solutions. *COPD: J. Chronic Obstr. Pulm. Dis.* **2005**, *2*, 57–62. [CrossRef] [PubMed]
30. Sefik, E.; Gunlusoy, B.; EKER, A.; Celik, S.; Ceylan, Y.; Koskderelioglu, A.; Basmaci, I.; Degirmenci, T. Anxiety and depression associated with a positive prostate biopsy result: A comparative, prospective cohort study. *Int. Braz. J. Urol.* **2020**, *46*, 993–1005. [CrossRef] [PubMed]
31. Dordoni, P.; Badenchini, F.; Alvisi, M.F.; Menichetti, J.; De Luca, L.; Di Florio, T.; Magnani, T.; Marenghi, C.; Rancati, T.; Valdagni, R.; et al. How do prostate cancer patients navigate the active surveillance journey? A 3-year longitudinal study. *Support. Care Cancer* **2021**, *29*, 645–651. [CrossRef]
32. Bloch, S.; Love, A.; MacVean, M.; Duchesne, G.; Couper, J.; Kissane, D. Psychological adjustment of men with prostate cancer: A review of the literature. *Biopsychosoc. Med.* **2007**, *1*, 2. [CrossRef]

33. Tanyi, Z.; Szluha, K.; Nemes, L.; Kovács, S.; Bugán, A. Positive consequences of cancer: Exploring relationships among post-traumatic growth, adult attachment, and quality of life. *Tumori* **2015**, *101*, 223–231. [CrossRef] [PubMed]
34. Kurian, C.J.; Leader, A.E.; Thong, M.S.Y.; Keith, S.W.; Zeigler-Johnson, C.M. Examining relationships between age at diagnosis and health-related quality of life outcomes in prostate cancer survivors. *BMC Public Health* **2018**, *18*, 1060. [CrossRef] [PubMed]
35. Farris, M.S.; Kopciuk, K.A.; Courneya, K.S.; McGregor, S.E.; Wang, Q.; Friedenreich, C.M. Identification and prediction of health-related quality of life trajectories after a prostate cancer diagnosis. *Int. J. Cancer* **2017**, *140*, 1517–1527. [CrossRef] [PubMed]
36. Punnen, S.; Cowan, J.E.; Chan, J.M.; Carroll, P.R.; Cooperberg, M.R. Long-term Health-related Quality of Life After Primary Treatment for Localized Prostate Cancer: Results from the CaPSURE Registry. *Eur. Urol.* **2015**, *68*, 600–608. [CrossRef]
37. Hoffman, K.E.; Penson, D.F.; Zhao, Z.; Huang, L.-C.; Conwill, R.; Laviana, A.A.; Joyce, D.D.; Luckenbaugh, A.N.; Goodman, M.; Hamilton, A.S.; et al. Patient-Reported Outcomes Through 5 Years for Active Surveillance, Surgery, Brachytherapy, or External Beam Radiation With or Without Androgen Deprivation Therapy for Localized Prostate Cancer. *JAMA* **2020**, *323*, 149–163. [CrossRef]
38. Donovan, J.L.; Hamdy, F.C.; Lane, J.A.; Mason, M.; Metcalfe, C.; Walsh, E.; Blazeby, J.M.; Peters, T.J.; Holding, P.; Bonnington, S.; et al. Patient-Reported Outcomes after Monitoring, Surgery, or Radiotherapy for Prostate Cancer. *N. Engl. J. Med.* **2016**, *375*, 1425–1437. [CrossRef]
39. Ferrer, M.; Guedea, F.; Suárez, J.F.; de Paula, B.; Macias, V.; Mariño, A.; Hervás, A.; Herruzo, I.; Ortiz, M.J.; de León, J.P.; et al. Quality of life impact of treatments for localized prostate cancer: Cohort study with a 5year follow-up. *Radiother. Oncol.* **2013**, *108*, 306–313. [CrossRef]
40. Vissers, P.A.J.; Falzon, L.; Van De Poll-Franse, L.V.; Pouwer, F.; Thong, M.S.Y. The impact of having both cancer and diabetes on patient-reported outcomes: A systematic review and directions for future research. *J. Cancer Surviv.* **2016**, *10*, 406–415. [CrossRef]
41. Hershey, D.S. Importance of glycemic control in cancer patients with diabetes: Treatment through end of life. *Asia-Pac. J. Oncol. Nurs.* **2017**, *4*, 313–318. [CrossRef]
42. Thong, M.S.; Van De Poll-Franse, L.; Hoffman, R.M.; Albertsen, P.C.; Hamilton, A.S.; Stanford, J.L.; Penson, D.F. Diabetes mellitus and health-related quality of life in prostate cancer: 5-year results from the Prostate Cancer Outcomes Study. *Br. J. Urol.* **2010**, *107*, 1223–1231. [CrossRef]
43. Reeve, B.B.; Chen, R.C.; Moore, D.T.; Deal, A.M.; Usinger, D.S.; Lyons, J.C.; Talcott, J.A. Impact of comorbidity on health-related quality of life after prostate cancer treatment: Combined analysis of two prospective cohort studies. *Br. J. Urol.* **2014**, *114*, E74–E81. [CrossRef] [PubMed]
44. Sureda, A.; Fumadó, L.; Ferrer, M.; Garín, O.; Bonet, X.; Castells, M.; Mir, M.C.; Abascal, J.M.; Vigués, F.; Cecchini, L.; et al. Health-related quality of life in men with prostate cancer undergoing active surveillance versus radical prostatectomy, external-beam radiotherapy, prostate brachytherapy and reference population: A cross-sectional study. *Health Qual. Life Outcomes* **2019**, *17*, 11. [CrossRef] [PubMed]
45. AIOM; AIRTUM S-I. *I Numeri del Cancro in Italia*; Intermedia Editore: Brescia, Italy, 2020.
46. Choi, E.P.; Wong, C.K.; Wan, E.Y.; Tsu, J.H.; Chin, W.Y.; Kung, K.; Yiu, M.K. The internal and external responsiveness of Functional Assessment of Cancer Therapy-Prostate (FACT-P) and Short Form-12 Health Survey version 2 (SF-12 v2) in patients with prostate cancer. *Qual. Life Res.* **2016**, *25*, 2379–2393. [CrossRef] [PubMed]

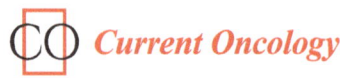 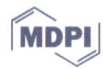

Article

Clinical Analysis of Perioperative Outcomes on Neoadjuvant Hormone Therapy before Laparoscopic and Robot-Assisted Surgery for Localized High-Risk Prostate Cancer in a Chinese Cohort

Guangyu Sun †, Zhengxin Liang †, Yuchen Jiang, Shenfei Ma, Shuaiqi Chen and Ranlu Liu *

Department of Urology, Tianjin Institute of Urology, The Second Hospital of Tianjin Medical University, Tianjin 300211, China
* Correspondence: ranluliu@126.com
† These authors contributed equally to this work.

Abstract: Objective: To analyze the perioperative outcomes of neoadjuvant hormone therapy (NHT) before laparoscopic and robot-assisted surgery for localized high-risk prostate cancer in a Chinese cohort. Methods: The clinical data of 385 patients with localized high-risk prostate cancer who underwent radical prostatectomy (RP) in our hospital from January 2019 to June 2021 were analyzed retrospectively, including 168 patients with preoperative NHT and 217 patients with simple surgery. Clinical characteristics were compared in the above two groups, the laparoscopic RP (LRP) cohort (n = 234) and the robot-assisted laparoscopic radical prostatectomy (RALP) cohort (n = 151), respectively. Results: In the overall cohort, compared with the control group, the NHT group had a shorter operative time, less blood loss, a lower positive surgical margin rate, and a higher proportion of Gleason score (GS) downgrading after the operation ($p < 0.05$). However, there was no significant difference in hospitalization time, biochemical recurrence, urine leakage, urinary continence, or prostate-specific antigen (PSA) progression-free survival ($p > 0.05$). In the LRP cohort, it was found that the NHT group also had shorter operative time, less blood loss, lower positive surgical margin rate, a higher proportion of GS downgrading after the operation, and faster recovery of urinary control than the control group ($p < 0.05$). There was no marked difference in hospitalization time, biochemical recurrence, urinary leakage, or PSA progression-free survival. However, in the RALP cohort, the NHT group had a significant difference in the GS downgrading after the operation compared with the control group ($p < 0.05$). In the overall cohort, multiple analyses showed that initial PSA level, GS at biopsy, clinical T stage, lymph node invasion, use of NHT, and surgical methods were significantly associated with positive surgical margin ($p < 0.05$) while NHT did not account for biochemical recurrence ($p > 0.05$). Conclusions: NHT can lower the difficulty of surgery, reduce positive surgical margin rate, and help recovery in short-term urinary control in patients with high-risk prostate cancer after LRP. However, we do not have evidence on the benefit of NHT in high-risk PCa patients treated with RALP. For these patients, surgery can be performed as early as possible.

Keywords: prostate cancer; neoadjuvant hormone therapy; laparoscopic radical prostatectomy; robot-assisted radical prostatectomy

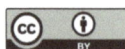

1. Introduction

Prostate cancer has the highest incidence and ranks second place in mortality among male cancers [1]. Due to the absence of early symptoms and sufficient prostate-specific antigen (PSA) screening, approximately 70% of patients in China are initially diagnosed with high-risk or even advanced prostate cancer [2,3]. Although each guideline differs slightly, comprehensive treatments are usually recommended, including surgery, radiation therapy, or new endocrine therapeutic drugs [4]. With the advantage of excellent control of local primary tumors, availability of accurate pathological staging, and the following guidance for adjuvant therapy, radical prostatectomy (RP) becomes one of the most effective treatments for low- and intermediate-risk prostate cancer and the main option for localized high-risk prostate cancer [5]. The European Association of Urology guidelines and the National Comprehensive Cancer Network guidelines also suggest that surgery should be one of the comprehensive treatments for high-risk prostate cancer [4]. However, in high-risk prostate cancer, pathologic findings reveal a relatively high proportion of positive surgical margins, suggesting that surgery may not be curative and therefore adjuvant therapy is necessary [6]. However, the clinical findings of neoadjuvant hormone therapy (NHT) before radical prostatectomy are inconsistent among various studies. Some studies have found that neoadjuvant hormone therapy prior to RP helps reduce the incidence of positive surgical margins and lymph node infiltration [7,8], but others have suggested that neoadjuvant hormone therapy prior to RP does not have a significant survival benefit for patients, including overall survival and disease-free survival [9], and therefore preoperative neoadjuvant therapy is not specifically recommended by current guidelines for patients with high-risk prostate cancer.

Currently, robotic-assisted radical prostatectomy (RALP) has become the main modality in prostate cancer surgery [10], and it has been reported that more than 85% of RP procedures in the United States are RALP [11]. Robotic-assisted systems have significant advantages over laparoscopic radical surgery in terms of improved ergonomics, a three-dimensional magnified view, and tremor filtration, with lower rates of urinary incontinence and biochemical recurrence [12]. However, the survival benefit of robotic-assisted radical surgery for patients with high-risk prostate cancer is not clear, especially in some patients who have undergone neoadjuvant hormonal therapy [13]. Our study retrospectively analyzed the perioperative outcomes of NHT in patients with high-risk prostate cancer and explored the benefits of NHT for patients with two different surgical approaches, RALP and LRP.

2. Materials and Methods

2.1. Patients and Treatments

The clinical data of 385 patients with localized high-risk prostate cancer treated in the second hospital of Tianjin Medical University from January 2019 to June 2021 were collected. Inclusion criteria: (1) localized high-risk prostate cancer diagnosed by pathology and imaging; (2) NHT cohort: NHT > 3 months; (3) LRP or RALP. Exclusion criteria: (1) incomplete relative data; (2) patients with metastatic lesions. High-risk prostate cancer was defined as clinical stage T3-4 and/or PSA > 20 ng/mL and/or Gleason score (GS) 8–10.

NHT includes oral administration of bicalutamide 50 mg once a day plus goserelin 3.6 mg or leuprorelin 3.75 mg subcutaneously or triptorelin 3.75 mg intramuscularly once a month. LRP or RALP were carried out by the same group of urologists.

All included cases underwent preoperative pelvic magnetic resonance imaging (MRI), thoracoabdominal CT and bone scan (ECT) to determine TNM staging (2017, AJCC). Pathological histological classification was performed using the Gleason scoring system (2016, WHO) for prostate cancer. All patients with adverse pathology received routine adjuvant hormone therapy ± external beam radiotherapy after surgery. Regular postoperative inpatient or outpatient reviews were performed regularly, with PSA every 1–3 months and ultrasound, MRI, and bone scan every 6–12 months, with a follow-up period of 12–36 months and a median follow-up of 25 months.

2.2. Perioperative Outcomes

The perioperative outcomes were observed and recorded, including operation time, intraoperative bleeding, postoperative urinary leakage, rate of positive surgical margin, GS downgrading, length of hospital stay, recovery of urinary control, biochemical recurrence, and PSA progression-free survival. Biochemical recurrence was determined using the

European Urological (EAU) criteria of two consecutive serum PSA levels > 0.2 ng/mL. Progression-free survival was defined as time from prostatectomy to biochemical recurrence.

2.3. Statistical Analysis

SPSS for Windows (Version 25.0) was used to conduct a statistical analysis of the data. The Kolmogorov–Smirnov test was used to judge the normal distribution of measurement data. The measurement data with normal distribution were expressed as mean ± standard deviation. Otherwise, the median ± interquartile range was used. The enumeration data were expressed as the number of cases and corresponding percentages. t-test or analysis of variance was used for component comparison of measurement data, and chi-square test or Fisher exact test were used for comparison between count data groups. Graphpad prism was used to analyze the PSA progression-free survival. Univariate and multiple logistic regression analyses were used to determine risk factors for positive surgical margins and biochemical recurrence. $p < 0.05$ was considered statistically significant.

3. Results

3.1. Comparison of General Clinical Characteristics and Perioperative Characteristics between the NHT and Control Group in the Overall Cohort

A total of 385 patients with localized high-risk prostate cancer were included in the overall cohort, including 234 cases treated with LRP and 151 cases treated with RALP. In the LRP cohort, 100 cases received NHT before operation and 134 cases were treated only by operation. In the RALP cohort, 68 cases received NHT before operation and 83 cases received simple surgical treatment.

In the overall cohort, there was no difference between the NHT group (168 patients) and the control group (217 patients) in age, BMI, PSA, prostate volume, Gleason score, T stage, or surgical methods ($p > 0.05$, Table 1). Compared with the control group, the NHT group had significantly shorter operative time, less blood loss, a lower positive surgical margin rate (28.6% vs. 38.3%), and a higher proportion of GS downgrading after the operation (24.4% vs. 13.8%), while there was no statistical significance in leakage rate (6% vs. 7.4%), biochemical recurrence rate (22.6% vs. 25.8%), or recovery time of urinary control (Table 2). No significant difference was found in PSA progression-free survival between the two groups (Table 2).

Table 1. Comparison of general clinical characteristics between the NHT and control groups in the overall cohort.

	NHT Group (n = 168)	Control Group (n = 217)	p-Value
Age (year-old)	67 ± 9	68 ± 9	0.100
BMI (kg/m^2)	22.45 ± 3.14	23.05 ± 2.92	0.057
Volume (mL)	39.33 ± 22.97	38.02 ± 24.53	0.261
Initial PSA (ng/mL)	23 ± 23.84	20 ± 12.26	0.075
GS at biopsy			0.917
GS = 7	8 (4.8%)	8 (3.6%)	
GS = 8	89 (53%)	118 (54.4%)	
GS = 9	53 (31.5%)	65 (30%)	
GS = 10	18 (10.7%)	26 (12%)	
Initial T stage			0.705
cT3	158 (94%)	206 (94.9%)	
cT4	10 (6%)	11 (5.1%)	
Lymph node invasion			0.560
N_0	127 (75.6%)	158 (72.8%)	
N_X	41 (24.4%)	59 (27.2%)	
surgical method			0.657
LRP	100 (59.5%)	134 (61.8%)	
RRP	68 (40.5%)	83 (38.2%)	

Table 2. Comparison of postoperative clinical characteristics between the NHT and control groups in overall cohort.

	NHT Group (n = 168)	Control Group (n = 217)	p-Value
Operative time (minutes)	108.99 ± 22.74	118.55 ± 24.71	0.007
Blood loss (mL)	110.76 ± 45.67	138.20 ± 48.17	<0.001
Urine leakage	10 (6%)	16 (7.4%)	0.582
Positive surgical margin	48 (28.6%)	83 (38.3%)	0.02
GS decreased after operation	41 (24.4%)	30 (13.8%)	0.008
Hospitalization (days)	7 ± 2	7 ± 2	0.086
Follow up time (months)	24 ± 7	25 ± 5	0.48
urinary continence			0.06
<1 month	101 (60.1%)	97 (44.7%)	
1–3 month	50 (29.8%)	98 (45.2%)	
>3 month	17 (10.1%)	22 (10.1%)	
BCR	38 (22.6%)	56 (25.8%)	0.47
PSA progression free survival (months)	23.5 ± 7	24 ± 5	0.152

3.2. Comparison of Postoperative Clinical Characteristics between the NHT and Control Groups in the LRP Cohort

In the LRP cohort, the same statistically significant trend was observed in the NHT group, including shorter operative time, less blood loss, lower positive surgical margin rate (34.00% vs. 49.3%), a higher proportion of GS decreasing after the operation (25.0% vs. 13.4%), and shorter recovery time of urinary control ($p < 0.05$, Table 3). There is no statistical significance in biochemical recurrence rate (24% vs. 29.9%), the leakage rate (7.0% vs. 9.0%) ($p = 0.26$, Table 3), or PSA progression-free survival ($p = 0.153$, Table 3).

Table 3. Comparison of postoperative clinical characteristics between the NHT and control groups in the LRP cohort.

	NHT Group (n = 100)	Control Group (n = 134)	p-Value
Operative time (minutes)	114 ± 29	128 ± 31	<0.001
Blood loss (mL)	112.65 ± 68.77	151.5 ± 33.8	<0.001
Urine leakage	7 (7%)	12 (9%)	0.26
Positive surgical margin	34 (34%)	66 (49.3%)	0.588
GS decreased after operation	25 (25%)	18 (13.4%)	0.024
Hospitalization (days)	7 ± 1	7 ± 1	0.957
Follow up time (months)	24 ± 8	25 ± 4	0.056
urinary continence			0.02
<1 month	58 (58%)	53 (39.6%)	
1–3 month	34 (34%)	65 (48.5%)	
>3 month	8 (8%)	16 (11.9%)	
BCR	24 (24%)	40 (29.9%)	0.321
PSA progression free survival (months)	23 ± 8	24 ± 5	0.153

3.3. Comparison of Postoperative Clinical Characteristics between the NHT and Control Groups in the RALP Cohort

In the RALP cohort, rather than the marked difference in the proportion of GS downgrading ($p < 0.05$, Table 4), other perioperative outcomes including operative time, blood loss, positive surgical margin rate, urinary control, biochemical recurrence rate, and PSA progression-free survival were not significantly different between NHT group and control group ($p > 0.05$, Table 4).

Table 4. Comparison of postoperative clinical characteristics between the NHT and control groups in RALP cohort.

	NHT Group (n = 68)	Control Group (n = 83)	p-Value
Operative time (minutes)	98.25 ± 18.6	100.5 ± 21.06	0.583
Blood loss (mL)	109.6 ± 19.62	105.15 ± 24.4	0.279
Urine leakage	3 (4.4%)	12 (4.8%)	0.906
Positive surgical margin	14 (20.6%)	17 (20.5%)	0.987
GS decreased after operation	20 (29.4%)	12 (14.5%)	0.025
Hospitalization (days)	5 ± 2	6 ± 2	0.208
Follow up time (months)	24 ± 6	25 ± 6	0.542
urinary continence			0.079
<1 month	43 (63.3%)	44 (53%)	
1–3 month	16 (23.5%)	33 (39.8%)	
>3 month	9 (13.2%)	6 (7.2%)	
BCR	14 (20.6%)	16 (19.3%)	0.84
PSA progression free survival (months)	24 ± 6	24 ± 6	0.592

3.4. Univariate and Multiple Logistic Regression Analysis of Positive Surgical Margins and Biochemical Recurrence in Overall Cohort

In the overall cohort, univariate analysis showed that volume of the prostate, initial PSA level, GS at biopsy, initial T stage, lymph node invasion, use of NHT and surgical method were significantly associated with positive surgical margins. Multiple analysis showed that initial PSA level, GS at biopsy, lymph node invasion, use of NHT, and surgical methods were significantly associated with positive surgical margin while NHT did not account for biochemical recurrence (Table 5).

Table 5. Univariate and multiple logistic regression analysis of positive surgical margins in the overall cohort.

	Univariate Analysis			Multiple Logistic Regression		
	OR	95%CI	p	OR	95%CI	p
Age (year-old)	0.982	0.952–1.012	0.227	-	-	-
BMI (kg/m^2)	1.093	0.989–1.206	0.08	-	-	-
Volume (mL)	1.02	1.004–1.036	0.012	1.003	0.981–1.025	0.797
Initial PSA (ng/mL)	1.084	1.061–1.107	<0.001	1.102	1.073–1.132	<0.001
GS at biopsy (GS7-8, GS9-10)	12.626	3.873–41.158	<0.001	5.220	2.688–10.134	<0.001
Initial T stage (T3, T4)	6.933	1.333–6.194	0.019	2.671	0.536–13.312	0.231
Lymph node invasion (N_0, N_X)	16.856	9.558–29.728	<0.001	5.443	2.378–12.462	<0.001
Treatment (Control, NHT)	0.646	0.419–0.995	0.047	0.365	0.190–0.700	0.002
surgical method (LRP, RALP)	0.346	0.216–0.555	<0.001	0.179	0.091–0.354	<0.001

Univariate analysis showed that volume of the prostate, initial PSA level, GS at biopsy, initial T stage, positive surgical margin, and lymph node invasion were significantly associated with biochemical recurrence. Multiple analysis of risk factors for biochemical recurrence in the overall cohort showed that only initial PSA levels, positive surgical margins, and lymph node invasion were independent risk factors for biochemical recurrence. (Table 6).

Table 6. Univariate and multiple logistic regression analysis of biochemical recurrence in the overall cohort.

	Univariate Analysis			Multiple Logistic Regression		
	OR	95%CI	p	OR	95%CI	p
Age (year-old)	1.033	0.998–1.07	0.068	-	-	-
BMI (kg/m^2)	1.091	0.978–1.216	0.118	-	-	-
Volume (mL)	1.034	1.016–1.053	<0.001	1.021	0.995–1.048	0.112
Initial PSA (ng/mL)	1.069	1.05–1.089	<0.001	1.027	1.020–1.066	0.018
GS at biopsy (GS7-8, GS9-10)	3.418	3.099–6.921	0.006	1.952	0.796–4.786	0.144
Initial T stage (T3, T4)	11.733	1.421–8.220	<0.001	1.862	0.487–7.112	0.363
Lymph node invasion (N_0, N_X)	37.712	19.938–71.331	<0.001	25.031	9.929–63.102	<0.001
Treatment (Control, NHT)	0.84	0.524–1.348	0.471	-	-	-
surgical method (LRP, RALP)	0.659	0.403–1.078	0.096	-	-	-
Positive surgical margin	11.885	6.861–20.586	<0.001	3.597	1.657–7.808	<0.001

4. Discussion

Traditionally, conservative treatments such as radiotherapy, surgery, and hormone therapy are preferred for high-risk prostate cancer [14]. However, with the continuous improvement of medical technology and minimally invasive surgical techniques, RP is considered the prior treatment choice for patients with localized high-risk prostate cancer [15,16]. NHT is widely used for the initial treatment of high-risk prostate cancer. However, the role of preoperative NHT in high-risk prostate cancer is still controversial due to potential drawbacks such as ineffectiveness, delayed access to surgery, and increased surgical complications [17]. In a prospective study in which investigators matched patients treated with/without NHT on a 1:2 basis, recipients of NHT groups had lower rates of positive surgical margins, seminal vesicle infiltration, and extracapsular extension than non-subjects, in addition to a lower rate of perioperative complications (7.4% vs. 18.4%) [18]. A meta-analysis conducted by Shelley showed that NHT treatment contributed to improved adverse pathologic outcomes [19]. Joung found that 6 (5.4%) of 111 postoperative specimens of high-risk prostate cancer patients treated with NHT were free of tumor residuals [20]. Our study likewise found a significantly lower rate of positive surgical margin in the NHT group (28.6% vs. 38.3%) and a higher rate of GS downgrading (24.4% vs. 13.8%) than in the control group. Another retrospective study found a significant decrease in operative time, blood loss, and positive surgical margins in the NHT group [21], consistent with the results of our analysis.

NHT could shrink the prostate volume and facilitate the surgery, significantly shortening the operative time and reducing intraoperative blood loss. As the prostate is relatively deep and fixed, the operative time and intraoperative bleeding are closely related to the adhesions around the tumor, thus bleeding is extremely easy when dealing with bilateral ligaments and freeing the vas deferens seminal vesicles, especially for patients with locally advanced prostate cancer [22]. With preoperative NHT, intraoperative anatomical structure was identified much more easily and the surgical difficulty was relatively low [23].

There are inconsistent results from various studies on whether neoadjuvant hormone therapy improves patients' prognosis. A multicenter study analyzed high-risk prostate cancer-related mortality after NHT in 1573 patients and found that preoperative NHT significantly reduced postoperative prostate cancer-related mortality [24]. Berglund concluded that NHT treatment improved progression-free and overall survival [25]. On the other hand, Scorieri concluded that NHT treatment did not benefit the survival of prostate cancer patients [26]. Our study found that NHT reduced the rate of positive surgical margin but there was no significant benefit in the NHT group in terms of biochemical recurrence and PSA progression-free survival by late follow-up ($p > 0.05$).

Currently, robot-assisted surgery is gradually replacing LRP as the preferred choice for the surgical treatment of localized prostate cancer [13]. Similarly, RALP is safe for patients with high-risk prostate cancer and has some advantages over general laparoscopic surgery in terms of operative time, hospital stay, and postoperative complication rate [27]. A meta-analysis by Ashutosh et al. related to the surgical approach to prostate cancer found lower positive surgical margins, less bleeding, less complications such as urinary incontinence and rectal injury for RALP compared to LRP and ORP, but no difference in biochemical recurrence [28], which is consistent with our findings. However, preoperative NHT is currently focused on laparoscopic surgery, and few studies have reported the clinical perioperative outcomes of ADT in robot-assisted surgery. However, side effects of neoadjuvant hormone therapy are also evident, most notably in cardiovascular risk. Neoadjuvant hormone therapy may increase the incidence of cardiovascular risk in patients, and therefore neoadjuvant hormone therapy for high-risk prostate cancer patients should be analyzed individually and risk stratified, which is subject to further study [29]. In this study, we subsequently performed a statistical analysis of the NHT group and the control group in the LRP cohort and the RALP cohort, respectively, and found that NHT was more efficient for laparoscopic surgery, with significant advantages in intraoperative bleeding, positive margin rate, GS downgrading, and recovery of urinary control ($p < 0.05$), consistent with the overall cohort. However, its effect on the RALP cohort was not that obvious. Therefore, we can conclude that the high accuracy of the robot-assisted system reduces the impact of prostate volume and stricture space during the procedure. we do not have evidence on the benefit of NHT in high-risk PCa patients treated with RALP. For these patients, surgery can be performed as early as possible.

Our study also has some limitations. First, our study is a retrospective study and inevitably suffers from selection bias, as the choice of neoadjuvant hormone therapy only included bicalutamide and not the latest new endocrine therapies such as enzalutamid, apalutamid and datolutamid. In addition, our surgical urethral reconstruction modalities are all standard, and other anastomotic modalities may have some impact on the postoperative observation index, which requires further refinement of subsequent studies [30]. Second, our study has a short follow-up period, which makes it difficult to find the ultimate benefit of patients; and finally, our study is a single-center study with a limited sample size, which needs to be confirmed by further multicenter prospective studies.

5. Conculsions

NHT can lower the difficulty of surgery, reduce positive surgical margin rate, and help recovery in short-term urinary control in patients with high-risk prostate cancer after LRP. However, we do not have evidence on the benefit of NHT in high-risk PCa patients treated with RALP. For these patients, surgery can be performed as early as possible.

Author Contributions: Conception, study design, writing—review and editing, G.S., S.M. and R.L.; collection of patient follow-up data, S.C. and Z.L.; data collation and verification, data analysis, Y.J. All authors have read and agreed to the published version of the manuscript.

Funding: This research was supported by Tianjin science and technology plan project (19ZXDBSY00050).

Institutional Review Board Statement: The study was conducted in accordance with the Declaration of Helsinki, and approved by Tianjin Medical University Ethics Committee (protocol code KY2021K118).

Informed Consent Statement: All enrolled individual participants in the study were provided with informed consent.

Data Availability Statement: The data presented in this study is available on request from the corresponding author.

Conflicts of Interest: The authors declare no conflict of interest.

References

1. Bray, F.; Ferlay, J.; Soerjomataram, I.; Siegel, R.L.; Torre, L.A.; Jemal, A. Global cancer statistics 2018: GLOBOCAN estimates of incidence and mortality worldwide for 36 cancers in 185 countries. *CA A Cancer J. Clin.* **2018**, *68*, 394–424. [CrossRef] [PubMed]
2. Zhu, Y.; Mo, M.; Wei, Y.; Wu, J.; Pan, J.; Freedland, S.J.; Zheng, Y.; Ye, D. Epidemiology and genomics of prostate cancer in Asian men. *Nat. Rev. Urol.* **2021**, *18*, 282–301. [CrossRef] [PubMed]
3. Chen, W.; Zheng, R.; Baade, P.D.; Zhang, S.; Zeng, H.; Bray, F.; Jemal, A.; Yu, X.Q.; He, J. Cancer statistics in China, 2015. *CA A Cancer J. Clin.* **2016**, *66*, 115–132. [CrossRef] [PubMed]
4. Chang, A.J.; Autio, K.A.; Roach, M., 3rd; Scher, H.I. High-risk prostate cancer-classification and therapy. *Nat. Rev. Clin. Oncol.* **2014**, *11*, 308–323. [CrossRef]
5. Devos, G.; Devlies, W.; De Meerleer, G.; Baldewijns, M.; Gevaert, T.; Moris, L.; Milonas, D.; Van Poppel, H.; Berghen, C.; Everaerts, W.; et al. Neoadjuvant hormonal therapy before radical prostatectomy in high-risk prostate cancer. *Nat. Rev. Urol.* **2021**, *18*, 739–762. [CrossRef]
6. Rosen, M.A.; Goldstone, L.; Lapin, S.; Wheeler, T.; Scardino, P.T. Frequency and location of extracapsular extension and positive surgical margins in radical prostatectomy specimens. *J. Urol.* **1992**, *148*, 331–337. [CrossRef]
7. Pignot, G.; Maillet, D.; Gross, E.; Barthelemy, P.; Beauval, J.B.; Constans-Schlurmann, F.; Loriot, Y.; Ploussard, G.; Sargos, P.; Timsit, M.O.; et al. Systemic treatments for high-risk localized prostate cancer. *Nat. Rev. Urol.* **2018**, *15*, 498–510. [CrossRef]
8. Sangkum, P.; Sirisopana, K.; Jenjitranant, P.; Kijvikai, K.; Pacharatakul, S.; Leenanupunth, C.; Kochakarn, W.; Kongchareonsombat, W. Neoadjuvant Androgen Deprivation Therapy Effects on Perioperative Outcomes Prior to Radical Prostatectomy: Eleven Years of Experiences at Ramathibodi Hospital. *Res. Rep. Urol.* **2021**, *13*, 303–312. [CrossRef]
9. Liu, W.; Yao, Y.; Liu, X.; Liu, Y.; Zhang, G.M. Neoadjuvant hormone therapy for patients with high-risk prostate cancer: A systematic review and meta-analysis. *Asian J. Androl.* **2021**, *23*, 429–436.
10. Porpiglia, F.; Fiori, C.; Bertolo, R.; Manfredi, M.; Mele, F.; Checcucci, E.; De Luca, S.; Passera, R.; Scarpa, R.M. Five-year Outcomes for a Prospective Randomised Controlled Trial Comparing Laparoscopic and Robot-assisted Radical Prostatectomy. *Eur. Urol. Focus* **2018**, *4*, 80–86. [CrossRef]
11. Autorino, R.; Porpiglia, F. Robotic surgery in urology: The way forward. *World J. Urol.* **2020**, *38*, 809–811. [CrossRef] [PubMed]
12. Minafra, P.; Carbonara, U.; Vitarelli, A.; Lucarelli, G.; Battaglia, M.; Ditonno, P. Robotic radical perineal prostatectomy: Tradition and evolution in the robotic era. *Curr. Opin. Urol.* **2021**, *31*, 11–17. [CrossRef] [PubMed]
13. Carbonara, U.; Srinath, M.; Crocerossa, F.; Ferro, M.; Cantiello, F.; Lucarelli, G.; Porpiglia, F.; Battaglia, M.; Ditonno, P.; Autorino, R. Robot-assisted radical prostatectomy versus standard laparoscopic radical prostatectomy: An evidence-based analysis of comparative outcomes. *World J. Urol.* **2021**, *39*, 3721–3732. [CrossRef] [PubMed]
14. Ohashi, T.; Yorozu, A.; Saito, S.; Momma, T.; Nishiyama, T.; Yamashita, S.; Shiraishi, Y.; Shigematsu, N. Combined brachytherapy and external beam radiotherapy without adjuvant androgen deprivation therapy for high-risk prostate cancer. *Radiat. Oncol.* **2014**, *9*, 13. [CrossRef]
15. Walz, J.; Joniau, S.; Chun, F.K.; Isbarn, H.; Jeldres, C.; Yossepowitch, O.; Chao-Yu, H.; Klein, E.A.; Scardino, P.T.; Reuther, A.; et al. Pathological results and rates of treatment failure in high-risk prostate cancer patients after radical prostatectomy. *BJU Int.* **2011**, *107*, 765–770. [CrossRef]
16. Sun, M.; Sammon, J.D.; Becker, A.; Roghmann, F.; Tian, Z.; Kim, S.P.; Larouche, A.; Abdollah, F.; Hu, J.C.; Karakiewicz, P.I.; et al. Radical prostatectomy vs radiotherapy vs observation among older patients with clinically localized prostate cancer: A comparative effectiveness evaluation. *BJU Int.* **2014**, *113*, 200–208. [CrossRef]
17. Yee, D.S.; Lowrance, W.T.; Eastham, J.A.; Maschino, A.C.; Cronin, A.M.; Rabbani, F. Long-term follow-up of 3-month neoadjuvant hormone therapy before radical prostatectomy in a randomized trial. *BJU Int.* **2010**, *105*, 185–190. [CrossRef]
18. Horwitz, E.M.; Bae, K.; Hanks, G.E.; Porter, A.; Grignon, D.J.; Brereton, H.D.; Venkatesan, V.; Lawton, C.A.; Rosenthal, S.A.; Sandler, H.M.; et al. Ten-year follow-up of radiation therapy oncology group protocol 92-02: A phase III trial of the duration of elective androgen deprivation in locally advanced prostate cancer. *J. Clin. Oncol.* **2008**, *26*, 2497–2504. [CrossRef]
19. Shelley, M.D.; Kumar, S.; Wilt, T.; Staffurth, J.; Coles, B.; Mason, M.D. A systematic review and meta-analysis of randomised trials of neo-adjuvant hormone therapy for localised and locally advanced prostate carcinoma. *Cancer Treat. Rev.* **2009**, *35*, 9–17. [CrossRef]
20. Joung, J.Y.; Kim, J.E.; Kim, S.H.; Seo, H.K.; Chung, J.; Park, W.S.; Hong, E.K.; Lee, K.H. The prevalence and outcomes of pT0 disease after neoadjuvant hormonal therapy and radical prostatectomy in high-risk prostate cancer. *BMC Urol.* **2015**, *15*, 82. [CrossRef]
21. Hu, J.C.; Hung, S.C.; Ou, Y.C. Assessments of Neoadjuvant Hormone Therapy Followed by Robotic-Assisted Radical Prostatectomy for Intermediate- and High-Risk Prostate Cancer. *Anticancer Res.* **2017**, *37*, 3143–3150. [PubMed]
22. Heidenreich, A.; Pfister, D.; Porres, D. Cytoreductive radical prostatectomy in patients with prostate cancer and low volume skeletal metastases: Results of a feasibility and case-control study. *J. Urol.* **2015**, *193*, 832–838. [CrossRef] [PubMed]
23. Spahn, M.; Briganti, A.; Capitanio, U.; Kneitz, B.; Gontero, P.; Karnes, J.R.; Schubert, M.; Montorsi, F.; Scholz, C.J.; Bader, P.; et al. Outcome predictors of radical prostatectomy followed by adjuvant androgen deprivation in patients with clinical high risk prostate cancer and pT3 surgical margin positive disease. *J. Urol.* **2012**, *188*, 84–90. [CrossRef] [PubMed]

24. Tosco, L.; Laenen, A.; Briganti, A.; Gontero, P.; Karnes, R.J.; Albersen, M.; Bastian, P.J.; Chlosta, P.; Claessens, F.; Chun, F.K.; et al. The survival impact of neoadjuvant hormonal therapy before radical prostatectomy for treatment of high-risk prostate cancer. *Prostate Cancer Prostatic Dis.* **2017**, *20*, 407–412. [CrossRef] [PubMed]
25. Berglund, R.K.; Tangen, C.M.; Powell, I.J.; Lowe, B.A.; Haas, G.P.; Carroll, P.R.; Canby-Hagino, E.D.; deVere White, R.; Hemstreet, G.P., 3rd; Crawford, E.D.; et al. Ten-year follow-up of neoadjuvant therapy with goserelin acetate and flutamide before radical prostatectomy for clinical T3 and T4 prostate cancer: Update on Southwest Oncology Group Study 9109. *Urology* **2012**, *79*, 633–637. [CrossRef]
26. Scolieri, M.J.; Altman, A.; Resnick, M.I. Neoadjuvant hormonal ablative therapy before radical prostatectomy: A review. Is it indicated? *J. Urol.* **2000**, *164*, 1465–1472. [CrossRef]
27. Autorino, R.; Zargar, H.; Mariano, M.B.; Sanchez-Salas, R.; Sotelo, R.J.; Chlosta, P.L.; Castillo, O.; Matei, D.V.; Celia, A.; Koc, G.; et al. Perioperative Outcomes of Robotic and Laparoscopic Simple Prostatectomy: A European-American Multi-institutional Analysis. *Eur. Urol.* **2015**, *68*, 86–94. [CrossRef]
28. Tewari, A.; Sooriakumaran, P.; Bloch, D.A.; Seshadri-Kreaden, U.; Hebert, A.E.; Wiklund, P. Positive surgical margin and perioperative complication rates of primary surgical treatments for prostate cancer: A systematic review and meta-analysis comparing retropubic, laparoscopic, and robotic prostatectomy. *Eur. Urol.* **2012**, *62*, 1–15. [CrossRef]
29. Nunzio, C.D.; Fiori, C.; Fusco, F.; Gregori, A.; Pagliarulo, V.; Alongi, F. Androgen deprivation therapy and cardiovascular risk in prostate cancer. *Minerva Urol. Nephrol.* **2022**, *74*, 508–517. [CrossRef]
30. Checcucci, E.; Pecoraro, A.; De Cillis, S.; Manfredi, M.; Amparore, D.; Aimar, R.; Piramide, F.; Granato, S.; Volpi, G.; Autorino, R.; et al. The importance of anatomical reconstruction for continence recovery after robot assisted radical prostatectomy: A systematic review and pooled analysis from referral centers. *Minerva Urol. Nephrol.* **2021**, *73*, 165–177. [CrossRef]

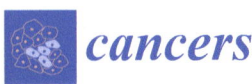

Article

Prognostic Evaluation of Metastatic Castration Resistant Prostate Cancer and Neuroendocrine Prostate Cancer with [^{68}Ga]Ga DOTATATE PET-CT

Mehmet Asim Bilen [1,2,*], Akinyemi Akintayo [3], Yuan Liu [2], Olayinka Abiodun-Ojo [3], Omer Kucuk [1,2], Bradley C. Carthon [1,2], David M. Schuster [3] and Ephraim E. Parent [3,4,*]

1 Department of Hematology and Medical Oncology, Emory University School of Medicine, Atlanta, GA 30322, USA
2 Winship Cancer Institute, Emory University, Atlanta, GA 30322, USA
3 Department of Radiology and Imaging Sciences, Emory University School of Medicine, Atlanta, GA 30322, USA
4 Department of Radiology, Mayo Clinic, Jacksonville, FL 32224, USA
* Correspondence: mehmet.a.bilen@emory.edu (M.A.B.); parent.ephraim@mayo.edu (E.E.P.); Tel.: +1-904-953-3270 (E.E.P.)

Citation: Bilen, M.A.; Akintayo, A.; Liu, Y.; Abiodun-Ojo, O.; Kucuk, O.; Carthon, B.C.; Schuster, D.M.; Parent, E.E. Prognostic Evaluation of Metastatic Castration Resistant Prostate Cancer and Neuroendocrine Prostate Cancer with [^{68}Ga]Ga DOTATATE PET-CT. *Cancers* **2022**, *14*, 6039. https://doi.org/10.3390/cancers14246039

Academic Editor: David Wong

Received: 7 November 2022
Accepted: 6 December 2022
Published: 8 December 2022

Publisher's Note: MDPI stays neutral with regard to jurisdictional claims in published maps and institutional affiliations.

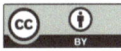

Copyright: © 2022 by the authors. Licensee MDPI, Basel, Switzerland. This article is an open access article distributed under the terms and conditions of the Creative Commons Attribution (CC BY) license (https://creativecommons.org/licenses/by/4.0/).

Simple Summary: Prostate cancer is the most common cancer in men and, along with the aggressive neuroendocrine variant of prostate cancer, is known to express high levels of the somatostatin receptor. This study explored the feasibility of using the somatostatin binding radiopharmaceutical, [^{68}Ga]Ga-DOTATATE PET/CT, to identify metastatic lesions in 17 men with known metastatic castrate resistant prostate cancer or neuroendocrine prostate cancer. All patients demonstrated [^{68}Ga]Ga-DOTATATE avid lesions corresponding to sites of disease as identified by CT. Additionally, we retrospectively correlated the degree of [^{68}Ga]Ga-DOTATATE to treatment response and found that men with marked [^{68}Ga]Ga-DOTATATE uptake in their metastatic deposits had significantly worse outcomes compared to those with moderate or mild [^{68}Ga]Ga-DOTATATE uptake. Conversely, men with only mild [^{68}Ga]Ga-DOTATATE uptake in their metastatic deposits had a favorable prognostic outcome.

Abstract: Objectives: Prostate cancer is well known to express high levels of somatostatin receptors and preliminary data suggests that PET imaging with the somatostatin analog, [^{68}Ga]Ga-DOTATATE, may allow for whole body staging of patients with metastatic castration resistant prostate cancer (mCRPC) and neuroendocrine prostate cancer (NePC). This study explores the utility of [^{68}Ga]Ga-DOTATATE PET-CT to identify metastatic deposits in men with mCRPC and NePC and prognosticate disease progression. Methods: [^{68}Ga]Ga-DOTATATE PET-CT was performed in 17 patients with mCRPC and of those, 2/17 had NePC. A semiquantitative analysis with standardized uptake values (SUV) (e.g., SUVmax, SUVmean) was performed for each metastatic lesion and reference background tissues. [^{68}Ga]Ga-DOTATATE uptake in metastatic deposits was further classified as: mild (less than liver), moderate (up to liver average), or marked (greater than liver). Serial prostate-specific antigen measurements and patient survival were followed up to 3 years after PET imaging to assess response to standard of care treatment. Results: All patients had at least one metastatic lesion with identifiable [^{68}Ga]Ga-DOTATATE uptake. Marked [^{68}Ga]Ga-DOTATATE uptake was found in 7/17 patients, including both NePC patients, and all were non-responders to systemic therapy and died within the follow up period, with a mean time to death of 8.1 months. Three patients had mild [^{68}Ga]Ga-DOTATATE uptake, and all were responders to systemic therapy and were alive 36 months after [^{68}Ga]Ga-DOTATATE imaging. Conclusions: [^{68}Ga]Ga-DOTATATE is able to identify mCRPC and NePC metastatic deposits, and lesions with [^{68}Ga]Ga-DOTATATE uptake > liver may portend poor outcomes in patients with mCRPC.

Keywords: DOTATATE; PET; prostate cancer; neuroendocrine prostate cancer

1. Introduction

Prostate cancer (PCa) is the most common cancer among men in the United States [1]. Androgen deprivation therapy (ADT) is the mainstay of treatment for advanced prostate cancer; however, most patients will eventually develop androgen-refractory disease, or metastatic castration resistant prostate cancer (mCRPC). While small cell neuroendocrine prostate carcinoma is rare, a subset of patients previously diagnosed with prostate adenocarcinoma may develop neuroendocrine features after ADT. Transformed neuroendocrine prostate cancer (NePC) has molecular and genetic changes making them resistant to traditional mCRPC therapies, including androgen receptor (AR) targeted therapies [2], and it has been hypothesized that some of the difficulty in treating patients with mCRPC may in fact be due to neuroendocrine differentiation [3]. The reported prevalence of NePC has varied between studies, possibly due to limitations in targeted tissue sampling and heterogeneous disease penetrance. For example, in a study of 450 patients with mCRPC by Perez et al., only 3 patients demonstrated NePC differentiation [4], whereas Jimenez et al. found NePC differentiation in 92/183 metastatic biopsies from 79 of 157 patients with mCRPC [5].

Somatostatin, a neuropeptide that suppresses prostate growth and neovascularization by inducing cell-cycle arrest and apoptosis, is highly expressed in NePC cells [6,7]. Somatostatin receptors, specifically SSTR2, have been shown to be upregulated in PCa and NePC [8,9]. [^{68}Ga]Ga-DOTATATE (NETSpot®) is a FDA-approved PET radiotracer with high affinity for SSTR2 [8]. Preliminary case reports suggest that [^{68}Ga]Ga-DOTA labeled somatostatin analogs may have high sensitivity in identifying sites of mCRPC in addition to NePC [10–13]. In a recent study involving 12 patients with mCRPC, all patients had at least 1 blastic neuroendocrine metastasis with increased radiotracer uptake [14]. Patients with multiple bone metastases also had significantly higher SUVmax when compared to patients with few metastases.

The goal of this study was to determine the feasibility of identifying mCRPC lesions, including patients with NePC, using noninvasive imaging and to assess whether such an early imaging biomarker can predict eventual progression in patients with mCRPC about to start first line treatment (abiraterone acetate or enzalutamide) for castration resistant disease.

We hypothesized that patients with higher levels of [^{68}Ga]Ga-DOTATATE uptake on an initial PET scan may have a shorter time to progression while on oral agents (abiraterone acetate or enzalutamide) due to resistance to antiandrogen based therapeutics [15] when compared to those with lower [^{68}Ga]Ga-DOTATATE uptake. We assessed for correlations between the degree and intensity of uptake of [^{68}Ga]Ga-DOTATATE with subsequent progression of disease, determined by standard of care whole body bone scans [16] and CT/MR imaging [17], as well as clinical parameters.

2. Materials and Methods

2.1. Patient Population

2.1.1. Subject Recruitment

Patients with biopsy proven PCa were recruited from the Winship Cancer Institute at Emory University from 18 April 2018 to 16 May 2019. All procedures performed in studies involving human participants were in accordance with the ethical standards of the institutional and/or national research committee and with the 1964 Helsinki declaration and its later amendments or comparable ethical standards. The recruitment protocol was approved by the Institutional Review Board (IRB) and complied with the Health Insurance Portability and Accountability Act (HIPAA). The data was collected as part of a feasibility trial for neuroendocrine prostate cancer imaging under the IRB title 'Molecular Imaging with [^{68}Ga]Ga-DOTATATE PET to Investigate Neuroendocrine Differentiation in Prostate Cancer Patients (IRB#99167)'. This study is listed on clinicaltrials.gov (NCT 03448458). The radiotracer was labeled using a provided NETSpot kit (Advanced Accelerator Applications USA, Inc. Millburn, NJ, USA) and generator produce [^{68}Ga]Ga (Eckert & Ziegler Radiopharma, Inc. Berlin, Germany). Safety monitoring during the drug infusion was performed, and no adverse events were recorded. Written informed consent was obtained from every study participant. This study did not interfere with standard patient evaluation or delayed therapy.

Male patients with known biopsy proven mCRPC were selected under the inclusion criteria of 18 years of age or older, with skeletal, visceral and/or nodal involvement, and able to undergo [^{68}Ga]Ga-DOTATATE PET-CT. Patients were previously treated with a combination of ADT ± antiandrogen therapy or chemotherapy prior to diagnosis of mCRPC and subsequently were treated with either hormonal therapy or chemotherapy after mCRPC status (Table 1). No intervention or tissue analysis was performed after the [^{68}Ga]Ga-DOTATATE PET-CT. In total, 17 patients were recruited and received at least one [^{68}Ga]Ga-DOTATATE PET-CT. One patient was subsequently found to have an additional metastatic pulmonary squamous cell carcinoma and was excluded from this analysis. These patients had a mean age of 62.8 years (range from 48y–87y) and were included per the inclusion criteria (Table 1). The two patients with biopsy proven NePC received platinum-based chemotherapy after [^{68}Ga]Ga-DOTATATE PET-CT. Of the 14 patients without NePC, 7/14 received enzalutamide or abiraterone, and 7/14 received taxane based chemotherapy after [^{68}Ga]Ga-DOTATATE PET-CT. The median PSA at time of imaging was 46.8 ng/mL (range: 4.44–1033.78 ng/mL).

Table 1. Patient demographics.

Gleason Grade	PSA at Time of PET/CT (ng/mL)	Index Lesions with [^{68}Ga]Ga DOTATATE Uptake	SUVmax Hottest Lesion	Systemic Treatments Prior to CRPC Diagnosis	Additional Systemic Treatments after CRPC Diagnosis
4	39.23	7	2.1	ADT alone	Enzalutamide
3	11.18	7	3.1	ADT alone	Enzalutamide
2	7.09	3	3.3	ADT alone	Enzalutamide
N/A *	48.08	6	6.2	ADT alone	Docetaxel
5	4.4	2	6.6	ADT alone	Enzalutamide
5	44.54	8	7.3	ADT alone	Docetaxel
5	38.99	9	8.3	ADT+ Docetaxel + anti-androgen therapy	Abiraterone
5	1033.87	7	8.6	ADT+ Abiraterone	cabazitaxol + carboplatin
5	28.76	9	8.9	ADT+ Docetaxel + anti-androgen therapy	Abiraterone
5	31.37	6	10.7	ADT alone	Docetaxel
5	115.45	5	11	ADT+ Docetaxel + anti-androgen therapy	Cabazitaxol
5 [†]	26.51	8	20.1	ADT + platinium/etoposide	Enzalutamide
4	128	6	20.2	ADT+ Abiraterone	Docetaxel
5	61.86	9	23.1	ADT alone	Enzalutamide
2	88.05	13	27	ADT+ Abiraterone	Docetaxel
N/A [‡]	<0.01	8	28.5	platinum+ etoposide	Cisplatin + etoposide

* Gleason grade not available. [†] Small cell neuroendocrine carcinoma and acinar adenocarcinoma. [‡] Small cell carcinoma.

2.1.2. Image Acquisition

All patients underwent [^{68}Ga]Ga-DOTATATE PET-CT of the whole body 55–70 min after intravenous bolus injection of 200 ± 11 MBq (5.4 ± 0.3 mCi) of [^{68}Ga]Ga-DOTATATE. PET-CT images were acquired on a GE Discovery-690 16 slice integrated PET-CT scanner (GE Healthcare) without IV contrast. CT scan of the skull base to proximal thighs (80–120 mA) was utilized for anatomic imaging and correction of emission data. PET images were acquired in 3-min scan time per bed position PET acquisition. Dead time, detector efficiency and scatter corrections were applied using the routines supplied by the manufacturer. The resulting images were quantitatively calibrated with 6 mm isotropic resolution. Images were reconstructed with the iterative technique and reviewed on a MimVista workstation (MIM Software, Version 7.2.1). Reconstruction parameters were VUE point FX with 3 iterations/24 subsets and 6.4 mm filter cutoff, and the reconstructed slice thickness was 3.75 mm.

2.1.3. Image Analysis

[^{68}Ga]Ga-DOTATATE PET-CT images were interpreted by a board-certified nuclear radiologist, blinded to details of clinical history (beyond inclusion criteria) and other imaging. Whenever possible, 3-dimensional PET-Edge conformational ROI were used to encompass the entire structure, otherwise conformational ROIs were utilized to record uptake in regions of physiologic and abnormal uptake. Up to 5 representative index lesions in each category were selected as markers of [^{68}Ga]Ga-DOTATATE uptake. If five lesions in each category could not be defined in a patient, all demonstrable lesions up to five were utilized. Lesions chosen were independent but may have coincided with index lesions on conventional imaging.

2.2. Semiquantitative PET and Visual Analysis

[^{68}Ga]Ga-DOTATATE in prostate/bed and extraprostatic sites such as lymph nodes, visceral organs, and the skeleton were quantified using maximum standardized uptake values (SUVmax) and mean standardized uptake values (SUVmean). SUV values and standard bi-dimensional size measurements of lesions were recorded for up to 5 bone and 5 soft tissue lesions in each patient. The SUVmax of pathological findings were compared with accumulation of the radiotracer (SUVmax and SUVmean) in the liver, bone marrow (L3), and blood pool as reference organs. Summation of [^{68}Ga]Ga-DOTATATE uptake parameters from all indexed lesions per patient was also recorded. In addition, visual comparison of the most [^{68}Ga]Ga-DOTATATE avid lesions was performed as a simple way to stratify the degree of uptake similar to that performed with Krenning scoring for patients with non-prostatic neuroendocrine carcinoma [18]. [^{68}Ga]Ga-DOTATATE PET uptake was visually classified with the lesion either having: (A) Mild [^{68}Ga]Ga-DOTATATE uptake (less than liver); defined as [^{68}Ga]Ga-DOTATATE uptake $\geq$ blood pool or L3 marrow < average liver (SUVmean) (Figure 1). (B) Moderate [^{68}Ga]Ga-DOTATATE uptake (equal to liver); defined as $\geq$average liver (SUVmean) and $\leq$ liver (SUVmax) (Figure 2). (C) Marked [^{68}Ga]Ga-DOTATATE uptake (greater than liver); defined as >liver (SUVmax) (Figure 3). For normal liver and bone marrow, SUVmean was determined by placing a spherical VOI (3.0 cm in diameter) in a representative healthy part of the organ. Whole blood uptake (SUVmean) was measured by placing a spherical VOI (1.0 cm in diameter) in the left ventricle of the heart. Lesions were determined to be equal to liver SUVmean if within 20% of the measured value.

[^{68}Ga]Ga-DOTATATE PET-CT uptake in metastatic deposits was correlated with response to subsequent standard of care therapy as identified by: Prostate-specific antigen (PSA) progression or PSA response (defined as a drop of >50%), change in clinical management, clinical progression as defined by their medical oncologist, progression free survival and patient mortality. Following [^{68}Ga]Ga-DOTATATE PET-CT, patients were treated according to standard of care per the clinician's discretion with oral agents (abiraterone acetate or enzalutamide) or other FDA-approved agents. The results of the [^{68}Ga]Ga-DOTATATE PET-CT did not influence the clinician's treatment decisions. Subsequent routine imaging and standard laboratory analysis (e.g., PSA level) were performed according to the clinician's discretion. Patients were followed in the context of this study (per clinical routine) for at least one-year after [^{68}Ga]Ga-DOTATATE PET-CT.

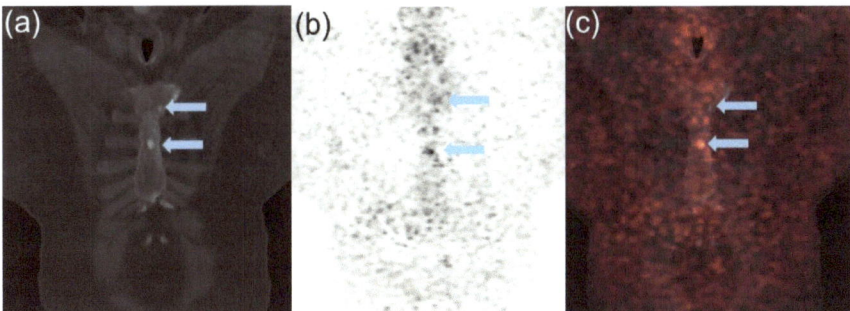

Figure 1. 64 year old male diagnosed with Gleason Score 4 + 3 = 7 prostate cancer in 2012. Was previously treated with Bicalutamide (Casodex) and currently maintained on Lupron. At time of [^{68}Ga]Ga-DOTATATE PET-CT, patient presented with rising PSA of 11.2 ng/mL with a doubling time of 1.8 months. Coronal images of CT (**a**) [^{68}Ga]Ga-DOTATATE PET (**b**) and fused [^{68}Ga]Ga-DOTATATE PET-CT (**c**) demonstrate mild [^{68}Ga]Ga-DOTATATE uptake in sclerotic lesions (blue arrows; SUVmax 3.1) greater than marrow but less than liver (SUVmax of 17.3). Patient was subsequently placed on Enzalutamide with subsequent PSA response to therapy and survived to the end of study.

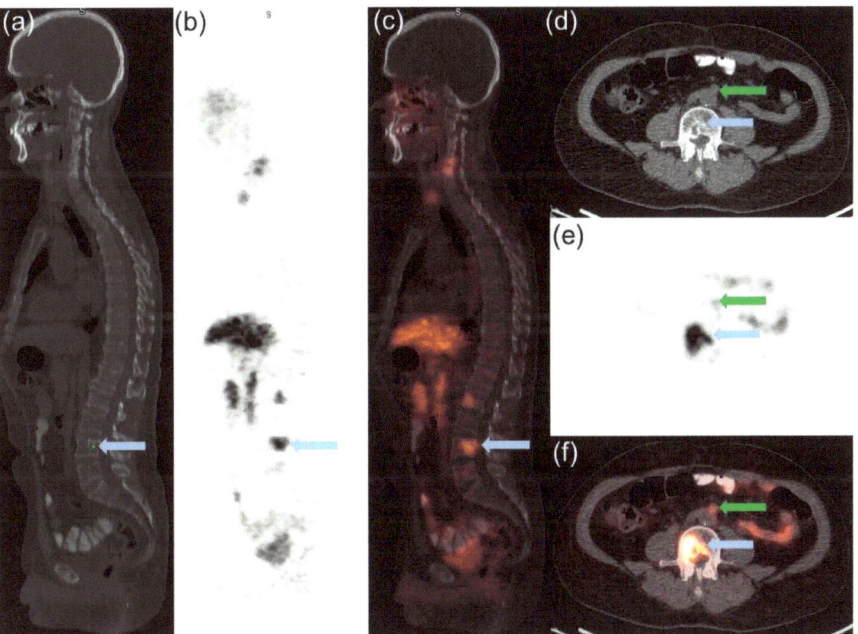

Figure 2. 51-year-old man with prostate cancer (Gleason score 9) maintained on ADT since 2011 and placed on enzalutamide four months prior to [^{68}Ga]Ga-DOTATATE PET-CT. Selected sagittal CT (**a**) [^{68}Ga]Ga-DOTATATE PET (**b**) and fused [^{68}Ga]Ga-DOTATATE PET-CT (**c**) images show moderate [^{68}Ga]Ga-DOTATATE uptake less than liver (SUVmax 11.8) in several osseus lesions, with the most avid L3 osseus lesion of SUVmax 10.7 (blue arrow). Transaxial CT (**d**) PET (**e**) and fused (**f**) [^{68}Ga]Ga-DOTATATE PET-CT views through the L3 vertebral deposit also demonstrates a preaortic lymph node (green arrow) with mild [^{68}Ga]Ga-DOTATATE uptake (SUVmax 3.4). Patient was switched to Docetaxel after [^{68}Ga]Ga-DOTATATE PET-CT with initial PSA response to therapy but eventually progressed and died 20 months after [^{68}Ga]Ga-DOTATATE PET-CT.

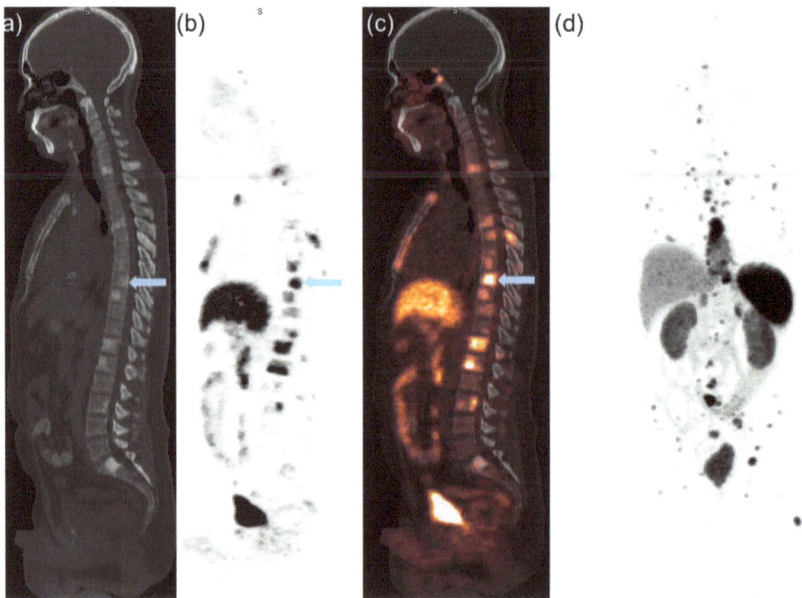

Figure 3. 47-year-old man with Gleason score 9, mixed prostate small cell neuroendocrine carcinoma and acinar adenocarcinoma. Patient was stated on ADT and cisplatin/etoposide prior to [^{68}Ga]Ga-DOTATATE PET-CT. Selected sagittal CT (**a**) [^{68}Ga]Ga-DOTATATE PET (**b**) and fused [^{68}Ga]Ga-DOTATATE PET-CT (**c**) images show marked [^{68}Ga]Ga-DOTATATE uptake greater than liver (SUVmax of 14.4) in several osseus lesions with the most avid T8 lesion having a SUVmax 20.1 (blue arrow). Anterior view of [^{68}Ga]Ga-DOTATATE PET MIP (**d**) demonstrates multiple [^{68}Ga]Ga-DOTATATE and nodal metastatic deposits. Patient did not demonstrate a PSA response to therapy and passed away 4 months after [^{68}Ga]Ga-DOTATATE PET-CT.

2.3. Statistical Analysis

Since this was a pilot study with the main goal to evaluate the feasibility, statistical power was not calculated.

3. Results

Semiquantitative PET and Visual Analysis

All patients had at least one lesion with identifiable [^{68}Ga]Ga-DOTATATE uptake as evidenced by abnormally increased focal [^{68}Ga]Ga-DOTATATE uptake with CT correlates (e.g., lymphadenopathy, sclerotic osseus lesions). Lesions with marked [^{68}Ga]Ga-DOTATATE uptake per visual and semiquantitative analysis were found in 7 of 16 patients analyzed and with a Gleason score range of 7–9. All patients with marked [^{68}Ga]Ga-DOTATATE uptake were non-responders to systemic therapy, all of which died within the follow up period, with a mean time to death of 8.1 months (range of 14.4–92.6 weeks). One patient was confirmed to be NePC and another with shown to have small cell neuroendocrine carcinoma and acinar adenocarcinoma on biopsy. Six of the 16 patients were found to have moderate [^{68}Ga]Ga-DOTATATE uptake and all had a Gleason score of 9. Of the patients with moderate [^{68}Ga]Ga-DOTATATE uptake, four died with a mean time of death of 13.3 months (range of 12.7–89.6 weeks). The two surviving patients with moderate [^{68}Ga]Ga-DOTATATE uptake both had an initial PSA response to therapy and no NePC was found. The three remaining patients with mild [^{68}Ga]Ga-DOTATATE uptake had a Gleason score range of 7–8. All patients were all still alive up to 36 months after [^{68}Ga]Ga-DOTATATE study and all had an initial PSA response to therapy (Figure 4).

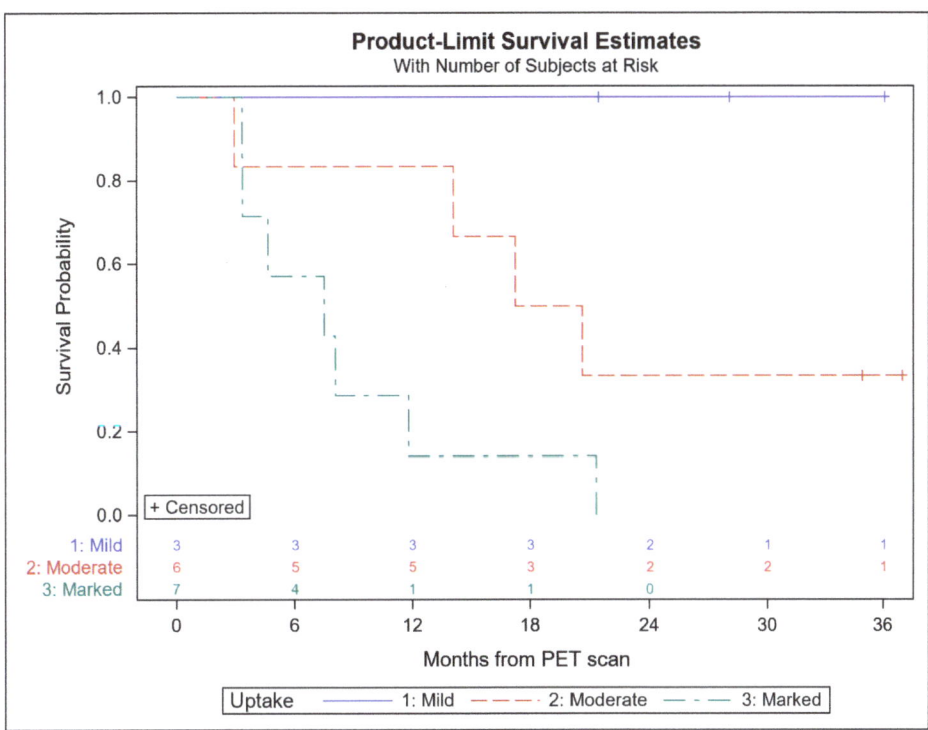

Figure 4. Kaplan-Meier Plots for mCRPC patients with mild, moderate, and marked [^{68}Ga]Ga-DOTATATE uptake with a log-rank p-value of 0.01.

On [^{68}Ga]Ga-DOTATATE PET, all patients had at least one lesion with a median number of seven lesions per patient. A total of 11/16 patients had bone and visceral/nodal lesions, 4/16 had only bone lesions, and one had only nodal disease. Summed SUVmax was significantly higher in the 2/16 patients with proven NePC compared to the 14/16 patients with non-neuroendocrine mCRPC (99.1 ± 16.5 ng/mL vs. 48.4 ± 40.6 ng/mL; $p = 0.04$). Generally, the patients with the highest summed SUVmax also had the highest lesion SUV and worse outcomes. However, there was no correlation between summed SUVmax and PSA. SUVmean lesion values followed similar trends to the reported SUVmax analysis; however, there was no easily identifiable comparable reference organ (e.g., liver, spleen) and for ease of analysis and reproducibility this analysis is limited to SUVmax. Next generation sequencing data was available from 6/16 patients. Of these, 1 patient without NePC had a BRCA2 mutation and also had the highest summed uptake in this study.

4. Conclusions

NePC is underdiagnosed, as biopsy of metastatic lesions after spread to soft tissue and bones, which is required for histologic confirmation, is rarely done [3,19]. Furthermore, the standard biopsy is subject to sampling error both within a lesion itself and on a global basis, and there is no established non-invasive imaging or biochemical marker to identify NePC. Almost all prostate cancers show focal neuroendocrine differentiation, but about 5–10% of patients with PCa, have a large number of clustered NE cells that are detected by chromogranin A immunostaining [20]. In tumors that can be classified as NePC, the neuroendocrine component usually comprises 5–30% of the tumor mass [21,22]. The mechanisms by which neuroendocrine cells influence prostate carcinogenesis are not fully understood. The transdifferentiation process from a typical epithelial-like to a neuroendocrine-like phenotype may be a consequence of the selective pressure induced by treatments that result in decreased androgen levels, stimulation of neuroendocrine and neural factors, and loss of tumor suppressors and genomic stability [23,24].

Definitive criteria defining high, moderate, and mild uptake have not been established. However, extrapolating a simple interpretation criteria based on literature examples [14] is as follows: (A) Mild [^{68}Ga]Ga-DOTATATE uptake defined as [^{68}Ga]Ga-DOTATATE uptake $\geq$ blood pool or L3 marrow < liver (SUVmean). (B) Moderate [^{68}Ga]Ga-DOTATATE uptake $\geq$ average liver (SUVmean) and $\leq$liver (SUVmax). (C) Marked [^{68}Ga]Ga-DOTATATE uptake > liver (SUVmax) [14]. We are not aware of any literature that has attempted to correlate [^{68}Ga]Ga-DOTATATE uptake to clinical outcomes in patients with prostate cancer. In this study, we showed that higher lesion ^{68}Ga DOTATATE uptake compared to physiologic background [^{68}Ga]Ga-DOTATATE uptake portends a worse prognosis, regardless of Gleason score, PSA, extent of disease, or systemic therapy. As expected, [^{68}Ga]Ga-DOTATATE uptake in lesions has been found to be higher in mCRPC patients with NePC. All patients with [^{68}Ga]Ga-DOTATATE uptake greater than liver (SUVmax) died within 2 years of imaging regardless of Gleason score, PSA value, or therapeutic management. This subgroup included the two patients with NePC differentiation. In patients with moderate [^{68}Ga]Ga-DOTATATE uptake, these also had a worse prognosis compared to patients with mild [^{68}Ga]Ga-DOTATATE uptake, who were all still alive at the conclusion of this study. We included in our study patients with mCRPC who were about to start the first line of treatment (abiraterone acetate or enzalutamide) for castration resistant disease. We believe that this inflection point best balances the early detection of potential neuroendocrine transdifferentiation with imaging, as these patients typically have higher ECOG (Eastern Cooperative Oncology Group) performance status than those further along the continuum of their treatment.

Case reports exist of increased [^{68}Ga]Ga-DOTATATE uptake in prostate adenocarcinoma as well as prostate carcinoma with neuroendocrine differentiation [25]. Typically, NePC does not express PSMA, but there are a few case reports of patients with known NePC also demonstrating several foci of increased PSMA PET uptake [12,26]. Prostate adenocarcinoma is known to upregulate somatostatin receptors resulting in [^{68}Ga]Ga-DOTATATE PET uptake, which does not imply by itself the transdifferentiation to a neuroendocrine pathway [14]. Benign conditions such as benign prostate hyperplasia have similarly been shown to have upregulated somatostatin and are [^{68}Ga]Ga-DOTATATE PET positive [27,28]. Patients with mCRPC and NePC and intense [^{68}Ga]Ga-DOTATATE uptake may be amenable to treatment with PRRT ([^{177}Lu]Lu-DOTATATE; Lutathera) [29,30]. [^{11}C]C-choline and [^{68}Ga]Ga-DOTATATE have been shown to have comparable detection rates for mCRPC [31].

There are several major limitations of our study. One major drawback of our study is the relatively small patient population for both mCRPC and NePC, with a total of 16 patients, including two with NePC. Additionally, this small group was heterogeneous in the Gleason grading and maintenance therapy prior to imaging with [^{68}Ga]Ga-DOTATATE. All patients were maintained on ADT prior to [^{68}Ga]Ga-DOTATATE PET-CT, but some patients were also maintained on oral agents or platinum chemotherapy. However, despite such a small and heterogeneous group of patients and lesions, we were able to identify differences in [^{68}Ga]Ga-DOTATATE uptake between the two groups and correlate uptake with outcomes. An additional limitation is that pathological confirmation was not available for most lesions and focal transformation to neuroendocrine differentiation was not able to be systemically evaluated. Moreover, this study was a feasibility study and was not powered to correlate [^{68}Ga]Ga-DOTATATE uptake to outcomes or neuroendocrine transdifferentiation. Additionally, there was no correlative molecular imaging performed on these patients such as with [^{68}Ga]Ga PMSA-11 (Locametz®) or [^{18}F]F PSMA DCFPyL (Pylarify®). This lack of correlative imaging limits the ability to further characterize potential transformation to neuroendocrine prostate cancer, as these typically have low PSMA uptake. Finally, it is not known if there is an optimal temporal point after beginning systemic therapy to discriminate either neuroendocrine transdifferentiation or clinical outcomes.

[^{68}Ga]Ga-DOTATATE PET provides high contrast images that are able to identify both mCRPC and NePC lesions. This study suggests that simple evaluation with SUV$_{max}$ may provide prognostic information to the treating physician and allow them to guide treatment accordingly. Further investigation with larger data sets is needed to confirm these preliminary findings and to further establish optimal [^{68}Ga]Ga-DOTATATE PET imaging parameters.

Author Contributions: M.A.B. and E.E.P. conceived the study, obtained funding, performed data analysis and drafted the manuscript. M.A.B., O.K. and B.C.C. recruited patients. A.A., O.A.-O. and D.M.S. helped write the first draft of the manuscript. Y.L. performed statistical analysis. All authors have read and agreed to the published version of the manuscript.

Funding: Funding was provided in part by grants to M.A.B. and E.E.P. from Advanced Accelerator Applications (Novartis) and Winship Cancer Institute of Emory University Winship (4165-17). The other authors declare that they have no competing interest.

Institutional Review Board Statement: The study was conducted in accordance with the Declaration of Helsinki, and approved by the Institutional Review Board of Emory University School of Medicine under the IRB title 'Molecular Imaging with [^{68}Ga]Ga-DOTATATE PET to Investigate Neuroendocrine Differentiation in Prostate Cancer Patients (IRB#99167)' for studies involving humans.

Informed Consent Statement: Written informed consent was obtained from all subjects involved in the study including consent to publish this paper.

Data Availability Statement: Data supporting the reported results can be obtained from the corresponding author.

Conflicts of Interest: The funders had no role in the design of the study; in the collection, analyses, or interpretation of data; in the writing of the manuscript, or in the decision to publish the results.

References

1. Siegel, R.L.; Miller, K.D.; Fuchs, H.E.; Jemal, A. Cancer Statistics, 2021. *CA Cancer J. Clin.* **2021**, *71*, 7–33. [CrossRef] [PubMed]
2. Santoni, M.; Scarpelli, M.; Mazzucchelli, R.; Lopez-Beltran, A.; Cheng, L.; Cascinu, S.; Montironi, R. Targeting prostate-specific membrane antigen for personalized therapies in prostate cancer: Morphologic and molecular backgrounds and future promises. *J. Biol. Regul. Homeost. Agents* **2014**, *28*, 555–563. [PubMed]
3. Parimi, V.; Goyal, R.; Poropatich, K.; Yang, X.J. Neuroendocrine differentiation of prostate cancer: A review. *Am. J. Clin. Exp. Urol.* **2014**, *2*, 273–285. [PubMed]
4. Perez, D.; Linares, E.; Almagro, E.; Cantos, B.; Mendez, M.; Maximiano, C.; Franco, F.; Rubio, J.; Palka, M.; Calvo, V.; et al. Neuroendocrine differentiation in carcinoma of the prostate: An institutional review. *J. Clin. Oncol.* **2014**, *15*, 32. [CrossRef]
5. Jimenez, R.E.; Nandy, D.; Qin, R.; Carlson, R.; Tan, W.; Kohli, M. Neuroendocrine differentiation patterns in metastases from advanced prostate cancer. *J. Clin. Oncol.* **2014**, *15*, 32. [CrossRef]
6. Nelson, E.C.; Cambio, A.J.; Yang, J.C.; Ok, J.H.; Lara, P.N., Jr.; Evans, C.P. Clinical implications of neuroendocrine differentiation in prostate cancer. *Prostate Cancer Prostatic. Dis.* **2007**, *10*, 6–14. [CrossRef]
7. Borre, M.; Nerstrom, B.; Overgaard, J. Association between immunohistochemical expression of vascular endothelial growth factor (VEGF), VEGF-expressing neuroendocrine-differentiated tumor cells, and outcome in prostate cancer patients subjected to watchful waiting. *Clin. Cancer Res.* **2000**, *6*, 1882–1890.
8. Morichetti, D.; Mazzucchelli, R.; Santinelli, A.; Stramazzotti, D.; Lopez-Beltran, A.; Scarpelli, M.; Bono, A.V.; Cheng, L.; Montironi, R. Immunohistochemical expression and localization of somatostatin receptor subtypes in prostate cancer with neuroendocrine differentiation. *Int. J. Immunopathol. Pharmacol.* **2010**, *23*, 511–522. [CrossRef]
9. Montironi, R.; Cheng, L.; Mazzucchelli, R.; Morichetti, D.; Stramazzotti, D.; Santinelli, A.; Moroncini, G.; Galosi, A.B.; Muzzonigro, G.; Comeri, G.; et al. Immunohistochemical detection and localization of somatostatin receptor subtypes in prostate tissue from patients with bladder outlet obstruction. *Cell Oncol.* **2008**, *30*, 473–482. [CrossRef]
10. Gabriel, M.; Decristoforo, C.; Kendler, D.; Dobrozemsky, G.; Heute, D.; Uprimny, C.; Kovacs, P.; Von Guggenberg, E.; Bale, R.; Virgolini, I.J. 68Ga-DOTA-Tyr3-octreotide PET in neuroendocrine tumors: Comparison with somatostatin receptor scintigraphy and CT. *J. Nucl. Med.* **2007**, *48*, 508–518. [CrossRef]
11. Alonso, O.; Gambini, J.P.; Lago, G.; Gaudiano, J.; Quagliata, A.; Engler, H. In vivo visualization of somatostatin receptor expression with Ga-68-DOTA-TATE PET/CT in advanced metastatic prostate cancer. *Clin. Nucl. Med.* **2011**, *36*, 1063–1064. [CrossRef] [PubMed]
12. Chen, S.; Cheung, S.K.; Wong, K.N.; Wong, K.K.; Ho, C.L. 68Ga-DOTATOC and 68Ga-PSMA PET/CT Unmasked a Case of Prostate Cancer With Neuroendocrine Differentiation. *Clin. Nucl. Med.* **2016**, *41*, 959–960. [CrossRef]

13. Todorovic-Tirnanic, M.V.; Gajic, M.M.; Obradovic, V.B.; Baum, R.P. Gallium-68 DOTATOC PET/CT in vivo characterization of somatostatin receptor expression in the prostate. *Cancer Biother. Radiopharm.* **2014**, *29*, 108–115. [CrossRef]
14. Gofrit, O.N.; Frank, S.; Meirovitz, A.; Nechushtan, H.; Orevi, M. PET/CT With 68Ga-DOTA-TATE for Diagnosis of Neuroendocrine: Differentiation in Patients With Castrate-Resistant Prostate Cancer. *Clin. Nucl. Med.* **2017**, *42*, 1–6. [CrossRef] [PubMed]
15. Hirano, D.; Okada, Y.; Minei, S.; Takimoto, Y.; Nemoto, N. Neuroendocrine differentiation in hormone refractory prostate cancer following androgen deprivation therapy. *Eur. Urol.* **2004**, *45*, 586–592, discussion 592. [CrossRef]
16. Scher, H.I.; Halabi, S.; Tannock, I.; Morris, M.; Sternberg, C.N.; Carducci, M.A.; Eisenberger, M.A.; Higano, C.; Bubley, G.J.; Dreicer, R.; et al. Design and end points of clinical trials for patients with progressive prostate cancer and castrate levels of testosterone: Recommendations of the Prostate Cancer Clinical Trials Working Group. *J. Clin. Oncol.* **2008**, *26*, 1148–1159. [CrossRef] [PubMed]
17. Schwartz, L.H.; Bogaerts, J.; Ford, R.; Shankar, L.; Therasse, P.; Gwyther, S.; Eisenhauer, E.A. Evaluation of lymph nodes with RECIST 1.1. *Eur. J. Cancer* **2009**, *45*, 261–267. [CrossRef]
18. Menon, B.K.; Kalshetty, A.; Bhattacharjee, A.; Basu, S. Standardized uptake values and ratios on 68Ga-DOTATATE PET-computed tomography for normal organs and malignant lesions and their correlation with Krenning score in patients with metastatic neuroendocrine tumors. *Nucl. Med. Commun.* **2020**, *41*, 1095–1099. [CrossRef]
19. Komiya, A.; Yasuda, K.; Watanabe, A.; Fujiuchi, Y.; Tsuzuki, T.; Fuse, H. The prognostic significance of loss of the androgen receptor and neuroendocrine differentiation in prostate biopsy specimens among castration-resistant prostate cancer patients. *Mol. Clin. Oncol.* **2013**, *1*, 257–262. [CrossRef]
20. di Sant'Agnese, P.A. Neuroendocrine differentiation in carcinoma of the prostate. Diagnostic, prognostic, and therapeutic implications. *Cancer* **1992**, *70*, 254–268. [CrossRef]
21. di Sant'Agnese, P.A. Neuroendocrine differentiation in prostatic carcinoma: An update on recent developments. *Ann. Oncol.* **2001**, *12* (Suppl. 2), S135–S140. [CrossRef] [PubMed]
22. Volante, M.; Rindi, G.; Papotti, M. The grey zone between pure (neuro)endocrine and non-(neuro)endocrine tumours: A comment on concepts and classification of mixed exocrine-endocrine neoplasms. *Virchows. Arch.* **2006**, *449*, 499–506. [CrossRef]
23. Beltran, H.; Tomlins, S.; Aparicio, A.; Arora, V.; Rickman, D.; Ayala, G.; Huang, J.; True, L.; Gleave, M.E.; Soule, H.; et al. Aggressive variants of castration-resistant prostate cancer. *Clin. Cancer Res.* **2014**, *20*, 2846–2850. [CrossRef] [PubMed]
24. Hu, C.D.; Choo, R.; Huang, J. Neuroendocrine differentiation in prostate cancer: A mechanism of radioresistance and treatment failure. *Front. Oncol.* **2015**, *5*, 90. [CrossRef]
25. Nisar, M.U.; Costa, D.N.; Jia, L.; Oz, O.K.; de Blanche, L. 68Ga-DOTATATE PET/CT Uptake in Prostate With an Incidental Finding of Prostatic Acinar Adenocarcinoma and Metastatic Neuroendocrine Cancer to the Liver. *Clin. Nucl. Med.* **2021**, *46*, e428–e430. [CrossRef] [PubMed]
26. Acar, E.; Kaya, G.C. 18F-FDG, 68Ga-DOTATATE and 68Ga-PSMA Positive Metastatic Large Cell Neuroendocrine Prostate Tumor. *Clin. Nucl. Med.* **2019**, *44*, 53–54. [CrossRef]
27. Wang, J. 68Ga-DOTATATE in Benign Prostate Hyperplasia. *Clin. Nucl. Med.* **2019**, *44*, 249–250. [CrossRef]
28. Schmidt, M.Q.; Trenbeath, Z.; Chin, B.B. Neuroendocrine prostate cancer or prostatitis? An unusual false positive on gallium-68 DOTA-Tyr3-octreotate positron emission tomography/computed tomography in a patient with known metastatic neuroendocrine tumor. *World J. Nucl. Med.* **2019**, *18*, 304–306. [CrossRef]
29. Assadi, M.; Pirayesh, E.; Rekabpour, S.J.; Zohrabi, F.; Jafari, E.; Nabipour, I.; Esmaili, A.; Amini, A.; Ahmadzadehfar, H. 177Lu-PSMA and 177Lu-DOTATATE Therapy in a Patient With Metastatic Castration-Resistant Prostate Cancer and Neuroendocrine Differentiation. *Clin. Nucl. Med.* **2019**, *44*, 978–980. [CrossRef]
30. Liu, C.; Liu, T.; Zhang, J.; Baum, R.P.; Yang, Z. Excellent Response to 177Lu-DOTATATE Peptide Receptor Radionuclide Therapy in a Patient With Progressive Metastatic Castration-Resistant Prostate Cancer With Neuroendocrine Differentiation After 177Lu-PSMA Therapy. *Clin. Nucl. Med.* **2019**, *44*, 876–878. [CrossRef]
31. Dos Santos, G.; Garcia Fontes, M.; Engler, H.; Alonso, O. Intraindividual comparison of (68)Ga-DOTATATE PET/CT vs. (11)C-Choline PET/CT in patients with prostate cancer in biochemical relapse: In vivo evaluation of the expression of somatostatin receptors. *Rev. Esp. Med. Nucl. Imagen Mol. Engl. Ed.* **2019**, *38*, 29–37. [CrossRef] [PubMed]

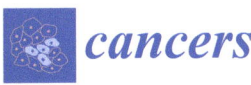

Article

A Single Dose of Novel PSMA-Targeting Radiopharmaceutical Agent [^{177}Lu]Ludotadipep for Patients with Metastatic Castration-Resistant Prostate Cancer: Phase I Clinical Trial

Dongho Shin [1], Seunggyun Ha [2], Joo Hyun O [2], Seung ah Rhew [1], Chang Eil Yoon [1], Hyeok Jae Kwon [1], Hyong Woo Moon [1], Yong Hyun Park [1], Sonya Youngju Park [2], Chansoo Park [3], Dae Yoon Chi [3], Ie Ryung Yoo [2,*] and Ji Youl Lee [1,*]

1 Department of Urology, Seoul St. Mary's Hospital, College of Medicine, The Catholic University of Korea, Seoul 06591, Republic of Korea
2 Department of Nuclear Medicine, Seoul St. Mary's Hospital, College of Medicine, The Catholic University of Korea, Seoul 06591, Republic of Korea
3 Research Institute of Labeling, FutureChem Co., Ltd., Seoul 04793, Republic of Korea
* Correspondence: iryoo@catholic.ac.kr (I.R.Y.); uroljy@catholic.ac.kr (J.Y.L.); Tel./Fax: +82-2-2258-1401 (I.R.Y.); +82-2-2258-1401 (J.Y.L.)

Simple Summary: Prostate specific membrane antigen (PSMA) is a transmembrane protein that is highly expressed in prostate cancer cells. For patients with metastatic castration-resistant prostate cancer (mCRPC) who do not respond to conventional treatment, PSMA targeting radiopharmaceutical therapy (RPT) has recently been in the spotlight. [^{177}Lu]Ludotadipep is a novel PSMA-targeting therapeutic agent designed with an albumin motif in order to increase the circulation time and uptake in the tumors. The safety and efficacy of [^{177}Lu]Ludotadipep were evaluated through a phase I trial.

Abstract: [^{177}Lu]Ludotadipep, which enables targeted delivery of beta-particle radiation to prostate tumor cells, had been suggested as a promising therapeutic option for mCRPC. From November 2020 to March 2022, a total of 30 patients were enrolled for single dose of [^{177}Lu]Ludotadipep RPT, 6 subjects in each of the 5 different activity groups of 1.9 GBq, 2.8 GBq, 3.7 GBq, 4.6 GBq, and 5.6 GBq. [^{177}Lu]Ludotadipep was administered via venous injection, and patients were hospitalized for three days to monitor for any adverse effects. Serum PSA levels were followed up at weeks 1, 2, 3, 4, 6, 8, and 12, and PSMA PET/CT with [^{18}F]Florastamin was obtained at baseline and again at weeks 4 and 8. The subjects required positive PSMA PET/CT prior to [^{177}Lu]Ludotadipep administration. Among the 29 subjects who received [^{177}Lu]Ludotadipep, 36 treatment emergent adverse events (TEAEs) occurred in 17 subjects (58.6%) and 4 adverse drug reactions (ADRs) in 3 subjects (10.3%). Of the total 24 subjects who had full 12-week follow-up data, 16 (66.7%) showed decrease in PSA of any magnitude, and 9 (37.5%) showed a decrease in PSA by 50% or greater. A total of 5 of the 24 patients (20.8%) showed disease progression (PSA increase of 25% or higher from the baseline) at the 12th week following single dose of [^{177}Lu]Ludotadipep. These data thus far suggest that [^{177}Lu]Ludotadipep could be a promising RPT agent with low toxicity in mCRPC patients who have not been responsive to conventional treatments.

Keywords: metastatic castration-resistant prostate cancer; lutetium-177; PSMA; radiopharmaceutical therapy

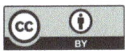

1. Introduction

Prostate cancer is the second most common cancer type in males; it is the leading cause of cancer death for men in the United States and the fifth leading cause of death for men in Republic of Korea [1]. Prostate cancer progresses relatively slowly, but biochemical recurrence occurs in about 35% of patients within 10 years after radical prostatectomy [2]. In the initial stage, androgen deprivation therapy is the primary treatment, but after duration of 18 months, only 75% of patients respond to the treatment with the rest converting to castration-resistant prostate cancer (CRPC) [3]. If CRPC is left untreated, the median survival is less than 12 months [4]. Distant metastases have been found in 84% of patients with CRPC, and one third of patients without distant metastases developed bone metastases within 2 years [5].

Prostate specific membrane antigen (PSMA) is a protein that is overexpressed in prostate cancer cells. It has a synergistic correlation with disease progression, and is recognized as a biomarker for diagnosis and treatment of prostate cancer [6]. PSMA protein has enzymatic activity that hydrolyzes N-acetyl-aspartyl-glutamate (NAAG) substrate in vivo to produce N-acetylaspartate and glutamate. A compound chemically modified to prevent degradation of NAAG, the in vivo substrate of PSMA, could become a substance that can specifically target PSMA [7]. Compounds based on glutamate-urea-lysine (GUL) structure are being studied for diagnosis and treatment of prostate cancer [8], and in particular compounds bound with radioisotopes are showing great promise.

Lutetium-177 is a radioactive isotope that emits high energy beta-type particles with the ability to destroy tumor cells. It has a half-life of 6.7 days and a beta energy of 490 keV. The amount of radiation reaching the surrounding normal tissue is relatively small due to the short tissue penetration range of maximum 1.6 mm, and makes Lutetium-177 a suitable radioisotope for therapeutic purposes [9]. Survival gains and patient benefits such as delayed time-to-skeletal-event and pain control were reported following RPT with the most widely studied [^{177}Lu]Lutetium-PSMA-617 [10,11], and this radiopharmaceutical was approved by the FDA for patients with mCRPC who progressed after androgen deprivation therapy and taxane based chemotherapy.

Numerous studies have explored various PSMA targeting compounds for diagnostic and therapeutic purposes [12,13]. In order to overcome the short circulation time of the small molecule based [^{177}Lu]Lutetium-PSMA-617, a compound was developed with an albumin motif to increase the circulation time and thus the total tumor uptake, [^{177}Lu]Ludotadipep, which is also based on the GUL structure. Preclinical treatment effect of this novel radiopharmaceutical on prostate cancer were published earlier [14]. High binding affinity and extended blood circulation time of the compound were observed and showed the potential as an effective RPT. In this prospective, phase I trial, we aimed to investigate the safety and efficacy of [^{177}Lu]Ludotadipep, a novel radiopharmaceutical, in patients with mCRPC unresponsive to standard treatment.

2. Materials and Methods

2.1. [^{177}Lu]Ludotadipep

[^{177}Lu]Ludotadipep (Figure 1) is a novel PSMA inhibitor labeled with Lu-177 and is characterized by a 4-iodophenyl butanoic group that can bind with albumin, allowing it to stay in the blood for a considerable time and be available longer to be taken up more in prostate cancer cells. [^{177}Lu]Ludotadipep was diluted with 0.9% NaCl 5 mL and slowly injected intravenously over 10 min, with 0.9% NaCl slowly administered for 90 min from 30 min before administration of [^{177}Lu]Ludotadipep to 60 min after administration. [^{177}Lu]Ludotadipep was manufactured and supplied from a GMP site (FutureChem, Seoul, Republic of Korea).

2.2. PSMA PET/CT

PSMA PET/CT was performed at screening (baseline), and again at the 4th and 8th weeks after [^{177}Lu]Ludotadipep RPT using the diagnostic radiopharmaceutical [^{18}F]Florastamin [15]. At 110 min after intravenous injection of 370 ± 37 MBq of [^{18}F]Florastamin (FutureChem, Seoul, Korea), PET/CT images were acquired. A focal uptake higher than the background level that was not associated with physiologic uptake or known pitfall was defined as positive.

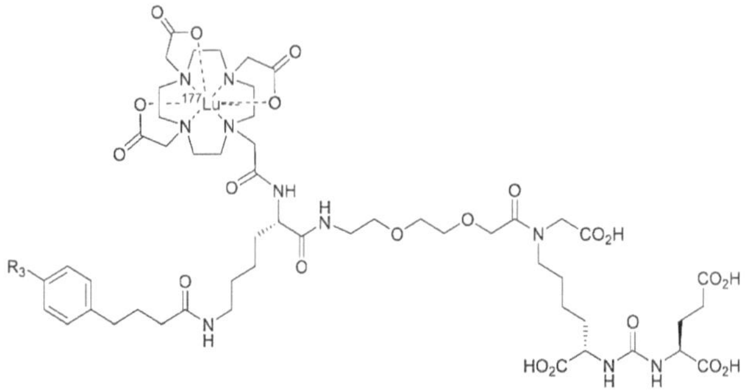

Figure 1. Structure of [^{177}Lu]Ludotadipep tested in phase I clinical trial. [^{177}Lu]Lutetium (III)2,2′,2″-(10-((4S,20S,24S)-20,24,26-tricarboxy-15-(carboxymethyl)-4-(4-(4-(4-iodophenyl)butanamido)butyl)-2,5,14,22-tetraoxo-9,12-dioxa-3,6,15,21,23-pentaazahexacosyl)-1,4,7,10-tetraazacyclododecane-1,4,7-triyl)triacetate.

2.3. Study Method

This was a prospective, single center, phase I open label study testing single administration of a radiopharmaceutical. Patients were required to have an Eastern Cooperative Oncology Group (ECOG) performance status score of 2 or lower. Subjects were screened with PSMA PET/CT for lesions showing PSMA-RADS 4 or 5 [16]. Five groups of up to six subjects were administered once with [^{177}Lu]Ludotadipep at doses of 1.9 GBq, 2.8 GBq, 3.7 GBq, 4.6 GBq, and 5.6 GBq. The dose was increased sequentially if two or less out of six subjects were confirmed with dose limiting toxicity (DLT). The subjects were hospitalized for three days following the administration of [^{177}Lu]Ludotadipep to monitor for any immediate adverse effect.

Serum prostate specific antigen (PSA) levels were tested 1, 2, 3, 4, 6, 8, and 12 weeks after administration of [^{177}Lu]Ludotadipep and compared with the baseline PSA measurements. We reviewed the occurrence of adverse events at the relevant time points in the outpatient clinics. At four and eight weeks after administration, the PSMA PET/CT was repeated for qualitative and quantitative comparison of the metastatic lesions.

2.4. Outcomes

The primary outcome was the DLT, defined as on common terminology criteria for adverse events (CTCAE) v5.0: grade 4 thrombocytopenia (platelet level < 25×10^9/L), grade 4 neutropenia (absolute neutrophil count, ANC < 0.5×10^9/L), grade 3 febrile neutropenia (ANC < 1.0×10^9/L with a body temperature exceeding 38.3 °C on at least 1 occasion or a body temperature above 38.0 °C persisting for 1 h), or grade 3 to 4 non-hematological toxicity resulting from [^{177}Lu]Ludotadipep that lasts more than five days. The maximum tolerated dose (MTD) for phase II was to be determined based on incidence of the DLT.

The secondary outcomes included (1) safety evaluation based on symptoms, physical examinations, and laboratory tests; (2) PSA level assessment; and (3) imaging assessment based on PSMA PET/CT.

2.5. Statistical Analysis

Statistical analyses were performed using SAS software version 9.4 (SAS institute, Cary, NC, USA). Demographic information, safety assessment, efficacy analyses based on PSA responses, and PET/CT findings are described from all subjects who received [^{177}Lu]Ludotadipep. DLT assessment was carried out in those who completed the follow up scheme. Median ± standard deviation (SD) are described for continuous parameters.

2.6. Ethical Statement

This study was approved by Seoul St. Mary's Hospital Institutional Review Board (IRB no. KC20MDSF0483) and the Korean Ministry of Food and Drug Safety (KMFDS). Written informed consent was obtained from all subjects, and the study was in compliance with the Helsinki Declaration and local regulations. (ClinicalTrials.gov Identifier: NCT04509557).

3. Results

3.1. Patient Characteristics

From November 2020 to March 2022, 42 men with mCRPC in whom disease had progressed after standard treatments were recruited for screening, and 12 men were excluded since they did not meet the inclusion/exclusion criteria (n = 6), withdrew consent (n = 2), or for other causes (n = 4; such as COVID19 quarantine). 30 patients were enrolled and 29 received [^{177}Lu]Ludotadipep (1 subject found to deviate from the inclusion/exclusion criteria after enrollment). A total of 24 subjects completed the follow-up protocol, while 5 patients withdrew after administration of [^{177}Lu]Ludotadipep (1 withdrawal of consent; 4 at the discretion of the investigator for other treatments including one subject admitted for treatment of COVID19 infection). Participants for the higher [^{177}Lu]Ludotadipep dose group were recruited after the DLT was confirmed from two or less of six subjects in a given dose group.

Mean age was 72.7 ± 8.1 years, and the mean PSA level prior to treatment was 681.3 ± 1139.9 ng/mL. The baseline characteristics of the 29 subjects who received the investigational RPT are shown in Table 1.

Table 1. Baseline characteristics.

Characteristics	N = 29
Age (years)	72.7 ± 8.1
Time from prostate cancer diagnosis (months)	67.0 ± 50.8
ECOG Performance Status	
0	26 (89.6%)
1	3 (10.34%)
PSA (ng/mL)	681.3 ± 1139.9
Gleason Score	
3 + 4	2 (6.9%)
4 + 3	2 (6.9%)
4 + 4	9 (31.0%)
4 + 5	9 (31.0%)
5 + 4	5 (17.2%)
5 + 5	2 (6.9%)
Bone metastasis	28 (96.6%)
Lymph node metastasis	18 (62.1%)
Liver metastasis	4 (13.8%)
Lung metastasis	5 (17.2%)
Radical prostatectomy	16 (55.2%)
Radiation Therapy	7 (24.1%)
Prior Systemic Treatment	
Androgen deprivation therapy only	7 (24.1%)
Docetaxel	3 (10.3%)
Abiraterone	7 (24.1%)
Enzalutamide	1 (3.4%)
Docetaxel then enzalutamide	4 (13.8%)
Docetaxel then abiraterone	3 (10.3%)
Degarelix then androgen deprivation therapy	1 (3.4%)
Abiraterone then docetaxel then enzalutamide	3 (10.3%)

3.2. Treatment Related Toxicity

Adverse events attributed to [^{177}Lu]Ludotadipep are shown in Table 2.

Table 2. Adverse events (AEs) depending on doses.

AEs/Dose	1.9 GBq (N = 6)	2.8 GBq (N = 6)	3.7 GBq (N = 6)	4.6 GBq (N = 6)	5.6 GBq (N = 5)
Hematologic					
Neutropenia	0	0	0	0	0
Febrile neutropenia	0	0	0	0	0
Anemia	1 (16.7%)	0	1 (16.7%)	0	1 (20.0%)
Thrombocytopenia	0	0	0	0	0
Non-hematologic					
Anorexia	0	1 (16.7%)	1 (16.7%)	0	1 (20.0%)
Dyspnea	0	0	0	0	0
Fatigue	0	0	0	0	0
Nausea	1 (16.7%)	1 (16.7%)	1 (16.7%)	0	2 (40.0%)
Stomatitis	0	0	0	0	0
Vomiting	0	0	0	0	0
Weight loss	0	0	0	0	0
Constipation	0	0	0	1 (16.7%)	1 (16.7%)
Xerostomia	1 (16.7%)	1 (16.7%)	1 (16.7%)	1 (16.7%)	2 (20.0%)

Total 24 subjects had full DLT assessment (4 from 1.9 GBq, 6 from 2.8 GBq, 6 from 3.7 GBq, 5 from 4.6 GBq, and 3 from 5.6 GBq group). No DLT occurred at any level of the 5 tested dose groups.

The treatment emergent adverse events (TEAEs) according to system organ class (SOC) and preferred term (PT) are also shown in Table 3. Among the 29 subjects, 36 TEAEs occurred in 17 subjects (58.6%) including 5 events that occurred in 4 subjects (66.7%) in the 1.9 GBq group, 3 events that occurred in 2 subjects (33.3%) in the 2.8 GBq group, 6 events that occurred in 3 subjects (50.0%) in the 3.7 GBq group, 9 events that occurred in 4 subjects (66.7%) in the 4.6 GBq group, and 13 events that occurred in 4 subjects (80.0%) in the 5.6 GBq group. In terms of severity, most of the TEAEs were grade 1 (29/36 events) or grade 2 (5/36 events). Two out of 36 TEAEs were grade 3, and they were not serious adverse events (SAE) and not related to the [^{177}Lu]Ludotadipep administration. A single SAE was reported by one subject in the [^{177}Lu]Ludotadipep 5.6 GBq group (asthenia), but it was considered not related to the [^{177}Lu]Ludotadipep administration and the severity was grade 1.

Adverse drug reactions (ADRs) according to SOC and PT are shown in Table 4. A total four ADRs occurred in three subjects, including one event that occurred in one subject each in the 1.9 GBq and 3.7 GBq groups and two events that occurred in one subject in the 2.8 GBq group. No ADR occurred in the [^{177}Lu]Ludotadipep 4.6 GBq and 5.6 GBq groups. In terms of severity, most of the ADRs were grade 1 (3/4 events) or grade 2 (1/4 events), and all were recovered (one recovering). No serious ADR was reported in any of the dose groups.

There were no adverse event or ADR leading to withdrawal from the study or death in any of the dose groups. Overall summary of TEAEs and ADRs are shown in Supplementary Tables S1 and S2.

3.3. Laboratory Changes

There were no significant changes in the serum hemoglobin (Hb), leukocyte, platelet, absolute neutrophil counts (ANC), and sodium levels (Supplementary Table S3) before and after the administration of [^{177}Lu]Ludotadipep.

Table 3. Treatment emergent adverse events (TEAEs) according to system organ class (SOC) and preferred term (PT).

	Total 29 Subjects
Subjects with TEAEs, n(%) [number of events]	**17(58.6) [36]**
Gastrointestinal disorders	**6(20.7) [8]**
Nausea	5(17.2) [5]
Constipation	2(6.9) [2]
Hematochezia	1(3.5) [1]
Blood and lymphatic system disorders	**3(10.3) [3]**
Anemia	3(10.3) [3]
Laboratory investigations	**3(10.3) [3]**
Alanine aminotransferase increased	1(3.5) [1]
Aspartate aminotransferase increased	1(3.5) [1]
Platelet count decreased	1(3.5) [1]
Metabolism and nutrition disorders	**3(10.3) [3]**
Decreased appetite	3(10.3) [3]
Nervous system disorders	**3(10.3) [3]**
Headache	2(6.9) [2]
Dizziness	1(3.5) [1]
General disorders and administration site conditions	**2(6.9) [3]**
Edema peripheral	1(3.5) [2]
Asthenia	1(3.5) [1]
Psychiatric disorders	**1(3.5) [2]**
Insomnia	1(3.5) [2]
Injury, poisoning and procedural complications	**1(3.5) [1]**
Procedural pain	1(3.5) [1]
Musculoskeletal and connective tissue disorders	**2(6.9) [1]**
Bone pain	1(3.5) [1]
Arthralgia	1(3.5) [1]
Renal and urinary disorders	**1(3.5) [1]**
Dysuria	1(3.5) [1]
Reproductive system and breast disorders	**1(3.5) [1]**
Scrotal pain	1(3.5) [1]
Dry mouth	**6(20.7) [6]**
Skin and subcutaneous tissue disorders	**1(3.5) [1]**
Dermatitis	1(3.5) [1]

Table 4. Adverse drug reactions (ADRs) according to SOC and PT.

	Total 29 Subjects
Subjects with ADRs, n(%) [number of events]	**3(10.3) [4]**
Gastrointestinal disorders	
Nausea	2(6.9) [2]
Metabolism and nutrition disorders	
Decreased appetite	1(3.5) [1]
Skin and subcutaneous tissue disorders	
Dermatitis	1(3.5) [1]

3.4. PSA Response

The detailed PSA levels at weeks 1, 2, 3, 4, 6, 8, and 12 after [^{177}Lu]Ludotadipep administration are shown in Supplementary Table S4. At 12 weeks, the 1.9 GBq and 2.8 GBq groups showed increases of 15.15 and 5.00 ng/mL in median absolute PSA levels, respectively, compared to baseline. In the 3.7 GBq and higher dose groups, decrease in median PSA level was observed compared to the baseline values. Among the dose groups, the 5.6 GBq treated group had the greatest drop in the median absolute PSA level of 87.00 ng/mL from baseline to 12 weeks.

Figure 2 shows waterfall plot for percentage change of each subject's best PSA response. Supplementary Figure S1 shows spider plots for PSA levels from baseline to 1, 2, 3, 4, 6, 8, and 12 weeks after [^{177}Lu]Ludotadipep administration.

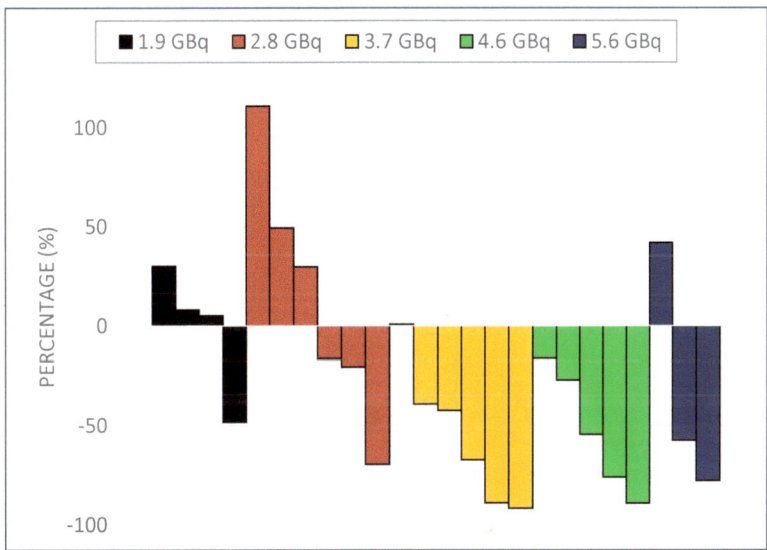

Figure 2. Waterfall plots by administered dose showing percentage change of best PSA response per subject.

Of the total 24 patients with full set of follow-up data for 12 weeks, 16 (66.7%) showed any decrease in PSA, 12 (50%) showed a decrease of PSA by more than 30%, and 9 (37.5%) showed a decrease in PSA by more than 50%. Overall, 5 out of 24 patients (20.8%) showed disease progression (25% or greater increase in PSA from the baseline) at the end of the study at the 12th week following [^{177}Lu]Ludotadipep administration.

3.5. Radiological Assessment

Three sets of PSMA PET/CT images, at baseline, 4 weeks and 8 weeks after [^{177}Lu] Ludotadipep administration were available in a total of 25 subjects. Mean (SD) of peak standardized uptake values corrected for lean body mass (SUL$_{peak}$) measured from PSMA PET/CT at baseline were 16.2 (12.0), 24.4 (22.0), 10.3 (5.9), 17.5 (11.9), and 20.1 (18.1) in the [^{177}Lu]Ludotadipep 1.9 GBq, 2.8 GBq, 3.7 GBq, 4.6 GBq, and 5.6 GBq groups, respectively. The mean SUL$_{peak}$ in the Week 4 and Week 8 PET/CT images decreased compared to baseline in all dose groups (Supplementary Figure S2). However, in the [^{177}Lu]Ludotadipep 1.9 GBq and 5.6 GBq groups, the week 8 PSMA PET/CT SUL$_{peak}$ drops were not greater than the week 4 drops.

No patient demonstrated complete response on either week 4 or week 8 PSMA PET/CT after single administration of [^{177}Lu]Ludotadipep. However, on week 8 PSMA PET/CT, 14 (56%) subjects had partial response and 10 subjects (40%) had stable disease (SD). One subject demonstrated progression on imaging. The overall objective response rate (ORR) was 40% at week 4 and 56% at week 8. The overall disease control rate (DCR) was 92% at week 4 and 96% at week 8 according to PSMA PET/CT findings. A case of a subject who received 3.7 GBq of [^{177}Lu]Ludotadipep is shown in Figure 3, and another case of a subject who received 4.6 GBq is shown in Figure 4.

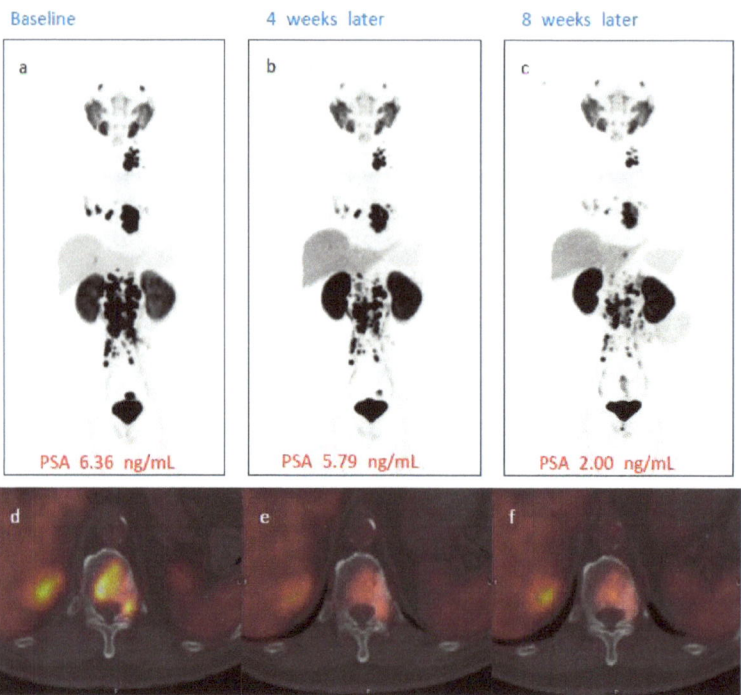

Figure 3. A case of a subject showing PSA response to [^{177}Lu]Ludotadipep. (**a,d**) Baseline [^{18}F]Florastamin PSMA PET/CT maximum intensity projection (MIP) and fused axial images with multiple bone and lymph node metastases. (**b,c**) PSMA PET/CT MIP images at four and eight weeks after administration of [^{177}Lu]Ludotadipep showing decreased tumor burden. (**e,f**) Axial fused PSMA PET/CT images at four and eight weeks show decreased uptake in metastatic lesion in the thoracic vertebra. The patient's PSA decreased from 6.36 to 2.00 ng/mL at 8 weeks.

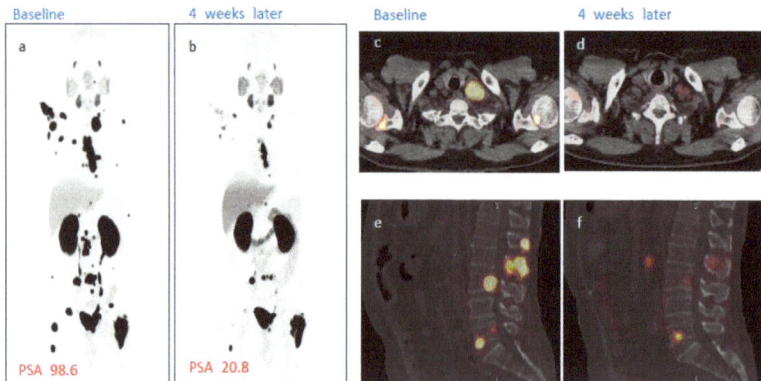

Figure 4. A case of a subject showing response to [^{177}Lu]Ludotadipep. (**a,c,e**) Baseline [^{18}F]Florastamin PSMA PET/CT MIP, fused axial and sagittal images. (**b,d,e**) PSMA PET/CT images four weeks after administration of [^{177}Lu]Ludotadipeps (**a,b**) MIP images show decreased tumor burden in the bone lesions and lymph nodes. (**c,d**) Axial fused PSMA PET/CT images show marked regression of left supraclavicular lymph node and bone metastases. (**e,f**) Sagittal PSMA PET/CT images show decreased uptake in the spine lesions.

4. Discussion

[^{177}Lu]Ludotadipep is a novel radiopharmaceutical based on the chemical structure of GUL (glutamate-urea-lysine), and is composed of relatively hydrophilic residues. It has a 4-iodophenyl butanoic group that interacts with serum albumin to elongate the circulation time of the compound and subsequently increase the uptake of the therapeutic radiopharmaceutical by prostate cancer cells.

Following single cycle of [^{177}Lu]Ludotadipep, PSA drop of 50% or greater was seen in 9 out of 24 subjects with full 12 weeks of follow-up data. In the TheraP trial, 66% of the patients showed PSA response after up to 6 cycles of [^{177}Lu]Lu-PSMA-617 RPT [10]. In the VISION Trial, the patients received 4 to 6 cycles of [^{177}Lu]Lu-PSMA-617 and PSA decrease of 50% or greater was seen in 46.0%, compared to the rate of 7.1% in the standard care alone group [11]. In this study, any decrease in PSA was noted in 12 of 14 (85.7%) subjects in the 3.7 to 5.6 GBq dose groups, and the overall radiological disease control rate was 96% on week 8 PSMA PET/CT. In this phase I study, the administered radiopharmaceutical activity was lower than the TheraP and VISION trials (doses of 6.0 to 8.5 GBq, and 7.4 GBq, respectively), and only single cycle rather than repeated cycles was tested. At all visits, the proportion of subjects showing PSA decrease was higher in the [^{177}Lu]Ludotadipep 3.7 to 5.6 GBq groups than in the [^{177}Lu]Ludotadipep 1.9 GBq and 2.8 GBq groups. Our results suggest favorable control rates compared to other early phase trials of novel PSMA targeting radiopharmaceuticals [17,18]. Though direct comparison with [^{177}Lu]Lu-PSMA-617 or other radiopharmaceuticals is not possible at this early stage, favorable PSA and PSMA PET/CT responses support further trials with repeated cycles of higher doses of [^{177}Lu]Ludotadipep.

As with [^{177}Lu]Lu-PSMA-617 [19], [^{177}Lu]Ludotadipep showed mostly renal clearance. Detailed biodistribution and dosimetry analyses for [^{177}Lu]Ludotadipep are ongoing for publication, and show kidneys and bone marrow to be the critical organs for [^{177}Lu]Ludotadipep. The serum creatinine levels did not show difference after administration, and no TEAEs or ADRs related to kidney injury occurred in this study. Grade 3 to 5 renal effects were comparable in the [^{177}Lu]Lu-PSMA-617 plus standard care group and standard care alone group (3.4% and 2.9%) in the VISION trial [11]. Though the incidence may not be high, nephrotoxicity was also observed after treatment with [^{177}Lu]Lu-Octreotate [20], and kidney damage should be monitored and investigated in upcoming clinical trials. Marrow suppression was observed with [^{177}Lu]Lu-PSMA-617 [11], but it could also be a manifestation in patients with extensive bone metastases in advanced prostate cancer. Longer follow-up of TheraP population did not raise additional safety issues [21]. Though severe marrow suppression did not develop during the 12 weeks of testing in this study, possibly due to the lower administered activity of the radiopharmaceutical, caution would be mandatory following higher activity RPT and with patients demonstrating high tumor burden in the skeletal lesions.

As could be expected from the high salivary gland uptake in the PSMA PET/CT images, xerostomia was the most frequent non-hematologic side effect in this study, though serum amylase level was not checked for the diagnosis. Previous studies have shown high uptake of the [^{177}Lu]Lu-PSMA-based radiopharmaceuticals by the salivary glands [8,22]. A recent study showed that mild xerostomia occurred in 2 out of 56 patients after 3 to 4 cycles of treatment but spontaneously resolved before 3 months [23] and was recoverable [24], and applying external cooling with ice packs may reduce the salivary gland uptakes [25]. It is necessary to learn how to further reduce xerostomia for futureapplications.

The lack of data on long-term safety, survival outcomes, and changes in patient reported bone pain or performance are among the limitations of this study, and will be addressed in future trials. In this pilot study of single cycle of [^{177}Lu]Ludotadipep, antitumor effects were observed in majority of the subjects. Phase II clinical trial with repeated cycles are ongoing, and the safety profile and therapeutic effect will be further assessed.

5. Conclusions

[^{177}Lu]Ludotadipep led to PSA drop of 50% or greater in 37.5% of subjects with mCRPC after single administration, and showed no serious treatment-related side effects. [^{177}Lu]Ludotadipep has the potential to be an effective option for mCRPC patients who have not responded to previous treatments, and phase II study of multi-cycle [^{177}Lu]Ludotadipep RPT is ongoing.

Supplementary Materials: The following supporting information can be downloaded at: https://www.mdpi.com/article/10.3390/cancers14246225/s1, Supplementary Table S1: Overall summary of TEAEs; Supplementary Table S2: Overall summary of ADRs; Supplementary Table S3: Change in hemoglobin, leukocyte, platelet, ANC; Supplementary Table S4. The PSA levels at Week 1, 2, 3, 4, 6, 8, and 12 after [^{177}Lu]Ludotadipep administration; Supplementary Figure S1: Spider plots for PSA level Week 1, 2, 3, 4, 6, 8, 12 after [^{177}Lu]Ludotadipep administration; Supplementary Figure S2: Waterfall plots of percent changes in SUL$_{peak}$ on PSMA PET/CT (a) at Week 4 after [^{177}Lu]Ludotadipep administration, and (b) at Week 8.

Author Contributions: Conceptualization, J.H.O., D.Y.C., I.R.Y. and J.Y.L.; methodology, J.H.O. and C.P.; validation, Y.H.P. and S.Y.P.; formal analysis, D.S. and S.H.; investigation, J.Y.L.; resources, D.Y.C.; data curation, S.H., J.H.O., S.a.R., C.E.Y., H.J.K., H.W.M. and Y.H.P.; writing—original draft preparation, D.S. and J.H.O.; writing—review and editing, D.S., J.H.O. and I.R.Y.; visualization, D.S. and J.H.O.; supervision, I.R.Y. and J.Y.L. All authors have read and agreed to the published version of the manuscript.

Funding: This research was supported by the National Research Foundation of Korea (Grant numbers: 2018R1D1A1A02086383, 2022R1A2C1009770, and 2022R1I1A1A01069887).

Institutional Review Board Statement: This study was approved by Seoul St. Mary's Hospital Institutional Review Board (IRB no. KC20MDSF0483).

Informed Consent Statement: Informed consent was obtained from all subjects involved in the study.

Data Availability Statement: The data presented in this study are available upon reasonable request.

Acknowledgments: The authors thank the study participants, the hospital staff for the care of our patients, and FutureChem for their scientific support.

Conflicts of Interest: Chansoo Park is an employee of FutureChem Co., Ltd., and Dae Yoon Chi is chief executive officer. The other authors declare no conflicts of interest.

References

1. Bray, F.; Ferlay, J.; Soerjomataram, I.; Siegel, R.L.; Torre, L.A.; Jemal, A. Global cancer statistics 2018: GLOBOCAN estimates of incidence and mortality worldwide for 36 cancers in 185 countries. *CA Cancer J. Clin.* **2018**, *68*, 394–424. [CrossRef] [PubMed]
2. Van den Broeck, T.; Van Den Bergh, R.C.N.; Arfi, N.; Gross, T.; Moris, L.; Briers, E.; Cumberbatch, M.; De Santis, M.; Tilki, D.; Fanti, S.; et al. Prognostic value of biochemical recurrence following treatment with curative intent for prostate cancer: A systematic review. *Eur. Urol.* **2019**, *75*, 967–987. [CrossRef] [PubMed]
3. Harris, W.P.; Mostaghel, E.A.; Nelson, P.S.; Montgomery, B. Androgen deprivation therapy: Progress in understanding mechanisms of resistance and optimizing androgen depletion. *Nat. Clin. Pract. Urol.* **2009**, *6*, 76–85. [CrossRef] [PubMed]
4. Sella, A.; Yarom, N.; Zisman, A.; Kovel, S. Paclitaxel, estramustine and carboplatin combination chemotherapy after initial docetaxel-based chemotherapy in castration-resistant prostate cancer. *Oncology* **2009**, *76*, 442–446. [CrossRef] [PubMed]
5. Kirby, M.; Hirst, C.; Crawford, E.D. Characterising the castration-resistant prostate cancer population: A systematic review. *Int. J. Clin. Pract.* **2011**, *65*, 1180–1192. [CrossRef] [PubMed]
6. Dong, L.; Su, Y.; Zhu, Y.; Markowski, M.C.; Xin, M.; Gorin, M.A.; Dong, B.; Pan, J.; Pomper, M.G.; Liu, J.; et al. The European Association of Urology biochemical recurrence risk groups predict findings on PSMA PET in patients with biochemically recurrent prostate cancer after radical prostatectomy. *J. Nucl. Med.* **2022**, *63*, 248–252. [CrossRef]
7. Neale, J.H.; Yamamoto, T. N-acetylaspartylglutamate (NAAG) and glutamate carboxypeptidase II: An abundant peptide neurotransmitter-enzyme system with multiple clinical applications. *Prog. Neurobiol.* **2020**, *184*, 101722. [CrossRef] [PubMed]
8. Bakht, M.K.; Hayward, J.J.; Shahbazi-Raz, F.; Skubal, M.; Tamura, R.; Stringer, K.F.; Meister, D.; Venkadakrishnan, V.B.; Xue, H.; Pillon, A.; et al. Identification of alternative protein targets of glutamate-ureido-lysine associated with PSMA tracer uptake in prostate cancer cells. *Proc. Natl. Acad. Sci. USA* **2022**, *119*, e2025710119. [CrossRef]
9. Ferdinandus, J.; Violet, J.; Sandhu, S.; Hofman, M.S. Prostate-specific membrane antigen theranostics: Therapy with lutetium-177. *Curr. Opin. Urol.* **2018**, *28*, 197–204. [CrossRef]

10. Hofman, M.S.; Emmett, L.; Sandhu, S.; Iravani, A.; Joshua, A.M.; Goh, J.C.; Pattison, D.A.; Tan, T.H.; Kirkwood, I.D.; Ng, S. [^{177}Lu] Lu-PSMA-617 versus cabazitaxel in patients with metastatic castration-resistant prostate cancer (TheraP): A randomised, open-label, phase 2 trial. *Lancet* **2021**, *397*, 797–804. [CrossRef]
11. Sartor, O.; De Bono, J.; Chi, K.N.; Fizazi, K.; Herrmann, K.; Rahbar, K.; Tagawa, S.T.; Nordquist, L.T.; Vaishampayan, N.; El-Haddad, G. Lutetium-177–PSMA-617 for metastatic castration-resistant prostate cancer. *New Engl. J. Med.* **2021**, *385*, 1091–1103. [CrossRef] [PubMed]
12. Lisney, A.R.; Leitsmann, C.; Strauß, A.; Meller, B.; Bucerius, J.A.; Sahlmann, C.-O. The Role of PSMA PET/CT in the Primary Diagnosis and Follow-Up of Prostate Cancer—A Practical Clinical Review. *Cancers* **2022**, *14*, 3638. [CrossRef] [PubMed]
13. Oh, S.W.; Suh, M.; Cheon, G.J. Current Status of PSMA-Targeted Radioligand Therapy in the Era of Radiopharmaceutical Therapy Acquiring Marketing Authorization. *Nucl. Med. Mol. Imaging* **2022**, *56*, 263–281. [CrossRef] [PubMed]
14. Lee, B.S.; Kim, M.H.; Chu, S.Y.; Jung, W.J.; Jeong, H.J.; Lee, K.; Kim, H.S.; Kim, M.H.; Kil, H.S.; Han, S.J.; et al. Improving Theranostic Gallium-68/Lutetium-177–Labeled PSMA Inhibitors with an Albumin Binder for Prostate CancerA Novel 177Lu-PSMA Ligand for Prostate Cancer Therapy. *Mol. Cancer Ther.* **2021**, *20*, 2410–2419. [CrossRef] [PubMed]
15. Lee, I.; Lim, I.; Byun, B.H.; Kim, B.I.; Choi, C.W.; Woo, S.-K.; Lee, K.C.; Kang, J.H.; Kil, H.S.; Park, C.; et al. A microdose clinical trial to evaluate [18F] Florastamin as a positron emission tomography imaging agent in patients with prostate cancer. *Eur. J. Nucl. Med. Mol. Imaging* **2021**, *48*, 95–102. [CrossRef] [PubMed]
16. Rowe, S.P.; Pienta, K.J.; Pomper, M.G.; Gorin, M.A. PSMA RADS version 1.0: A step towards standardizing the interpretation and reporting of PSMA-targeted PET imaging studies. *Eur. Urol.* **2018**, *73*, 485–487. [CrossRef]
17. Tagawa, S.T.; Vallabhajosula, S.; Christos, P.J.; Jhanwar, Y.S.; Batra, J.S.; Lam, L.; Osborne, J.; Beltran, H.; Molina, A.M.; Goldsmith, S.J.; et al. Phase 1/2 study of fractionated dose lutetium-177–labeled anti–prostate-specific membrane antigen monoclonal antibody J591 (177Lu-J591) for metastatic castration-resistant prostate cancer. *Cancer* **2019**, *125*, 2561–2569. [CrossRef]
18. Zang, J.; Fan, X.; Wang, H.; Liu, Q.; Wang, J.; Li, H.; Li, F.; Jacobson, O.; Niu, G.; Zhu, Z.; et al. First-in-human study of 177Lu-EB-PSMA-617 in patients with metastatic castration-resistant prostate cancer. *Eur. J. Nucl. Med. Mol. Imaging* **2019**, *46*, 148–158. [CrossRef]
19. Kratochwil, C.; Giesel, F.L.; Stefanova, M.; Benešová, M.; Bronzel, M.; Afshar-Oromieh, A.; Mier, W.; Eder, M.; Kopka, K.; Haberkorn, U. PSMA-targeted radionuclide therapy of metastatic castration-resistant prostate cancer with 177Lu-labeled PSMA-617. *J. Nucl. Med.* **2016**, *57*, 1170–1176. [CrossRef]
20. Bergsma, H.; Konijnenberg, M.W.; van der Zwan, W.A.; Kam, B.L.; Teunissen, J.J.; Kooij, P.P.; Mauff, K.A.; Krenning, E.P.; Kwekkeboom, D.J. Nephrotoxicity after PRRT with 177Lu-DOTA-octreotate. *Eur. J. Nucl. Med. Mol. Imaging* **2016**, *43*, 1802–1811. [CrossRef]
21. Hofman, M.S.; Emmett, L.; Sandhu, S.; Iravani, A.; Joshua, A.M.; Goh, J.C.; Pattison, D.A.; Tan, T.H.; Kirkwood, I.D.; Francis, R.J. *TheraP: 177Lu-PSMA-617 (LuPSMA) Versus Cabazitaxel in Metastatic Castration-Resistant Prostate Cancer (mCRPC) Progressing after Docetaxel—Overall Survival after Median Follow-Up of 3 Years (ANZUP 1603)*; American Society of Clinical Oncology: Chicago, IL, USA, 2022.
22. Van Kalmthout, L.W.M.; van der Sar, E.C.A.; Braat, A.J.A.T.; de Keizer, B.; Lam, M.G.E.H. Lutetium-177-PSMA therapy for prostate cancer patients-a brief overview of the literature. *Tijdschr. Voor Urol.* **2020**, *10*, 141–146. [CrossRef]
23. Baum, R.P.; Kulkarni, H.R.; Schuchardt, C.; Singh, A.; Wirtz, M.; Wiessalla, S.; Schottelius, M.; Mueller, D.; Klette, I.; Wester, H.-J. Lutetium-177 PSMA radioligand therapy of metastatic castration-resistant prostate cancer: Safety and efficacy. *J. Nucl. Med.* **2016**, *57*, 1006–1013. [CrossRef] [PubMed]
24. Heynickx, N.; Herrmann, K.; Vermeulen, K.; Baatout, S.; Aerts, A. The salivary glands as a dose limiting organ of PSMA-targeted radionuclide therapy: A review of the lessons learnt so far. *Nucl. Med. Biol.* **2021**, *98–99*, 30–39. [CrossRef] [PubMed]
25. Van Kalmthout, L.W.M.; Lam, M.G.E.H.; de Keizer, B.; Krijger, G.C.; Ververs, T.F.T.; de Roos, R.; Braat, A.J.A.T. Impact of external cooling with icepacks on 68Ga-PSMA uptake in salivary glands. *EJNMMI Res.* **2018**, *8*, 56. [CrossRef] [PubMed]

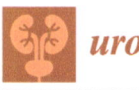 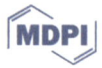

Communication

PARP Inhibitors in the Management of BRCA-Positive Prostate Cancer: An Overview

Islam Kourampi [1,*], Ioannis-Panagiotis Tsetzan [1], Panagiota Kappi [1] and Nityanand Jain [2,3,*]

[1] Department of Medicine, National and Kapodistrian University of Athens, Mikras Asias 75, 11527 Athens, Greece
[2] Faculty of Medicine, Riga Stradiņš University, Dzirciema Street 16, LV-1007 Riga, Latvia
[3] Joint Microbiology Laboratory, Pauls Stradiņš Clinical University Hospital, Pilsoņu Street 13, Zemgales Priekšpilsēta, LV-1002 Riga, Latvia
* Correspondence: kourampiislam@gmail.com (I.K.); nityapkl@gmail.com (N.J.)

Abstract: Prostate cancer is the second most common form of cancer in men and the fifth leading cause of death among men worldwide. Men with metastatic castration-resistant prostate cancer (mCRPC) often have BRCA-1 or BRCA-2 gene mutations which can make them sensitive to poly-(ADP-ribose) polymerase inhibitors or PARP inhibitors (PARPi), such as Olaparib, Rucaparib, and Niraparib. Although significant advances have been made with PARPi and the prognosis of patients with mCRPC has improved dramatically, resistance often constitutes a challenge that frequently results in tumor escape. This present communication paper explores the role of PARPi in BRCA-positive prostate cancer and sheds light on numerous published and ongoing clinical trials that will determine the future of PARPi at various tumor stages as a monotherapy or polytherapy regime.

Keywords: prostate cancer; BRCA; PARP; treatment; resistance; inhibitors

1. Introduction

Prostate cancer is the second most common form of cancer in men and the fifth leading cause of death among men worldwide. In 2020 alone, about 1.4 million new cases of prostate cancer were reported globally, accounting for 7.3% of all malignancies in males. The incidence of prostate cancer varies greatly from country to country, especially amongst countries with a high HDI (human development index) and those with a low HDI (37.5 and 11.3 per 100,000, respectively). Geographically, Europe accounts for more than a third of all registered prostate cancer cases, followed by Asia (24%), Northern America (19%), Latin America and the Caribbean (14%) and Africa (4%) [1]. It is predicted that for every 14 years of life, the prevalence of cancer doubles with age, and this proves to be one of the most significant prognostic factors for determining the prevalence of prostate cancer [2]. Furthermore, patients over 65 years old experience an independently higher predictive risk of mortality from prostate cancer [3]. In terms of mortality, the Caribbean has the highest death rate (27.9 per 100,000), while South-Central Asia has the lowest death rate (3.1 per 100,000) [1].

Despite the high incidence rates of prostate cancer worldwide, most cases are identified at an early stage, thus drastically affecting the overall survival rate. Men with a diagnosis of prostate cancer in the US are predicted to have a 5-year survival rate of 98% (all SEER—Surveillance, Epidemiology and End Result stages combined), which rises to almost 100% when the disease is diagnosed at an early stage (localized and regional stages) [4]. The data from the EUROCARE-5 study revealed a life expectancy of fatal cases for patients with prostate cancer aged 65–74 years of 7.7 years, with an overall 5-year survival rate in Europe of 83% [5].

Carcinogenesis is a complex multistage and multistep molecular cascade triggered either by the activation of oncogenes or by the suppression of tumor suppression genes.

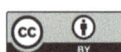

These genes are responsible for controlling genome stability, cellular proliferation, and apoptosis. Among those controlling genomic stability, BRCA-1 and BRCA-2 genes are of considerable importance. These tumor suppressor genes are involved in the homologous repair of the double-stranded breaks. Mutations in these BRCA genes can cause genomic instability that leads to the transformation of non-cancerous cells into cancer cells [6].

The type of BRCA mutation that an individual has can play an important role in choosing a personalized and efficient treatment [6]. BRCA-1 is an 1863 amino-acids-long protein with approximately 300 mutations that have been described to date [7]. These mutations predispose an individual to breast, ovarian, and prostate cancer, as well as cancer of the GI tract. The BRCA-2 protein on the other hand, is made of 3418 amino acids, with more than 1800 mutations that have been detected so far. As with BRCA-1 mutations, BRCA-2 mutations are mainly linked to breast, ovarian, and prostate cancer. However other malignancies, such as melanoma, pancreatic, gallbladder, bile duct, and stomach cancers, should also be taken into consideration [6].

2. Methods

For the purposes of this narrative review, we carried out a MEDLINE search for all articles published in the English language using the following terms: "BRCA" and "prostate cancer" and "therapy" or "PARP inhibitor" from January 2014 through November 2022. Relevant articles were searched in the American Society of Clinical Oncology (ASCO) and the European Society for Medical Oncology (ESMO) annual meetings. We also used relevant data from the American Cancer Society (ACS) website. A total of 144 articles were retrieved and checked for inclusion. From these 144 articles, we deemed 22 articles to be fit for inclusion in the present study (the exclusion of papers was based on insufficient data, papers describing prostate cancer with negative BRCA gene mutation, or lack of clarity about the status of BRCA gene mutation, and other review papers). Trial data was obtained from the U.S. National Library of Medicine's clinicaltrial.gov website (https://clinicaltrials.gov/; accessed 10 January 2023).

3. PARP Inhibitors (PARPi)

Back in 1995, the spread of prostate cancer to the regional lymph nodes was considered end-stage, and radiation was administered, since the function of the PSA (prostate specific antigen) was not yet well understood. With few systemic treatment options available, mitoxantrone was mostly used, a chemotherapy drug for the treatment of androgen independent (hormone refractory) metastatic prostate cancer. The drug gave patients a median survival of fewer than six months [8]. As a result, there have been significant changes in the way that localized prostate cancer is treated, with advancements having taken place in all aspects of therapeutic care. More recently, poly-ADP-ribose polymerase (PARP) inhibitors have dramatically improved the prognosis of patients with metastatic prostate cancer carrying BRCA genes abnormalities. The accumulation of DNA lesions has also been observed to result in a considerable rise in PARP levels in the cells, thereby providing evidence for a crucial role for PARP in DNA repair. When single-stranded DNA breaks occur, base excision repair (BER) is performed by the PARP [9]. The most well-known member of this family of enzymes, PARP-1, is essential for identifying and repairing DNA breaks. When single strand DNA damage is localized, PARP-1 produces poly-ADP-ribose (PAR) and transfers it to acceptor proteins, after which it brings in additional crucial repair enzymes to the damaged DNA spot [10].

Numerous studies have revealed a high correlation between advanced prostate cancer and common deleterious germline mutations in DNA damage repair (DDR) genes, which established the rationale for using PARP inhibitors to treat this condition. Inhibiting PARP should increase the susceptibility of malignant cells to chemotherapy and other therapeutics, since tumor cells with DDR gene mutations depend largely on PARP to repair DNA breaks and mismatches [10]. PARPi act by blocking the enzymes' ability to catalyze reactions and by binding the PARP on DNA at the locations of single-strand breaks [11].

Due to their synthetic lethality, PARP inhibitors are the first-line treatment indicated for the treatment of mCRPC (metastatic castration-resistant prostate cancer) [11].

4. PARPi Clinical Trials

Men with mCRPC often have BRCA-1 or BRCA-2 mutations, which can make them sensitive to poly-(ADP-ribose) polymerase inhibitors or PARP inhibitors (PARPi) [12]. PARP inhibitors are, hence, being investigated in numerous clinical trials for prostate cancer, either as a monotherapy or as a component of combination therapy (Table 1).

Table 1. Clinical trials investigating PARP inhibitors for prostate cancer.

Clinical Trial	Phase	Intervention	Condition/Disease	Recruitment Status	ClinicalTrials.gov Identifier
BRCAAway	II	Olaparib	mCRPC and DNA-Repair Defects	Recruiting	NCT03012321
COMRADE	I/II	Olaparib + Ra 223 dichloride	mCRPC	Recruiting	NCT03317392
GALAHAD	II	Niparib	mCRPC and DNA-Repair Anomalies	Active, not recruiting	NCT02854436
IMANOL	II	Olaparib after docetaxel	mCRPC	Completed	NCT03434158
LuPARP	I	Olaparib + 177Lu-PSMA in mCRPC	mCRPC	Recruiting	NCT03874884
MAGNITUDE	III	Niraparib + Abiraterone Acetate + Prednisone vs. Abiraterone Acetate + Prednisone	mCRPC	Active, not recruiting	NCT03748641
NCT02893917	II	Olaparib + Cediranib vs. Olaparib monotherapy	mCRPC	Active, not recruiting	NCT02893917
NCT03263650	II	Olaparib after Cabazitaxel + Carboplatin	AVPC	Active, not recruiting	NCT03263650
NCT03338790	II	Rucaparib + Nivolumab + Docetaxel or Enzalutamide	mCRPC	Active, not recruiting	NCT03338790
NCT03516812	II	Olaparib + Testosterone	CRPC	Active, not recruiting	NCT03516812
NCT03572478	I/II	Rucaparib + Nivolumab	mCRPC and metastatic Endometrial Cancer	Terminated due to lack of efficacy	NCT03572478
NCT03834519	III	Olaparib + Pemprolizumab vs. Abiraterone Acetate or Enzalutamide	mCRPC	Active, not recruiting	NCT03834519
NCT03840200	I	Rucaparib + Ipatasertib	Advanced prostate, breast, ovarian cancer	Completed	NCT03840200
NCT04019327	I/II	Talazoparib + Temozolamide	Prostate cancer	Recruiting	NCT04019327
NCT04824937	II	Talazoparib + Telaglenastat	mCRPC	Not yet recruiting	NCT04824937
NCT04846478	I	Talazoparib + Tazemetostat	mCRPC	Recruiting	NCT04846478
NiraRad	IB	Niraparib + Radium-223	mCRPC	Completed	NCT03076203
PLATI-PARP	II	Rucaparib + Carboplatin + Docetaxel	mCRPC with homologous recombination DNA repair anomalies	Recruiting	NCT03442556
ProFOUND	III	Olaparib vs. Enzalutamide or Abiraterone Acetate	mCRPC	Active, not recruiting	NCT02987543
PROpel	III	Olaparib + Abiraterone	mCRPC	Active, not recruiting	NCT03732820
QUEST	I/II	Niraparib Combination Therapies	mCRPC	Active, not recruiting	NCT03431350
RAMP	I	RUCAPARIB + other anticancer agents	mCRPC	Active, not recruiting	NCT04179396

Table 1. Cont.

Clinical Trial	Phase	Intervention	Condition/Disease	Recruitment Status	ClinicalTrials.gov Identifier
TALAPRO-1	II	Talazoparib	Metastatic Castration Resistant Prostate Cancer and DNA-Repair Anomalies	Active, not recruiting	NCT03148795
TALAPRO-2	III	Talazoparib + Enzalutamide vs. Enzalutamide Monotherapy	mCRPC	Active, not recruiting	NCT03395197
TOPARP A	II	Olaparib	Advanced prostate cancer	Unknown	-
TOPARP B	II	Olaparib	mCRPC and DDR alterations	Unknown	NCT01682772
TRAP	II	Olaparib + AZD6738	mCRPC	Active, not recruiting	NCT03787680
TRITON 2	II	Rucaparib	mCRPC	Completed	NCT02952534
TRITON 3	III	Rucaparib	mCRPC	Active, not recruiting	NCT02975934

Note—mCRPC (metastatic Castration-resistant prostate cancer); AVPC (aggressive-variant prostate cancer); CRPC (castration-resistant prostate cancer); DDR (DNA damage response).

The first PARP inhibitor authorization took place on 15 May 2020 (Figure 1). Rubraca® had been granted FDA approval. Its effectiveness was examined by the TRITON 2 (NCT02952534) clinical trial, which included 115 patients with BRCA-mutated (germline and/or somatic) mCRPC who had received androgen receptor-directed treatment and taxane-based chemotherapy. Rucaparib showed potential benefit in individuals with mCRPC and a germline or somatic BRCA or other DDR gene mutation; 43.9% of these patients experienced an objective response, and 52% reported a documented PSA response. Rucaparib's safety profile was comparable with earlier reports in cases of ovarian and prostate cancer [13].

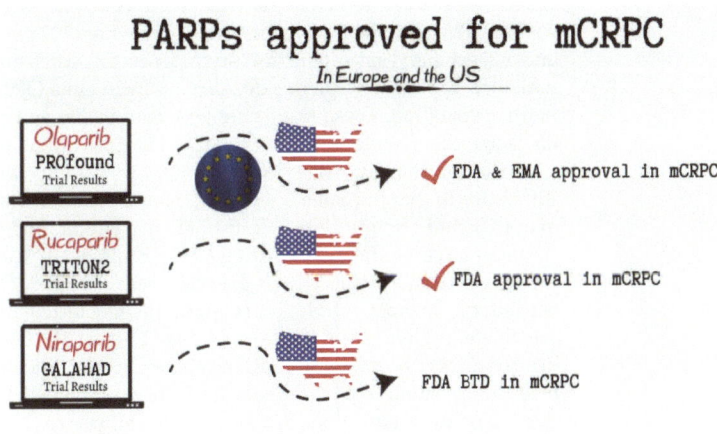

Figure 1. PARP inhibitors approved for the treatment of mCRPC across the globe.

In the ProFOUND study, men with mCRPC who had disease progression despite hormonal treatment were included. This phase III randomized, open-label clinical trial included a total of 387 patients who were divided into two cohorts of 245 patients (cohort A) with BRCA-1, BRCA-2, or ATM mutations and 142 patients (cohort B) having all other DDR gene alterations. Subjects were divided in a 2:1 ratio to take either Olaparib or prednisolone and an AR signaling inhibitor (enzalutamide or abiraterone) as part of the control group. The primary endpoint was progression-free survival that was proven radiologically. Cohort A had a median duration of overall survival of 19.1 months with Olaparib compared to the control group, which had a median overall survival of 14.7 months (hazard ratio for death, 0.69; 95% confidence interval [CI], 0.50 to 0.97; $p = 0.02$). In cohort B, the median survival was 14.1 months with Olaparib and 11.5 months with the control therapy. In the overall population (cohorts A and B), the corresponding durations were 17.3 months and 14.0 months, respectively. Overall, 66% of the subjects in the control group crossed over to receive Olaparib (56 of 83 patients [67%] in cohort A). A sensitivity analysis that adjusted for crossover to Olaparib showed hazard ratios for death of 0.42 (95% CI, 0.19 to 0.91) in cohort A, 0.83 (95% CI, 0.11 to 5.98) in cohort B, and 0.55 (95% CI, 0.29 to 1.06) in the overall population. Based on the initial findings, the Food and Drug Administration (FDA), in May of 2020, approved Olaparib for mCRPC patients with deleterious HR gene mutations with disease progression following therapy with androgen receptor-signaling inhibitors [14].

A phase II trial called GALAHAD is currently being conducted on 165 patients with mCRPC, 81 of whom had germline mutations (46 BRCA and 35 non-BRCA), and 47% of whom had organ metastases. A total of 300 mg of Niraparib was administered once a day to patients who were included in this trial and whose mCRPC cancer has progressed despite receiving taxane-based chemotherapy and an AR signaling inhibitor as first-line therapy. When compared to patients without BRCA mutations, the findings showed that patients with BRCA-1 or BRCA-2 mutations had a composite rate of 63% whereas those without BRCA mutations had a CRR of 17% [15]. Trials including GALAHAD, MAGNITUDE, and QUEST continue to assess the effectiveness and safety of niraparib in patients with mCRPC and DDR mutations [16]. It is significant to highlight that, whereas the TRITON-1 and ProFOUND studies investigated patients with mono- and bi-allelic mutations, respectively, the GALAHAD study validated patient eligibility with bi-allelic mutations [17].

TALAPRO-1 was an open-label, phase II trial that assessed the efficiency of Talazoparib against mCRPC cancer. Eligibility criteria included men at the age of 18 years old or above, with progressive mCRPC and mono- or bi-allelic alterations of the DDR-HR genes, who received chemotherapy (taxane) and one or more NHT (enzalutamide, abiraterone or both). Eligible individuals received oral Talazoparib (1 mg daily). From October 18, 2017, to March 20, 2020, 128 individuals were recruited, from whom 127 got at least one dose of Talazoparib, and 104 exhibited soft-tissue disease. After 16.4 months, the odds ratio was 29.8% (31/104 patients). The most frequent side effects were anemia (31%), thrombocytopenia (9%) and neutropenia (8%). These results are very convincing and demonstrate a high anti-tumor efficacy for men with mCRPC with DDR-HR gene mutations [18].

The safety profile of PARP inhibitors in patients with mCRPC is of insignificant difference to that in patients with other solid tumors. The most often reported adverse events include fatigue, gastrointestinal side effects, and myelosuppression. The most frequent adverse effects, according to the ProFOUND trial, were nausea (41%), anemia (46%), and fatigue (41%). The drug dosage was reduced in 22% of the patients because of the side effects. Anemia, which occurs approximately in 22% of the cases, is the most frequent adverse effect, according to the GALAHAD and TRITON2 trials [15]. Myelodysplastic syndrome may be linked to PARP inhibitors in combination therapy, according to Nitecki et al., however, this complication is rare. There was no related hepatic or renal impairment, despite frequent elevations in alanine transaminase (ALT), aspartate transaminase (AST), and creatinine [19].

5. Resistance to PARPi

Although PARPi are very effective in everyday clinical practice, the increasing application of these medications in clinical settings has brought up the problem of PARPi resistance [20]. Multiple mechanisms for resistance have been proposed. Firstly, the restoration of homologous recombination (HR) may occur through a variety of different events, including intragenic mutations or the reversion of the epigenome that activates the open reading frame, thereby restoring the functionality of BRCA-1 or BRCA-2 proteins. Additionally, HR could also be recovered by other DNA repair-related proteins, such as p53-binding protein 1 (53BP1). This protein collaborates with BRCA-1 in balancing the HR and blocks the CtIP-mediated DNA end resection, which promotes DNA repair towards non-homologous end joining (NHEJ). When this protein is under-expressed in the cells that lack BRCA, it draws RAD51 and restores HR. The RAD51 protein is crucial to HR restoration, since it is placed on single and double-stranded DNA with the help of BRCA-2 to create a nuclease-resistant filament that, thus, encourages HR and PARPi resistance [21].

Secondly, an upregulation of ATP-binding cassette (ABC) transporters, which can be caused by the overexpression of the respective genes, is shown to increase the drug efflux and thus reduce the amount of the drug available intracellularly [22]. Thirdly, the accumulation of unrepaired single stranded breaks and the slowed progression of replication forks are significant causes of cell death, and PARPi capacity for PARP trapping exemplifies this. Recent research has shown that the emergence of PARPi resistance is functionally related to the suppression of PARP trapping activity [23]. In tumor samples that were resistant to PARPi, a mutation in PARP-1 (R591C) was frequently noted, which was connected to a decreased PARP-1 trapping action on DNA. In addition, the PAR glycohydrolase (PARG) enzyme participates in PARP-1 trapping action by reverting PARylation to avoid poly-ADP-ribose (PAR) buildup. Loss of the PARG causes cells that have been exposed to PARP to accumulate PAR, which is then used to restore PARP-1-dependent DNA damage signaling. PARP-1 trapping activity is hence reduced, which ultimately leads to PARPi resistance [20].

Fourthly, in halted replication fork protection, BRCA-1 and BRCA-2 genes play a crucial role. The nucleases MRE1164 and MUS8165 can target replication forks that have stalled in tumor cells with BRCA1 or BRCA-2 deficiency, thus leading to fork collapse and chromosomal abnormalities as a result. Some nucleases that can stabilize the replication fork act as a mechanism to prevent DNA replication fork disintegration when PARPi resistance develops. Particularly, the activity of EZH2 (enhancer of zeste 2 polycomb repressive complex 2 subunit) and PTIP (PAX transcription activation domain interacting protein 1-like) at the fork are suppressed in the BRCA-1 or BRCA-2 deficient cells, thereby reducing the recruitment of nucleases and promoting fork protection. Since it is known that PARPi causes unprotected replication forks to degrade, enhanced replication fork stabilization creates resistance to PARPi. Resistance to PARPi can also be mediated by several molecular signaling mechanisms controlling cell division. By being able to stimulate the PARP-1 enzymatic activity (by phosphorylation), the proto-oncogene mesenchymal-epithelial transition tyrosine kinase lowers the binding capacity of the PARPi. A considerable increase in the PI3K/AKT pathway has also been seen after using PARPi, which has the added benefit of promoting cell growth and proliferation. Lastly, the activation of the ATM/ATR pathway is also related to PARPi resistance. It serves as a crucial step in the DNA damage response pathway because it may attract DNA repair complexes by phosphorylating histone H2A. Inhibiting this route might be a future tactic to combat PARPi resistance, because it results in HR restoration [20].

6. PARPi and Immunotherapy

There is mounting evidence that immune checkpoint inhibitors and PARP inhibitors work synergistically. The programed death ligand-1 (PD-L1) plays a role in tumor immunosuppression and is activated in prostate cancer. Thus, suppression of the PD-L1 may enable efficient T-cell activation against cancerous cells. Additionally, PARP inhibition leads to the higher expression of PD-L1 in cells that express BRCA-2 in low amounts. Many ongoing clinical trials combine PARP inhibitors with PD1 blockers, such as pembrolizumab and nivolumab, and PD-L1 blockers, such as durvalumab. According to Karzai et al., mCRPC patients who received a combination of Olaparib and Durvalumab experienced a PSA drop of over 50% in most of the cases, with the median radiographic progression-free survival being 16.1 months as opposed to 4.8 months for those who did not have DDR abnormalities [24].

7. Conclusions

The PARP inhibitors are emerging as very useful treatment modalities in the management of prostate tumors caused by mutations in the HR system. Their use is associated with positive effects, including prolonged survival rates in patients with BRCA-1 or BRCA-2 gene mutations. However, the growing usage of PARP inhibitors in clinical practice sheds light on a rising clinical problem characterized by increasing resistance. There is a need for future studies investigating biomarkers other than BRCA to predict the efficacy of PARP inhibitors, given that the current clinical trials assess the utility and applicability of combination therapy in circumventing PARPi resistance.

Author Contributions: I.K., I.-P.T. and P.K. conceptualized the present paper, while all authors were involved in data collection and the preparation of the manuscript. Supervision was done by I.K. and N.J. All authors have read and agreed to the published version of the manuscript.

Funding: This research received no external funding.

Institutional Review Board Statement: Not applicable.

Informed Consent Statement: Not applicable.

Data Availability Statement: Not applicable.

Conflicts of Interest: The authors declare no conflict of interest.

References

1. Sung, H.; Ferlay, J.; Siegel, R.L.; Laversanne, M.; Soerjomataram, I.; Jemal, A.; Bray, F. Global Cancer Statistics 2020: GLOBOCAN Estimates of Incidence and Mortality Worldwide for 36 Cancers in 185 Countries. *CA Cancer J. Clin.* **2021**, *71*, 209–249. [CrossRef] [PubMed]
2. Bell, K.J.; Del Mar, C.; Wright, G.; Dickinson, J.; Glasziou, P. Prevalence of incidental prostate cancer: A systematic review of autopsy studies. *Int. J. Cancer.* **2015**, *137*, 1749–1757. [CrossRef] [PubMed]
3. Knipper, S.; Pecoraro, A.; Palumbo, C.; Rosiello, G.; Luzzago, S.; Deuker, M.; Tian, Z.; Shariat, S.F.; Saad, F.; Tilki, D.; et al. The effect of age on cancer-specific mortality in patients with prostate cancer: A population-based study across all stages. *Cancer Causes Control* **2020**, *31*, 283–290. [CrossRef] [PubMed]
4. American Cancer Society. Survival Rates for Prostate Cancer [Online]. Available online: https://www.cancer.org/cancer/prostate-cancer/detection-diagnosis-staging/survival-rates.html (accessed on 20 November 2022).
5. Dal Maso, L.; Panato, C.; Tavilla, A.; Guzzinati, S.; Serraino, D.; Mallone, S.; Botta, L.; Boussari, O.; Capocaccia, R.; Colonna, M.; et al. Cancer cure for 32 cancer types: Results from the EUROCARE-5 study. *Int. J. Epidemiol.* **2020**, *49*, 1517–1525. [CrossRef]
6. Gorodetska, I.; Kozeretska, I.; Dubrovska, A. BRCA Genes: The Role in Genome Stability, Cancer Stemness and Therapy Resistance. *J. Cancer* **2019**, *10*, 2109–2127. [CrossRef] [PubMed]
7. Mehrgou, A.; Akouchekian, M. The importance of BRCA1 and BRCA2 genes mutations in breast cancer development. *Med. J. Islam. Repub. Iran* **2016**, *30*, 369.
8. Dorff, T.B.; O'Neil, B.; Hoffman, K.E.; Lin, D.W.; Loughlin, K.R.; Dall'Era, M. 25-year perspective on prostate cancer: Conquering frontiers and understanding tumor biology. *Urol. Oncol.* **2021**, *39*, 521–527. [CrossRef] [PubMed]
9. Morales, J.; Li, L.; Fattah, F.J.; Dong, Y.; Bey, E.A.; Patel, M.; Gao, J.; Boothman, D.A. Review of poly (ADP-ribose) polymerase (PARP) mechanisms of action and rationale for targeting in cancer and other diseases. *Crit. Rev.™ Eukaryot. Gene Expr.* **2014**, *24*, 15–28. [CrossRef]
10. Grewal, K.; Grewal, K.; Tabbara, I.A. PARP Inhibitors in Prostate Cancer. *Anticancer. Res.* **2021**, *41*, 551–556. [CrossRef]
11. Murai, J.; Zhang, Y.; Morris, J.; Ji, J.; Takeda, S.; Doroshow, J.H.; Pommier, Y. Rationale for poly(ADP-ribose) polymerase (PARP) inhibitors in combination therapy with camptothecins or temozolomide based on PARP trapping versus catalytic inhibition. *J. Pharmacol. Exp. Ther.* **2014**, *349*, 408–416. [CrossRef]
12. Abida, W.; Patnaik, A.; Campbell, D.; Shapiro, J.; Bryce, A.H.; McDermott, R.; Sautois, B.; Vogelzang, N.J.; Bambury, R.M.; Voog, E.; et al. Rucaparib in Men With Metastatic Castration-Resistant Prostate Cancer Harboring a BRCA1 or BRCA2 Gene Alteration. *J. Clin. Oncol.* **2020**, *38*, 3763–3772. [CrossRef] [PubMed]
13. Abida, W.; Campbell, D.; Patnaik, A.; Sautois, B.; Shapiro, J.; Vogelzang, N.; Bryce, A.; Mcdermott, R.; Ricci, F.; Rowe, J.; et al. ESMO 2019: Preliminary Results from the TRITON2 Study of Rucaparib in Patients with DNA Damage Repair-Deficient mCRPC: Updated Analyses. UroToday.com and 2019 European Society for Medical Oncology Annual Meeting, ESMO 2019 #ESMO19, 27 Sept–1 Oct 2019 in Barcelona, Spain. Available online: https://www.urotoday.com/conference-highlights/esmo-2019/esmo-2019-prostate-cancer/115264-esmo-2019-preliminary-results-from-the-triton2-study-of-rucaparib-in-patients-with-dna-damage-repair-deficient-mcrpc-updated-analyses.html (accessed on 20 November 2022).

14. Hussain, M.; Mateo, J.; Fizazi, K.; Saad, F.; Shore, N.; Sandhu, S.; Chi, K.N.; Sartor, O.; Agarwal, N.; Olmos, D.; et al. Survival with Olaparib in Metastatic Castration-Resistant Prostate Cancer. *N. Engl. J. Med.* **2020**, *383*, 2345–2357. [CrossRef]
15. Shah, S.; Rachmat, R.; Enyioma, S.; Ghose, A.; Revythis, A.; Boussios, S. BRCA Mutations in Prostate Cancer: Assessment, Implications and Treatment Considerations. *Int. J. Mol. Sci.* **2021**, *22*, 12628. [CrossRef] [PubMed]
16. Smith, M.R. ESMO 2019: GALAHAD—A Phase 2 Study of Niraparib in Patients with mCRPC and Biallelic DNA-Repair Gene Defects, A Pre-Specified Interim Analysis. UroToday.com and 2019 European Society for Medical Oncology Annual Meeting, ESMO 2019 #ESMO19, 27 Sept–1 Oct 2019 in Barcelona, Spain. Available online: https://www.urotoday.com/conference-highlights/esmo-2019/esmo-2019-prostate-cancer/115258-esmo-2019-galaha-a-phase-2-study-of-niraparib-in-patients-with-mcrpc-and-biallelic-dna-repair-gene-defects-a-pre-specified-interim-analysis.html (accessed on 20 November 2022).
17. Messina, C.; Cattrini, C.; Soldato, D.; Vallome, G.; Caffo, O.; Castro, E.; Olmos, D.; Boccardo, F.; Zanardi, E. BRCA Mutations in Prostate Cancer: Prognostic and Predictive Implications. *J. Oncol.* **2020**, *2020*, 4986365. [CrossRef]
18. de Bono, J.S.; Mehra, N.; Scagliotti, G.V.; Castro, E.; Dorff, T.; Stirling, A.; Stenzl, A.; Fleming, M.T.; Higano, C.S.; Saad, F.; et al. Talazoparib monotherapy in metastatic castration-resistant prostate cancer with DNA repair alterations (TALAPRO-1): An open-label, phase 2 trial. *Lancet Oncol.* **2021**, *22*, 1250–1264, Erratum in *Lancet Oncol.* **2022**, *23*, e207. Erratum in *Lancet Oncol.* **2022**, *23*, e249. [CrossRef] [PubMed]
19. Nitecki, R.; Melamed, A.; Gockley, A.A.; Floyd, J.; Krause, K.J.; Coleman, R.L.; Matulonis, U.A.; Giordano, S.H.; Lu, K.H.; Rauh-Hain, J.A. Incidence of myelodysplastic syndrome and acute myeloid leukemia in patients receiving poly-ADP ribose polymerase inhibitors for the treatment of solid tumors: A meta-analysis of randomized trials. *Gynecol. Oncol.* **2021**, *161*, 653–659. [CrossRef]
20. Giudice, E.; Gentile, M.; Salutari, V.; Ricci, C.; Musacchio, L.; Carbone, M.V.; Ghizzoni, V.; Camarda, F.; Tronconi, F.; Nero, C.; et al. PARP Inhibitors Resistance: Mechanisms and Perspectives. *Cancers* **2022**, *14*, 1420. [CrossRef]
21. Mweempwa, A.; Wilson, M.K. Mechanisms of resistance to PARP inhibitors—An evolving challenge in oncology. *Cancer Drug Resist.* **2019**, *2*, 608–617. [CrossRef]
22. Noordermeer, S.M.; van Attikum, H. PARP Inhibitor Resistance: A Tug-of-War in BRCA-Mutated Cells. *Trends Cell Biol.* **2019**, *29*, 820–834. [CrossRef]
23. Gogola, E.; Duarte, A.A.; de Ruiter, J.R.; Wiegant, W.W.; Schmid, J.A.; de Bruijn, R.; James, D.I.; Llobet, S.G.; Vis, D.J.; Annunziato, S.; et al. Selective Loss of PARG Restores PARylation and Counteracts PARP Inhibitor-Mediated Synthetic Lethality. *Cancer Cell* **2019**, *35*, 950–952, Erratum in *Cancer Cell* **2018**, *33*, 1078–1093.e12. [CrossRef]
24. Karzai, F.; VanderWeele, D.; Madan, R.A.; Owens, H.; Cordes, L.M.; Hankin, A.; Couvillon, A.; Nichols, E.; Bilusic, M.; Beshiri, M.L.; et al. Activity of durvalumab plus olaparib in metastatic castration-resistant prostate cancer in men with and without DNA damage repair mutations. *J. Immunother. Cancer* **2018**, *6*, 141. [CrossRef] [PubMed]

Disclaimer/Publisher's Note: The statements, opinions and data contained in all publications are solely those of the individual author(s) and contributor(s) and not of MDPI and/or the editor(s). MDPI and/or the editor(s) disclaim responsibility for any injury to people or property resulting from any ideas, methods, instructions or products referred to in the content.

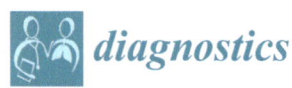

Article

Research of Prostate Cancer Urinary Diagnostic Biomarkers by Proteomics: The Noteworthy Influence of Inflammation

Elisa Bellei [1], Stefania Caramaschi [2], Giovanna A. Giannico [3], Emanuela Monari [1], Eugenio Martorana [4], Luca Reggiani Bonetti [2] and Stefania Bergamini [1,*]

[1] Department of Surgery, Medicine, Dentistry and Morphological Sciences with Transplant Surgery, Oncology and Regenerative Medicine Relevance, Proteomic Lab, University of Modena and Reggio Emilia, 41124 Modena, Italy; elisa.bellei@unimore.it (E.B.); emanuela.monari@unimore.it (E.M.)

[2] Department of Medical and Surgical Sciences for Children and Adults, University of Modena and Reggio Emilia, AOU Policlinico di Modena, 41124 Modena, Italy; stefania.caramaschi@unimore.it (S.C.); luca.reggianibonetti@unimore.it (L.R.B.)

[3] Department of Pathology, Microbiology and Immunology, Vanderbilt University Medical Center, Nashville, TN 37232, USA; giovanna.giannico@vumc.org

[4] Division of Urology, New Civilian Hospital of Sassuolo, 41049 Modena, Italy; eugeniomartorana@gmail.com

* Correspondence: stefania.bergamini@unimore.it; Tel.: +39-0592055362

Abstract: Nowadays, in the case of suspected prostate cancer (PCa), tissue needle biopsy remains the benchmark for diagnosis despite its invasiveness and poor tolerability, as serum prostate-specific antigen (PSA) is limited by low specificity. The aim of this proteomic study was to identify new diagnostic biomarkers in urine, an easily and non-invasively available sample, able to selectively discriminate cancer from benign prostatic hyperplasia (BPH), evaluating whether the presence of inflammation may be a confounding parameter. The analysis was performed by two-dimensional gel electrophoresis (2-DE), mass spectrometry (LC-MS/MS) and Enzyme-Linked Immunosorbent Assay (ELISA) on urine samples from PCa and BPH patients, divided into subgroups based on the presence or absence of inflammation. Significant quantitative and qualitative differences were found in the urinary proteomic profile of PCa and BPH groups. Of the nine differentially expressed proteins, only five can properly be considered potential biomarkers of PCa able to discriminate the two diseases, as they were not affected by the inflammatory process. Therefore, the proteomic research of novel and reliable urinary biomarkers of PCa should be conducted considering the presence of inflammation as a realistic interfering element, as it could hinder the detection of important protein targets.

Keywords: prostate cancer; benign prostatic hyperplasia; diagnostic biomarkers; proteomics; urine; inflammation

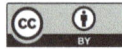

1. Introduction

To date, prostate cancer (PCa) is the second most common male malignancy, according to the estimated number of incident cases worldwide [1]. An increase in the number of new cases is expected in the coming years [2]. Rising incidence is secondary to longer life expectancy, population preventive strategies, and serum prostate-specific antigen (PSA) screening [3]. Presently, PCa appears as the fifth most common global cause of death from cancer in men [4]. Survival is 88% at 5 years after diagnosis and is increasing over time [5]. The pathogenesis of PCa is multifactorial due to the interaction of different risk factors, such as age, geographic area, familiarity, lifestyle, environmental agents, and genetic factors [6], while its etiology is not yet fully understood.

Current screening strategies for PCa diagnosis include prostatic digital rectal examination (DRE) and PSA measurement. However, neither can reliably differentiate a benign prostate condition from a cancerous one. PSA is an organ-specific and not a tumor-specific marker. A high PSA level can also be found in other non-malignant prostate conditions, such as benign prostatic hyperplasia (BPH) or prostatitis [7], and after prostate instrumentation or cystoscopy. Therefore, at present, the diagnostic gold standard is prostate needle biopsy (PBx), which is performed following an abnormal DRE and/or PSA. Unfortunately, this is an invasive technique associated with various side effects. Furthermore, about two-thirds of biopsies performed following elevated PSA were unneeded [8], underscoring the low specificity of this marker, which can lead to over-diagnosis of PCa and unnecessary treatment [9].

Hence, there is a pressing need for selective and noninvasive biomarkers for an accurate diagnosis and management of PCa. In this regard, urine is one of the most attractive biofluids in clinical proteomics, as it can be collected non-invasively, easily, inexpensively and in the large amount [10]. Moreover, compared to other biological specimens, such as plasma and serum, urine has a quite simple composition, as it contains a relatively lower number of proteins. This characteristic is a great advantage in the proteomic analysis [11]. Beyond urine, another encouraging and emerging strategy to deepen the knowledge of PCa is liquid biopsy, as it represents the tumor microenvironment, thus allowing overall information for the disease diagnosis, prognosis, monitoring and treatment [12]. In this regard, it has recently been reported that BRCA germline mutations have important implications in assessing the risk of developing PCa, as well as in the prognosis and treatment of the disease, proving their relevance in the clinical setting [13].

In the last few years, growing numbers of promising biomarkers have been described for different urological tumors, such as bladder cancer, renal cell carcinoma, and PCa, by urine-based proteomics studies [14,15]. Therefore, this approach could have the potential to limit tissue biopsy sampling, thus reducing the number of patients undergoing PBx.

Inflammation is an inherent and important component of cancer disease, with a substantial impact on studies aimed at the discovery and validation of biomarkers. Despite its crucial aspect, inflammation is frequently overlooked in most cancer biomarker studies [16,17]. Notably, our prior proteomic study conducted on serum samples from PCa and BPH patients has focused on the presence of inflammation, demonstrating that it can be a confounding parameter for protein biomarker discovery [18].

In the present study, new potential urinary diagnostic biomarkers of PCa were searched by two-dimensional gel electrophoresis (2-DE) associated with mass spectrometry analysis (LC-MS/MS). Significantly, the urinary proteomic profiles of PCa and BPH were compared, considering the presence or absence of inflammation.

2. Materials and Methods

2.1. Patients Selection and Classification

Patient enrollment was conducted at the Urology Department of the University Hospital Policlinico di Modena (Italy). All procedures followed in the study were approved by the Provincial Ethics Committee of Modena, Italy (Project identification code 57/08). The enrolled subjects provided written informed consent to participate in the study, which was conducted according to the ethical principles of the Helsinki Declaration (2013, last edition).

Inclusion criteria were age between 58 and 81 years, elevated serum PSA, and palpable lesions on DRE in patients who underwent PBx. Exclusion criteria were the presence of systemic diseases, renal disorders, diabetes, proteinuria from a routine clinical laboratory test, significant clinical events occurring within 6 months of enrollment, hormonal treatment, radiotherapy, and chemotherapy.

Patients with histopathologic diagnosis of PCa and BPH were included in the study in two separate groups: the PCa group (comprising all patients diagnosed with PCa) and the BPH group (comprising all patients diagnosed with BPH) [19]. Each group was further divided into two subgroups considering the absence or presence of inflammation, assessed during histological examination by the occurrence of pathological infiltration of the prostatic tissue by inflammatory cells, namely aggregations of lymphocytes and plasma cells. All slides were stained with hematoxylin and eosin (H&E) and were re-reviewed and graded by a pathologist according to the 2014 Modified Gleason System [20]. Therefore, the urinary proteome analysis was performed on six groups: (1) all cases of PCa (PCa group, n = 30), (2) PCa without inflammation (noI-PCa group, n = 10), (3) PCa with inflammation (I-PCa group, n = 20), (4) all cases of BPH (BPH group, n = 30), (5) BPH without inflammation (noI-BPH group, n = 11), and (6) BPH with inflammation (I-BPH group, n = 19).

2.2. Urinary Samples Preparation

Morning urine samples (10 mL, midstream) were collected before the biopsy. After centrifugation (800× g, 4 °C, 10 min) to remove any cellular debris and contamination, they were stored in aliquots at −80 °C for proteomic analysis. Urine samples were then pooled for each group (4 mL/pool), desalted, and concentrated to a final volume of 100/120 µL with Desalting Spin Columns (cut-off 3 kDa MW, Amicon Ultra-4, Merck Millipore, Milan, Italy) following the manufacturer's instructions.

2.3. Proteins Quantification

Protein content from each concentrated pool was quantified by the Bradford method [21] using the Protein Assay Dye Reagent (Bio-Rad Laboratories, Hercules, CA, USA) and bovine serum albumin (Sigma-Aldrich, Milan, Italy) as colorimetric reagent and calibration standard, respectively. Optical density (OD) reading was performed at 595 nm using a microplate reader (Multiskan™ FC, Thermo Fisher Scientific, Waltham, MA, USA).

2.4. Proteomic Analysis

The 2-DE analysis was performed on concentrated urinary pools. The proteins of each group (80 µg) were solubilized with rehydration buffer (6 M urea, 2 M thiourea, 4% 3-[(3-Cholamidopropyl)-dimethylammonio]-propane-sulfonate, CHAPS, 25 mM dithiothreitol, 0.2% ampholytes) and subjected to the first-dimension separation using 17 cm Immobilized pH Gradient strips (IPG strip, Bio-Rad Laboratories, Hercules, CA, USA), narrow pH range 4–7, and 8–16% polyacrylamide gradient gels in the second-dimension separation, as previously fully described [18].

After 2-DE, gels were stained with a silver nitrate protocol [22], then the gel images were acquired by a calibrated densitometer (series GS-800, Bio-Rad Laboratories, Hercules, CA, USA). The PDQuest 2-D Image analysis software program, version 7.3.1 (Bio-Rad Laboratories, Hercules, CA, USA) (accessed on 4 May 2022), was used to evaluate the spot intensity as OD (mean value) × area (mm^2). The difference in protein expression (fold-change) among the groups was obtained by the ratio between the values of spot intensity: variations $\geq$ 1.5 were considered statistically significant.

The different spots were manually removed from the gels and subjected to "in-gel trypsin digestion" for subsequent protein identification by LC-MS/MS, using a 1200 Nano HPLC/Chip microfluidic device (Agilent Technologies Inc., Santa Clara, CA, USA) associated with a 6520 Accurate-Mass ElectroSprayIonization-Quadrupole-Time-of-Flight mass spectrometer (ESI-Q-ToF, Agilent Technologies Inc., Santa Clara, CA, USA), as previously described [22]. Triptych digests were first resuspended in 10 µL of 3% acetonitrile (ACN)/0.1% formic acid (FA), then MS analysis was performed at a flow rate of 0.4 µL/min with a mobile phase composed of 95% ACN/5% water/0.1% FA, using a Chip enrichment column (Zorbax C18, 4 mm × 5 µm i.d., Agilent Technologies Inc., Santa Clara, CA, USA) and a separation column (Zorbax C18, 43 mm × 75 µm i.d., Agilent Technologies Inc., Santa Clara, CA, USA), with nitrogen as the nebulizer gas.

Protein characterization was performed using the SwissProt database and the search engine Mascot MS/MS Ion Search (accessed on 13 May 2022), specifying the following parameters: species Homo sapiens (Human), two possibilities of trypsin failure, peptide tolerance ± 20 ppm, MS/MS error tolerance ± 0.1 Da, carbamidomethylation of cysteines as fixed modifications and methionine oxidation as variable modifications.

2.5. Enzyme-Linked Immunosorbent Assay (ELISA)

The commercial Human Prostaglandin D Synthase (Lipocalin-Type) ELISA kit (BioVendor, TEMA Ricerca S.r.l., Castenaso, BO, Italy) It was used to validate and quantify Prostaglandin-H2 D-isomerase (PTGDS) in urine samples of patients from the four subgroups. Diluted urine samples (1:100) were analyzed in duplicate following the manufacturer's recommendations. The absorbance of the final product was measured at 450 nm using a microplate reader (Multiskan FC, Thermo Fisher Scientific), and protein concentration was calculated from a standard curve generated by the stock solution furnished with the kit.

2.6. Statistical Analysis

The patient's age and PSA levels are reported as the median. Total protein content in each group and PTGDS concentrations are provided as mean ± standard deviation (SD). The statistical analysis was carried out using the parametric Student's t-test, considering p-values ≤ 0.05 as statistically significant.

3. Results

3.1. Histological Examination

PCa was characterized by atypical glands or nests of irregular epithelial cells with amphophilic cytoplasm, enlarged hyperchromatic nuclei, and prominent nucleoli. BPH was diagnosed when were observed increases in epithelial and/or stromal cells and typical nodular and expansive growth without evidence of atypia. PCa and BPH patients were stratified into 4 subgroups based on the absence or presence of inflammation, determined by the presence of inflammatory cells infiltrating the prostate tissue. Representative H&E slides for the different tissue conditions are shown in Figure 1.

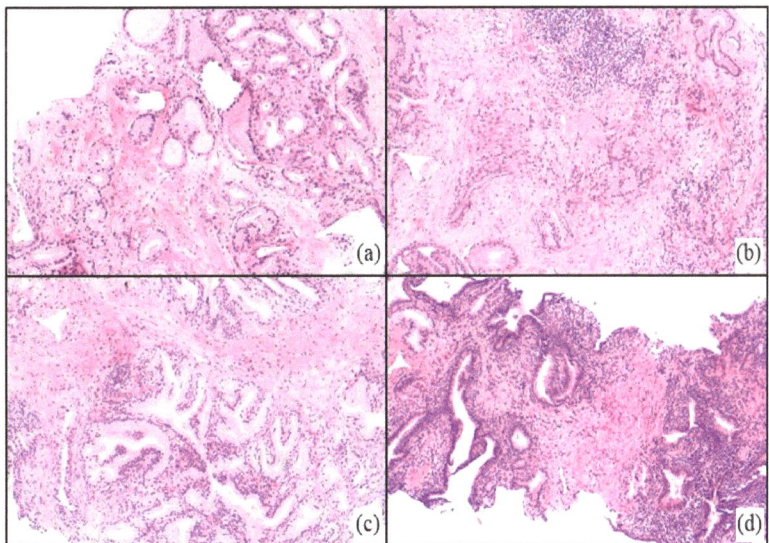

Figure 1. Representative histological slides displaying the different tissue conditions for the four subgroups: (**a**) noI-PCa; (**b**) I-PCa; (**c**) noI-BPH; (**d**) I-BPH.

3.2. Clinical Data

The median age of the enrolled patients was 68 years (range 59–73) for the PCa group and 68 years (range 59–81) for the BPH group, denoting no significant differences between the two groups, as well as among the relative subgroups. Within noI-PCa, five patients showed Grade Group (G) < 7 and 5 patients G $\geq$ 7. Within I-PCa, nine patients showed

G < 7, and 11 cases showed G ≥ 7. PSA values were significantly higher in PCa vs. BPH ($p = 0.03$) and in noI-PCa vs. noI-BPH ($p = 0.02$) (Table 1).

Table 1. Clinical data of selected patients.

Groups	Age (Years) Median (Range)	Grade Group	PSA (ng/mL) Median (Range)	PSA Comparisons
PCa ($n = 30$)	68 (59–73)	G < 7 ($n = 14$) G ≥ 7 ($n = 16$)	5.80 (0.80–34.36)	PCa vs. BPH, $p = 0.03$
noI-PCa ($n = 10$)	68.5 (62–73)	G < 7 ($n = 5$) G ≥ 7 ($n = 5$)	5.95 (4.49–34.00)	noI-PCa vs. noI-BPH, $p = 0.02$
I-PCa ($n = 20$)	67 (59–73)	G < 7 ($n = 9$) G ≥ 7 ($n = 11$)	5.49 (0.80–34.36)	I-PCa vs. I-BPH, $p > 0.05$ I-PCa vs. noI-PCa, $p > 0.05$
BPH ($n = 30$)	68 (59–81)	- -	3.60 (0.20–25.00)	
noI-BPH ($n = 11$)	67 (59–77)	- -	3.65 (0.20–6.80)	
I-BPH ($n = 19$)	69 (60–81)	- -	3.60 (0.40–25.00)	I-BPH vs. noI-BPH, $p > 0.05$

Statistical analysis was performed by Student's t-test ($p \leq 0.05$ is considered statistically significant).

3.3. Protein Concentration

The spectrophotometric quantification of urinary protein content is illustrated in Table 2. PCa groups showed a significantly lower total protein concentration than BPH groups, regardless of inflammation (PCa vs. BPH, $p < 0.001$; noI-PCa vs. noI-BPH, $p \leq 0.05$; I-PCa vs. I-BPH, $p \leq 0.05$). When comparing the same group with and without inflammation, total protein content was found to be significantly higher in I-BPH vs. noI-BPH ($p \leq 0.05$), while the result was not significantly different in Pca ($p > 0.05$).

Table 2. Protein concentration of urinary pools.

Groups	Concentration (µg/µL)	Group Comparisons	p-Value
Pca	1.57 ± 0.48	Pca vs. BPH	$p < 0.001$
noI-Pca	1.74 ± 0.49	noI-Pca vs. noI-BPH	$p \leq 0.05$
I-Pca	1.49 ± 0.26	I-Pca vs. I-BPH	$p \leq 0.05$
		I-Pca vs. noI-PCa	$p > 0.05$
BPH	4.06 ± 0.57		
noI-BPH	2.72 ± 0.34		
I-BPH	4.77 ± 1.22	I-BPH vs. noI-BPH	$p \leq 0.05$

Protein content is expressed as mean ± SD. Statistical analysis was performed by Student's t-test.

3.4. Proteomic Comparisons

The urinary protein maps obtained by 2-DE analysis for each group are shown in Figure 2.

3.4.1. Urinary Protein Expression in PCa and BPH Regardless Inflammation

The comparison of the urinary proteomic profiles of PCa and BPH, regardless of the presence or absence of inflammation, showed 18 differentially expressed protein spots, corresponding to 9 unique proteins. Specifically, three spots, two of which related to Alpha-1-microglobulin (AMBP[1] and AMBP[2]), and one identified as Ganglioside GM2 activator (SAP3) were increased in PCa (Figure 2a) compared to BPH (Figure 2b). In the same comparison, 15 spots resulted decreased: Alpha-1-antichymotrypsin (spots AACT[1] and AACT[2]), Alpha-1-beta-glycoprotein (A1BG), Serotransferrin (TRFE), six isoforms of Alpha-1-antitrypsin (A1AT[1]-A1AT[6]), two spots recognized as Haptoglobin (HPT[1] and

HPT[2]), two spots corresponding to Apolipoprotein A1 (APOA1[1] and APOA1[2]), and Transthyretin (TTHY).

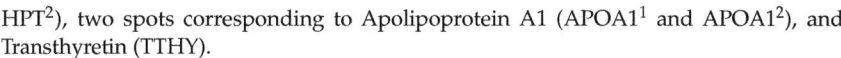

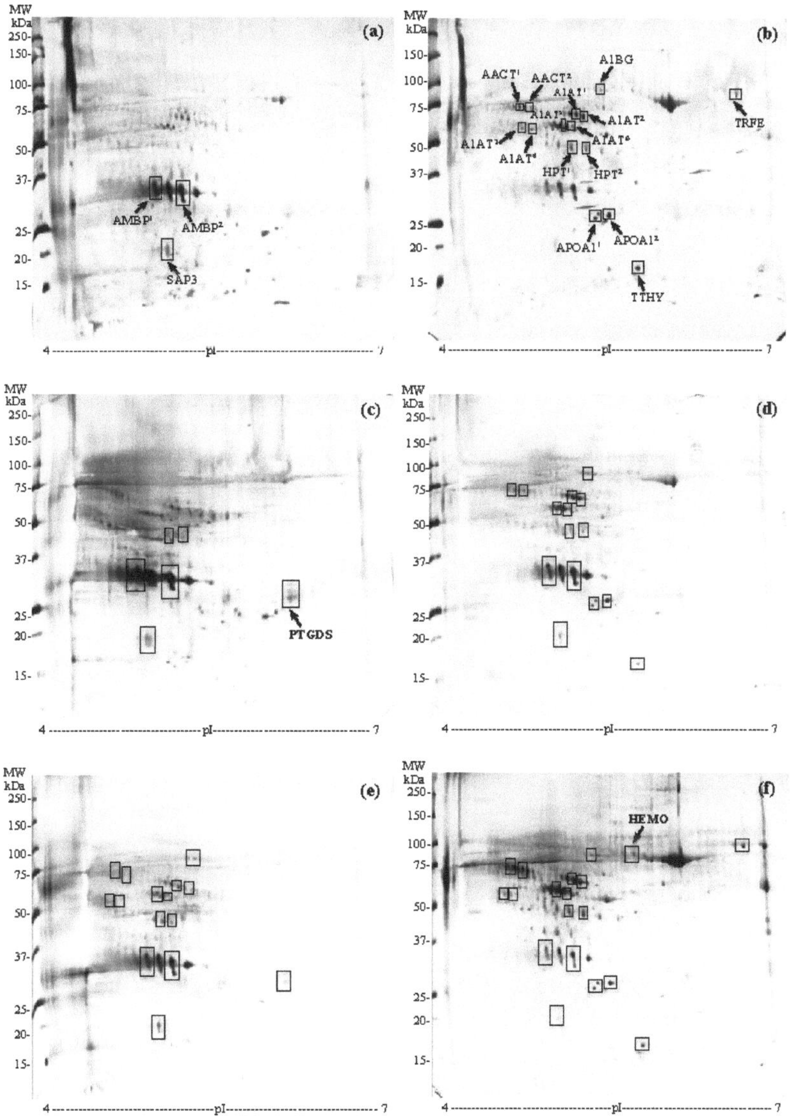

Figure 2. Representative urinary 2D gels; (**a**) PCa group (all PCa patients with and without inflammation); (**b**) BPH group (all BPH patients with and without inflammation); (**c**) noI-PCa group (PCa patients without inflammation); (**d**) noI-BPH group (BPH patients without inflammation); (**e**) I-PCa group (PCa patients with inflammation); (**f**) I-BPH group (BPH patients with inflammation). The significantly different spots are enclosed in rectangles, and in panels (**a–c,f**) are included the protein entry names, corresponding to those reported in Table 3. AMBP, Alpha-1-microglobulin; SAP3, Ganglioside GM2 activator; AACT, Alpha-1-antichymotrypsin; A1BG, Alpha-1-beta-glicoprotein; TRFE, Serotransferrin; A1AT, Alpha-1-antitrypsin; HPT, Haptoglobin; APOA1, Apolipoprotein A1; TTHY, Transthyretin; PTGDS, Prostaglandin-H2 D-isomerase; HEMO, Hemopexin.

Table 3. Urinary proteins identified by ESI-Q-ToF-MS/MS analysis.

Entry Name [a]	Protein Name [b]	Acc. No. [c]	MW (Da) [d]	Fold-Change of Protein Expression [e]			
				PCa vs. BPH [e1]	noI-PCa vs. noI-BPH [e2]	I-PCa vs. noI-Pca [e3]	I-BPH vs. noI-BPH [e4]
AMBP[1]	Alpha-1-microglobulin	P02760	39,886	+4.40	+2.39	−1.51	−2.28
AMBP[2]	Alpha-1-microglobulin	P02760	39,886	+2.06	+2.70	−1.64	−1.83
SAP3	Ganglioside GM2 activator	P17900	21,281	+3.80	+2.18	−1.53	−2.09
AACT[1]	Alpha-1-antichymotrypsin	P01011	47,792	−7.91	−5.39	−1.77	+4.23
AACT[2]	Alpha-1-antichymotrypsin	P01011	47,792	−1.50	/	−2.78	+3.99
A1BG	Alpha-1-beta-glicoprotein	P04217	54,790	−5.44	−2.60	+4.50	+6.69
TRFE	Serotransferrin	P02787	79,294	−2.18	ND	ND	+2.14
A1AT[1]	Alpha-1-antitrypsin	P01009	46,878	−6.02	/	/	+2.19
A1AT[2]	Alpha-1-antitrypsin	P01009	46,878	−6.31	−1.91	+2.11	+6.35
A1AT[3]	Alpha-1-antitrypsin	P01009	46,878	−2.57	ND	+1.75	+2.53
A1AT[4]	Alpha-1-antitrypsin	P01009	46,878	−1.50	ND	+1.86	/
A1AT[5]	Alpha-1-antitrypsin	P01009	46,878	−10.90	−2.55	+3.56	+10.3
A1AT[6]	Alpha-1-antitrypsin	P01009	46,878	−2.32	−2.30	+10.8	+1.61
HPT[1]	Haptoglobin	P00738	45,861	−3.34	/	+2.27	+2.16
HPT[2]	Haptoglobin	P00738	45,861	−2.02	/	+1.61	+3.11
APOA1[1]	Apolipoprotein A1	P02647	30,759	−6.67	/	ND	/
APOA1[2]	Apolipoprotein A1	P02647	30,759	−10.40	−3.68	ND	/
TTHY	Transthyretin	P02766	15,991	−3.45	/	ND	+3.46
PTGDS	Prostaglandin-H2 D-isomerase	P41222	21,243	ND	+6.53	−2.79	/
HEMO	Hemopexin	P02790	52,385	ND	ND	ND	+2.52

[a] Protein entry names from UniProtKB database (all with extension -HUMAN), corresponding to those reported in proteins maps (Figure 2); [b] Protein complete names; [c] Protein accession number from UniProtKB database; [d] MW, theoretical molecular weight (Da, Dalton); [e] Fold-change of protein expression among groups, (+) increased expression, (−) decreased expression in [e1] PCa vs. BPH, [e2] noI-PCa vs. noI-BPH, [e3] I-PCa vs. noI-Pca, [e4] I-BPH vs. noI-BPH. ND: protein spot not detectable. (/): not significant comparison (<1.5).

3.4.2. Urinary Protein Expression in Specimens without Inflammation

Similar to the previous comparison, AMBP[1], AMBP[2], and SAP3 were overexpressed, while AACT, A1BG, A1AT, and APOA1 were decreased in noI-PCa (Figure 2c) vs. noI-BPH (Figure 2d). Otherwise, no expression difference was revealed for HPT and TTHY, while TRFE was not detectable. Noteworthy, a novel spot was significantly detected in noI-PCa, identified as PTGDS.

3.4.3. Urinary Protein Expression in PCa with and without Inflammation

AMBP[1], AMBP[2,] SAP3, AACT[1] and AACT[2] spots were decreased, while A1BG, A1AT and HPT were increased in I-PCa (Figure 2e) vs. noI-PCa (Figure 2c). TRFE, APOA1, and TTHY were not detectable. Remarkably, PTGDS was found to be downregulated in the presence of inflammation.

3.4.4. Urinary Protein Expression in BPH with and without Inflammation

AMBP[1], AMBP[2] and SAP3 were decreased, while AACT, A1BG, TRFE, A1AT, HPT, and TTHY resulted in an increase in I-BPH (Figure 2f) compared to noI-BPH (Figure 2d). APOA1 and PTGDS showed no significant expression difference. Additionally, a new protein spot, identified as Hemopexin (HEMO), was revealed only in I-BPH.

The values of fold-change in expression obtained by each comparison are reported in Table 3, as well as the complete list of proteins identified by LC-MS/MS analysis. All proteins presented the highest ion scores obtained with the MASCOT search engine (ranging from 2686 to 51), indicating the observed correspondence between the experimental data and the theoretical data. Moreover, the number of significant sequences, that is, the number of significant peptides that matched the identified proteins, were at least >2, and the protein coverage, namely the percentage of amino acids sequenced for each detected protein, ranged from a minimum of 13% up to 66%.

In addition, were pointed out the main functions of each protein (Figure 3). As evidenced, most of the detected proteins (64%) were acute-phase proteins (APPs). However, these proteins play other roles, including antioxidant, radical scavenging, and tissue repair (AMBP), proteolysis (AACT, A1AT), antioxidant and antibacterial activity (HPT), iron binding and transport (TRFE), hormone binding and transport (TTHY), heme and metal ion binding (HEMO). Other proteins (36%) were involved in further biological actions, namely lipid transport (SAP3), steroid metabolism and cholesterol transport (APOA1), binding of lipophilic molecules and scavenging of harmful hydrophobic constituents (PTGDS), as inferred by the UniProtKB and The Human Protein Atlas databases (accessed on 30 May 2022).

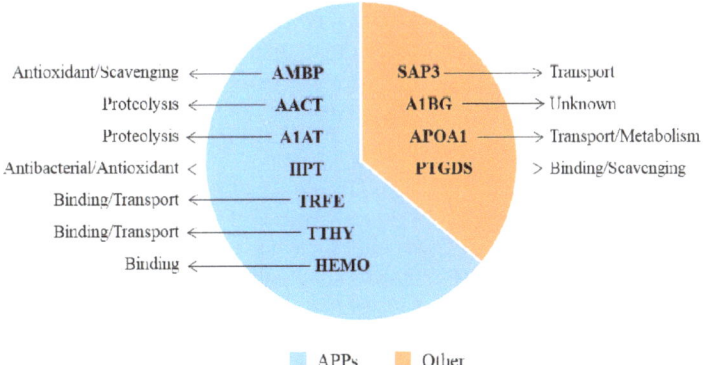

Figure 3. Principal roles of the differentially expressed proteins. The majority (64%) were acute-phase response proteins (APPs) involved in various biological processes, while the others (36%) were proteins with similar or different molecular functions.

3.5. PTGDS Quantification by ELISA

The urinary concentration of PTGDS was significantly higher in noI-PCa (1156.8 ± 276.2 ng/mL) compared to: I-PCa (595.6 ± 338.3 ng/mL) ($p = 0.03$), noI-BPH (712.6 ± 285.8 ng/mL), ($p = 0.02$) and I-BPH (593.2 ± 229.3 ng/mL) ($p = 0.05$) (Figure 4). Conversely, no significant differences were found between I-PCa and I-BPH, and I-BPH vs. noI-BPH ($p > 0.05$).

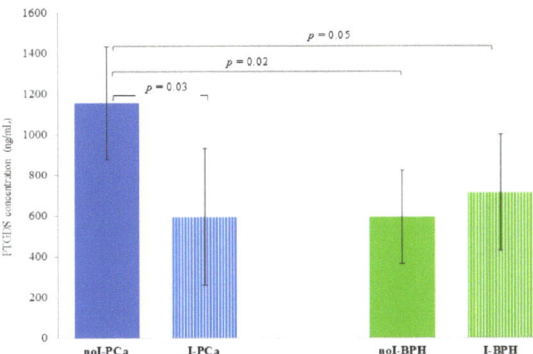

Figure 4. PTGDS quantification by ELISA. Protein concentrations are expressed as mean ± SD. Significant comparisons are highlighted by connecting lines, each showing the p-value obtained by Student's t-test ($p \leq 0.05$ are considered as statistically significant).

4. Discussion

Currently, the gold standard for the detection of clinically significant PCa is MRI-targeted or standard transrectal prostate biopsy [23]. Serum PSA lacks the specificity to discriminate between benign prostatic diseases (such as BPH and prostatitis) and PCa, being organ rather than cancer-specific [24,25]. Hence, there is a reasonable need for novel and unambiguous biomarkers of clinical utility for PCa diagnosis, prognosis, and beneficial treatment strategies [26]. Proteomics proves to be a promising approach for protein biomarkers discovery aimed at improving the management of PCa patients [27]. Furthermore, samples obtained through non-invasive procedures, such as urine, are a suitable target for proteomics [28].

In this study, we analyzed the urinary proteome of patients with PCa and BPH, addressing, for the first time to our knowledge, the role of inflammation as a potential confounding element. We revealed both quantitative and qualitative differences in the urinary protein content between PCa and BPH. Particularly, PCa samples showed a significantly lower protein content than BPH, regardless of inflammation. This could be due to the disease-related modifications of the molecular pathways that cause the adjustment of the metabolic profile observed in PCa and promote the adaptability of the prostate cells to the cancer microenvironment. According to the literature, the changes occurring in PCa can affect the entire central metabolism, and it seems that the prostate has a unique metabolism not found in other types of tissues [29]. When the same disease was compared, taking into account the presence or absence of inflammation, total protein content was significantly lower in I-PCa vs. noI-PCa, while resulting in significantly higher in I-BPH vs. noI-BPH. It is important to underline that inflammation is a pivotal process associated with benign and malignant prostate diseases [30]. Inflammation activates hyperproliferative systems in BPH and creates an appropriate microenvironment for cancer growth and progression [31]. Consequently, this study was performed considering the inflammatory process as a common denominator of both conditions.

Qualitative variations in protein expression were detected by 2-DE and LC-MS/MS analysis through the comparison among the groups. The comparison of the urinary proteome between PCa and BPH, without taking into consideration the presence/absence of inflammation, showed nine deregulated proteins in PCa patients. Specifically, AMBP and SAP3 were found to be upregulated, while AACT, A1BG, TRFE, A1AT, HPT, APOA1 and TTHY resulted in significantly downregulated. As inflammation can affect potential PCa biomarkers in proteomic research [18], PCa and BPH were compared, excluding samples with evident histological signs of inflammation (noI-PCa vs. noI-BPH). In this case, both AMBP spots and SAP3 were increased in PCa, but only AACT, A1BG, A1AT, and APOA1 were decreased. TRFE was not detectable, while HPT and TTHY showed no significant expression difference. Remarkably, in the absence of inflammation was identified the PTGDS protein in PCa samples was not detected in the previous comparison, namely in PCa and BPH groups regardless of inflammation.

AMBP is an acute phase protein (APP) previously revealed as a promising diagnostic biomarker for PCa [32]. Moreover, it has already been proven to be a potential biomarker of other cancer types, such as non-small-cell lung carcinoma [33] and pancreatic cancer [34]. SAP3 is a ganglioside with supported roles in mediating tumor-induced growth and progression [35] and cancer cell migration, as reported by a proteomic analysis of the breast cancer secretome [36]. It is proven that, in tumor cells, the expression levels of gangliosides positively or negatively regulate the signaling of cancer cells, promoting the malignancy of the disease [37]. SAP3 is also implicated in lipids transport. It is well established that lipid metabolism has a key role in PCa progression due to its interactions with androgens and its close involvement in the interactivity between immune and tumor cells [38]. The carcinomic prostate tissue becomes dependent on the use of lipids to survive and proliferate; this could explain the higher expression of SAP3 revealed in PCa vs. BPH. Both AMBP and SAP3 were found to increase also in our previous proteomic study conducted on urine samples from PCa patients with different risks of cancer progression [39]. The glycoprotein AACT is a serine protease inhibitor involved in the acute phase response and proteolysis (UniProtKB). Its dysregulation and glycosylation levels are associated with tumor progression and recurrence [40]. A1BG, another glycoprotein belonging to the immunoglobulin superfamily, was found overexpressed by proteomics in various forms of cancer, such as pancreatic ductal adenocarcinoma [41], cervical intraepithelial neoplasia [42] and bladder cancer [43]. Additionally, A1BG has been found to be associated with tumor heterogeneity and malignancy in an animal model of breast cancer [44]. Recently, its key role in tumorigenesis has been confirmed, suggesting that A1BG could be a promising target for cancer diagnosis, prognosis, and therapy [40]. Regarding A1AT, its high levels have been positively correlated with unfavorable clinical outcomes in cancer [45]. In support of our findings, Dong and co-authors reported a close association between urinary glycoproteins, including A1AT, and an aggressive form of PCa [46]. Furthermore, the higher expression of APOA1 in BPH versus PCa was previously shown in other proteomic studies, thus consolidating our current results [9,32,47].

To evaluate the changes induced in the urinary proteome by inflammation, PCa and BPH with and without inflammation were further compared with each other. In I-PCa vs. noI-PCa comparison, AMBP, SAP3 and AACT appeared under-expressed, while A1BG, A1AT and HPT were overexpressed. TRFE was confirmed not detectable, endorsing the result obtained from the previous comparison (noI-PCa vs. noI-BPH), together with APOA1 and TTHY. On the contrary, PTGDS was found downregulated in I-PCa samples, so it is reasonable to infer that its detection is sensibly affected by the presence of inflammation. The ELISA test confirmed this finding, as PTGDS concentration resulted significantly different only in PCa free of inflammation. Accordingly, PTGDS cannot be considered a candidate biomarker of PCa due to its influence on inflammation. Besides, in our previous study, this protein was identified in the urine of PCa patients with low, intermediate, and high progression risk, so it cannot even be considered an index of tumor aggressiveness [39]. Finally, AMBP, SAP3 and PTGDS were confirmed downregulated, and A1BG, A1AT, and HPT were proved to be upregulated in I-BPH vs. noI-BPH, like the previous comparison concerning PCa. Particularly, HPT was found downregulated in the PCa group in the first comparison (PCa vs. BPH), while the same comparison in the absence of inflammation was not significant. Then, HPT was found to have a significant increase in both conditions in the presence of inflammation, so it cannot be a feasible biomarker of PCa but rather a protein characterizing the urinary proteome of both diseases when present inflammation. Likewise, high levels of HPT were also evidenced in serum samples from PCa and BPH in the presence of inflammation [18], strengthening the assumption that this is more an inflammation-linked protein rather than a disease-associated protein. Peculiarly, the 2 "negative" acute phase proteins TRFE and TTHY, not detectable in previous comparisons, and HEMO, identified exclusively in this comparison, resulted in an increase in the I-BPH group. So, we can assume that these proteins could be associated with the benign disease rather than with the PCa, as well as with the presence of inflammation. Notable, HEMO, a "positive" APP, was also increased in the serum of BPH patients compared to PCa patient groups [18]. Moreover, consistent with our results, HEMO was found to be downregulated in the urine of PCa vs. BPH in a comparative proteomic analysis by Devalieva et al. [48]. In agreement, it is today widely recognized that high-grade prostatic inflammation is significantly more common in subjects with BPH rather than in those with PCa, contributing to the promotion of the disease development [49].

In summary, only five proteins, namely AMBP, SAP3, AACT, A1BG, and A1AT, could be rightly considered potential PCa biomarkers, as they are not affected by the inflammatory process. Moreover, they could discriminate cancer from BPH. Some of these proteins have already been reported in the literature as possible targets of PCa [32,39,46], while others are thought to be promising biomarkers for different types of malignant diseases [33,34,41–44]. In the future, once validated and endorsed for clinical practice, these new biomarkers could be proposed as a complementary analysis after a PSA-positive scenario to differentiate between PCa and BPH. Furthermore, this set of targeted urinary proteins could be combined in a multi-panel assay to develop a routine diagnostic test for the screening of PCa. Otherwise, TRFE, TTHY and HEMO were found to be closely associated with inflammation and BPH rather than cancer, and therefore, they are unlikely candidate biomarkers for PCa. A similar result was obtained for APOA1, as its expression was linked to BPH. Additionally, HPT results are primarily related to inflammation in both PCa and BPH and, as such, not a likely candidate marker of PCa. Finally, PTGDS expression was affected by the presence of inflammation.

This study has some limitations, including the small sample size in each subgroup. On the other hand, this is a preliminary proteomic investigation conducted on urine samples considering, for the first time, the possible interference of inflammation during the search for protein biomarkers. Future studies with a larger sample size will be needed to validate these initial results. Secondly, only the most questionable protein, PTGDS, was further verified/quantified by a complementary method, i.e., the ELISA test, which has the benefit of being the gold standard procedure to confirm potential protein biomarkers in urine thanks to its high throughput, simplicity, specificity, and sensitivity [15].

5. Conclusions

Considering the presence of inflammation as a real confounding element, a promising pattern of diagnostic biomarkers of PCa was identified in urine samples by a proteomic approach. A reliable urinary profile of PCa-associated protein biomarkers, combined with clinical and histopathological information, could represent an integrative diagnostic tool for early cancer screening, ensuring the best selection of patient candidates for biopsy, as well as enhancing patient stratification or setting up a personalized therapeutic strategy, with the potential to improve the clinical management of PCa.

Author Contributions: Conceptualization, E.B., S.C., L.R.B. and S.B.; methodology, E.B., S.C., E.M. (Emanuela Monari) and S.B.; software, E.B., S.C., L.R.B. and S.B.; validation, E.B., E.M. (Emanuela Monari) and S.B.; formal analysis, E.B., S.C., E.M. (Emanuela Monari), E.M. (Eugenio Martorana), L.R.B. and S.B.; investigation, E.B., S.C., G.A.G., E.M. (Emanuela Monari), E.M. (Eugenio Martorana), L.R.B. and S.B.; data curation, E.B., S.C. and S.B.; writing—original draft preparation, E.B., S.C., G.A.G. and S.B.; writing—review and editing, E.B., S.C., G.A.G., E.M. (Emanuela Monari), E.M. (Eugenio Martorana), L.R.B. and S.B.; supervision, E.B., S.C., G.A.G. and S.B.; project administration, E.B., S.C. and S.B. All authors have read and agreed to the published version of the manuscript.

Funding: This research received no external funding.

Institutional Review Board Statement: The study was conducted in accordance with the Declaration of Helsinki and approved by the Provincial Ethics Committee of Modena, Italy (protocol code 57/08, date of approval 1 April 2008).

Informed Consent Statement: Informed consent was obtained from all subjects involved in the study. Written informed consent has been obtained from the patients to publish this paper.

Data Availability Statement: All data considered in this study are reported in this article.

Acknowledgments: We thank the Fondazione Cassa di Risparmio di Modena, which financed the purchase of the ESI-Q-ToF mass spectrometer used in this study, and Diego Pinetti and Filippo Genovese (CIGS, University of Modena and Reggio Emilia, Italy) for their technical assistance during MS analysis.

Conflicts of Interest: The authors declare no conflict of interest.

Abbreviations

A1AT	Alpha-1-antitrypsin
A1BG	Alpha-1-beta-glicoprotein
AACT	Alpha-1-antichymotrypsin
AMBP	Alpha-1-microglobulin
APOA1	Apolipoprotein A1

APPs	Acute phase proteins
BPH	Benign prostatic hyperplasia
2-DE	Two-dimensional gel electrophoresis
H&E	Hematoxylin and eosin stain
HEMO	Hemopexin
HPT	Haptoglobin
I-BPH	BPH group with inflammation
I-PCa	PCa group with inflammation
noI-BPH	BPH group without inflammation
noI-PCa	PCa group without inflammation
PBx	Prostate needle biopsy
PCA	Prostate Cancer
PSA	Prostate-specific antigen
PTGDS	Prostaglandin-H2 D-isomerase
SAP3	Ganglioside GM2 activator
TRFE	Serotransferrin
TTHY	Transthyretin

References

1. GLOBOCAN 2020, Cancer Today. International Agency for Research on Cancer. 2023. Available online: http://bit.ly/41XKskq (accessed on 16 March 2023).
2. GLOBOCAN 2020, Cancer Tomorrow. International Agency for Research on Cancer. 2023. Available online: http://bit.ly/3YHDZYk (accessed on 16 March 2023).
3. Hassanipour-Azgomi, S.; Mohammadian-Hafshejani, A.; Ghoncheh, M.; Towhidi, F.; Jamehshorani, S.; Salehiniya, H. Incidence and mortality of prostate cancer and their relationship with the Human Development Index worldwide. *Prostate Int.* **2016**, *4*, 118–124. [CrossRef] [PubMed]
4. GLOBOCAN 2020, Cancer Today. International Agency for Research on Cancer. 2023. Available online: http://bit.ly/3ymcAjT (accessed on 16 March 2023).
5. Ferlay, J.; Soerjomataram, I.; Dikshit, R.; Eser, S.; Mathers, C.; Rebelo, M.; Parkin, D.M.; Forman, D.; Bray, F. Cancer incidence and mortality worldwide: Sources, methods and major patterns in GLOBOCAN 2012. *Int. J. Cancer.* **2015**, *136*, E359–E386. [CrossRef]
6. Paulo, P.; Maia, S.; Pinto, C.; Pinto, P.; Monteiro, A.; Peixoto, A.; Teixeira, M.R. Targeted next generation sequencing identifies functionally deleterious germline mutations in novel genes in early-onset/familial prostate cancer. *PLoS Genet.* **2018**, *14*, e1007355. [CrossRef] [PubMed]
7. Jia, G.; Dong, Z.; Sun, C.; Wen, F.; Wang, H.; Guo, H.; Gao, X.; Xu, C.; Xu, C.; Yang, C.; et al. Alterations in expressed prostate secretion-urine PSA N-glycosylation discriminate prostate cancer from benign prostate hyperplasia. *Oncotarget* **2017**, *8*, 76987–76999. [CrossRef]
8. Rigau, M.; Olivan, M.; Garcia, M.; Sequeiros, T.; Montes, M.; Colas, E.; Llaurado, M.; Planas, J.; de Torres, I.; Morote, J.; et al. The present and future of prostate cancer urine biomarkers. *Int. J. Mol. Sci.* **2013**, *14*, 12620–12649. [CrossRef]
9. McNally, C.J.; Ruddock, M.W.; Moore, T.; McKenna, D.J. Biomarkers that differentiate benign prostatic hyperplasia from prostate cancer: A literature review. *Cancer Manag. Res.* **2020**, *12*, 5225–5241. [CrossRef]
10. Decramer, S.; Gonzalez de Peredo, A.; Breuil, B.; Mischak, H.; Monsarrat, B.; Bascands, J.-L.; Schanstra, J.P. Urine in clinical proteomics. *Mol. Cell. Proteomics* **2008**, *7*, 1850–1862. [CrossRef]
11. Gopalan, G.; Rao, V.S.; Kakkar, V.V. An overview of urinary proteomics applications in human diseases. *Int. J. High. Throughput Screen.* **2010**, *1*, 183–192. [CrossRef]
12. Crocetto, F.; Russo, G.; Di Zazzo, E.; Pisapia, P.; Mirto, B.F.; Palmieri, A.; Pepe, F.; Bellevicine, C.; Russo, A.; La Civita, E.; et al. Liquid biopsy in prostate cancer management—Current challenges and future perspectives. *Cancers* **2022**, *14*, 3272. [CrossRef] [PubMed]
13. Crocetto, F.; Barone, B.; Caputo, V.F.; Fonatana, M.; de Cobelli, O.; Ferro, M. BRCA germline mutations in prostate cancer: The future is tailored. *Diagnostics* **2021**, *11*, 908. [CrossRef]
14. Swensen, A.C.; He, J.; Fang, A.C.; Ye, Y.; Nicora, C.D.; Shi, T.; Liu, A.Y.; Sigdel, T.K.; Sarwal, M.M.; Qian, W.-J. A comprehensive urine proteome database generated from patients with various renal conditions and prostate cancer. *Front. Med.* **2021**, *8*, 548212. [CrossRef]
15. Jedinak, A.; Loughlin, K.R.; Moses, M.A. Approaches to the discovery of non-invasive urinary biomarkers of prostate cancer. *Oncotarget* **2018**, *9*, 32534–32550. [CrossRef] [PubMed]
16. Kowalewska, M.; Nowak, R.; Chechlinska, M. Implications of cancer-associated systemic inflammation for biomarkers study. *Biochim. Biophys. Acta* **2010**, *1806*, 163–171. [CrossRef] [PubMed]
17. Chechlinska, M.; Kowalewska, M.; Nowak, R. Systemic inflammation as a confounding factor in cancer biomarker discovery and validation. *Nat. Rev. Cancer* **2010**, *10*, 2–3. [CrossRef] [PubMed]

18. Bergamini, S.; Bellei, E.; Reggiani Bonetti, L.; Monari, E.; Cuoghi, A.; Borelli, F.; Sighinolfi, M.C.; Bianchi, G.; Ozben, T.; Tomasi, A. Inflammation: An important parameter in the search of prostate cancer biomarkers. *Proteome Sci.* **2014**, *12*, 32. [CrossRef]
19. Epstein, J.I.; Magi-Galluzzi, C.; Zhou, M.; Cubilla, A.L. *Tumors of the Prostate Gland, Seminal Vesicles, Penis, and Scrotum*; AFIP-ATLAS of Tumor and Non-Tumor Pathology; Series 5; American Registry of Pathology: Washington, DC, USA, 2020. [CrossRef]
20. Epstein, J.I.; Amin, M.B.; Reuter, V.E.; Humphrey, P.A. Contemporary Gleason grading of prostatic carcinoma: An update with discussion on practical issues to implement the 2014 International Society of Urological Pathology (ISUP) Consensus Conference on Gleason Grading of Prostatic Carcinoma. *Am. J. Surg. Pathol.* **2017**, *41*, e1–e7. [CrossRef]
21. Bradford, M.M. A rapid and sensitive method for the quantitation of microgram quantities of protein utilizing the principle of protein-dye binding. *Anal. Biochem.* **1976**, *72*, 248–254. [CrossRef]
22. Bellei, E.; Bergamini, S.; Monari, E.; Fantoni, L.I.; Cuoghi, A.; Ozben, T.; Tomasi, A. High-abundance proteins depletion for serum proteomic analysis: Concomitant removal of non-targeted proteins. *Amino Acids* **2011**, *40*, 145–156. [CrossRef] [PubMed]
23. Eklund, M.; Jäderling, F.; Discacciati, A.; Bergman, M.; Annerstedt, M.; Aly, M.; Glaessgen, A.; Carlsson, S.; Grönberg, H.; Nordström, T. MRI-targeted or standard biopsy in prostate cancer screening. *N. Engl. J. Med.* **2021**, *385*, 908–920. [CrossRef]
24. Descotes, J.-L. Diagnosis of prostate cancer. *Asian J. Urol.* **2019**, *6*, 129–136. [CrossRef]
25. Prensner, J.R.; Rubin, M.A.; Wei, J.T.; Chinnaiyan, A.M. Beyond PSA: The next generation of prostate cancer biomarkers. *Sci. Transl. Med.* **2012**, *4*, 127rv3. [CrossRef]
26. Matuszczak, M.; Schalken, J.A.; Salagierski, M. Prostate cancer liquid biopsy biomarkers' clinical utility in diagnosis and prognosis. *Cancers* **2021**, *13*, 3373. [CrossRef] [PubMed]
27. Pin, E.; Fredolini, C.; Petricoin III, E.F. The role of proteomics in prostate cancer research: Biomarker discovery and validation. *Clin. Biochem.* **2013**, *46*, 524–538. [CrossRef] [PubMed]
28. Haj-Ahmad, T.A.; Abdalla, M.A.K.; Haj-Ahmad, Y. Potential urinary protein biomarker candidates for the accurate detection of prostate cancer among benign prostatic hyperplasia patients. *J. Cancer* **2014**, *5*, 103–114. [CrossRef] [PubMed]
29. Sousa, A.P.; Costa, R.; Alves, M.G.; Soares, R.; Baylina, P.; Fernandes, R. The impact of metabolic syndrome and type 2 diabetes mellitus on prostate cancer. *Front. Cell. Dev. Biol.* **2022**, *10*, 843458. [CrossRef]
30. De Nunzio, C.; Kramer, G.; Marberger, M.; Montironi, R.; Nelson, W.; Schröder, F.; Sciarra, A.; Tubaro, A. The controversial relationship between benign prostatic hyperplasia and prostate cancer: The role of inflammation. *Eur. Urol.* **2011**, *60*, 106–117. [CrossRef]
31. Kruslin, B.; Tomas, D.; Dzombeta, T.; Milkovic-Perisa, M.; Ulamec, M. Inflammation in prostatic hyperplasia and carcinoma—Basic scientific approach. *Front. Oncol.* **2017**, *7*, 77. [CrossRef]
32. Davalieva, K.; Kiprijanovska, S.; Komina, S.; Petrusevska, G.; Chokrevska Zografska, N.; Polenakovic, M. Proteomics analysis of urine reveals acute phase response proteins as candidate diagnostic biomarkers for prostate cancer. *Proteome Sci.* **2015**, *13*, 2. [CrossRef]
33. Di Domenico, M.; Pozzi, D.; Palchetti, S.; Digiacomo, L.; Iorio, R.; Siciliano, C.; Pinto, F.; Settembre, G.; Pierdiluca, M.; Santini, M.; et al. Alpha-1-microglobulin/bikunin (AMBP) protein corona (PPC) as biomarker for early diagnosis in non-small-cell-lung carcinomas (NSCLC) patients: A case report. *Meta Gene* **2018**, *17*, S19. [CrossRef]
34. Saraswat, M.; Joenväärä, S.; Seppänen, H.; Mustonen, H.; Haglund, C.; Renkonen, R. Comparative proteomic profiling of the serum differentiates pancreatic cancer from chronic pancreatitis. *Cancer Med.* **2017**, *6*, 1738–1751. [CrossRef]
35. Kundu, M.; Mahata, B.; Banerjee, A.; Chakraborty, S.; Debnath, S.; Ray, S.S.; Ghosh, Z.; Biswas, K. Ganglioside GM2 mediates migration of tumor cells by interacting with integrin and modulating the downstream signaling pathway. *Biochim. Biophys. Acta* **2016**, *1863*, 1472–1489. [CrossRef]
36. Shin, M.; Kim, G.; Lee, J.W.; Lee, J.E.; Kim, Y.S.; Yu, J.-H.; Lee, S.-T.; Ahn, S.H.; Kim, H.; Lee, C. Identification of ganglioside GM2 activator playing a role in cancer cell migration through proteomic analysis of breast cancer secretomes. *Cancer Sci.* **2016**, *107*, 828–835. [CrossRef]
37. Sasaki, N.; Toyoda, M.; Ishiwata, T. Gangliosides as signaling regulators in cancer. *Int. J. Mol. Sci.* **2021**, *22*, 5076. [CrossRef]
38. Siltari, A.; Syvälä, H.; Lou, Y.R.; Gao, Y.; Murtola, T.J. Role of lipids and lipid metabolism in prostate cancer progression and the tumor's immune environment. *Cancers* **2022**, *14*, 4293. [CrossRef] [PubMed]
39. Bergamini, S.; Caramaschi, S.; Monari, E.; Martorana, E.; Salviato, T.; Mangogna, A.; Balduit, A.; Tomasi, A.; Canu, P.; Bellei, E. Urinary proteomic profiles of prostate cancer with different risk of progression and correlation with histopathological features. *Ann. Diagn. Pathol.* **2021**, *51*, 151704. [CrossRef]
40. Jin, Y.; Wang, W.; Wang, Q. Alpha-1-antichymotrypsin as a novel biomarker for diagnosis, prognosis, and therapy prediction in human diseases. *Cancer Cell. Int.* **2022**, *22*, 156. [CrossRef]
41. Tian, M.; Cui, Y.Z.; Song, G.-H.; Zong, M.-J.; Zhou, X.-Y.; Chen, Y.; Han, J.-X. Proteomic analysis identifies MMP-9, DJ-1 and A1BG as overexpressed proteins in pancreatic juice from pancreatic ductal adenocarcinoma patients. *BMC Cancer* **2008**, *8*, 241. [CrossRef] [PubMed]
42. Canales, N.A.G.; Marina, V.M.; Castro, J.S. A1BG and C3 are overexpressed in patients with cervical intraepithelial neoplasia III. *Oncol. Lett.* **2014**, *8*, 939–947. [CrossRef]
43. Kreunin, P.; Zhao, J.; Rosser, C.; Urquidi, V.; Lubman, D.M.; Goodison, S. Bladder cancer associated glycoprotein signatures revealed by urinary proteomic profiling. *J. Proteome Res.* **2007**, *6*, 2631–2639. [CrossRef] [PubMed]

44. Cordeiro, Y.G.; Mulder, L.M.; van Zeijl, R.J.M.; Paskoski, L.B.; van Veelen, P.; de Ru, A.; Strefezzi, R.F.; Heijs, B.; Fukumasu, H. Proteomic analysis identifies FNDC1, A1BG, and antigen processing proteins associated with tumor heterogeneity and malignancy in a canine model of breast cancer. *Cancers* **2021**, *13*, 5901. [CrossRef]
45. Janciauskiene, S.; Wrenger, S.; Günzel, S.; Gründing, A.R.; Golpon, H.; Welte, T. Potential roles of acute phase proteins in cancer: Why do cancer cells produce or take up exogenous acute phase protein alpha-1-antitrypsin? *Front. Oncol.* **2021**, *11*, 622076. [CrossRef] [PubMed]
46. Dong, M.; Lih, T.M.; Chen, S.-Y.; Cho, K.-C.; Eguez, R.V.; Höti, N.; Zhou, Y.; Yang, W.; Mangold, L.; Chan, D.W.; et al. Urinary glycoproteins associated with aggressive prostate cancer. *Theranostics* **2020**, *10*, 11892–11907. [CrossRef]
47. Alaiya, A.A.; Al-Mohanna, M.; Aslam, M.; Shinwari, Z.; Al-Mansouri, L.; Al-Rodayan, M.; Al-Eid, M.; Ahmad, I.; Hanash, K.; Tulbah, A.; et al. Proteomics-based signature for human benign prostate hyperplasia and prostate adenocarcinoma. *Int. J. Oncol.* **2011**, *38*, 1047–1057. [CrossRef] [PubMed]
48. Davalieva, K.; Kiprijanovska, S.; Kostovska, I.M.; Stavridis, S.; Stankov, O.; Komina, S.; Petrusevska, G.; Polenakovic, M. Comparative proteomics analysis of urine reveals down-regulation of acute phase response signaling and LXR/RXR activation pathways in prostate cancer. *Proteomes* **2018**, *6*, 1. [CrossRef] [PubMed]
49. Falagario, U.; Selvaggio, O.; Carrieri, G.; Barret, E.; Sanguedolce, F.; Cormio, L. Prostatic inflammation is associated with benign prostatic hyperplasia rather than prostate cancer. *J. Gerontol. Geriatr.* **2018**, *66*, 178–182.

Disclaimer/Publisher's Note: The statements, opinions and data contained in all publications are solely those of the individual author(s) and contributor(s) and not of MDPI and/or the editor(s). MDPI and/or the editor(s) disclaim responsibility for any injury to people or property resulting from any ideas, methods, instructions or products referred to in the content.

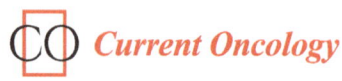 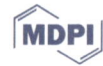

Article

Head-to-Head Comparison of [^{18}F]F-choline and Imaging of Prostate-Specific Membrane Antigen, Using [^{18}F]DCFPyL PET/CT, in Patients with Biochemical Recurrence of Prostate Cancer

Laura García-Zoghby [1], Cristina Lucas-Lucas [2], Mariano Amo-Salas [3], Ángel María Soriano-Castrejón [1] and Ana María García-Vicente [1,*]

[1] Nuclear Medicine Department, University Hospital of Toledo, 45007 Toledo, Spain; lgarciaz@sescam.jccm.es (L.G.-Z.); asoriano@sescam.org (Á.M.S.-C.)
[2] Nuclear Medicine Department, University General Hospital of Ciudad Real, 13005 Ciudad Real, Spain; clucasl@sescam.jccm.es
[3] Department of Mathematics, Castilla-La Mancha University, 13071 Ciudad Real, Spain; mariano.amo@uclm.es
* Correspondence: amgarcia@sescam.jccm.es; Tel./Fax: +34-925-269200

Abstract: Purpose: To analyse diagnostic and therapeutic impact of molecular imaging TNM (miTNM) stage obtained with [^{18}F]DCFPyL versus [^{18}F]F-choline in head-to-head comparison in biochemical recurrence (BCR) of prostate cancer (PCa). Material and methods: Patients with BCR of PCa after radical treatment with previous [^{18}F]F-choline-PET/CT (negative or oligometastatic disease) were recruited to [^{18}F]DCFPyL-PET/CT. Patients were classified according to: grade group, European Association of Urology classification, PSA, PSA doubling time (PSAdt) and PSA velocity (PSAvel). The overall detection rate (DR) and miTNM stage according to PROMISE criteria were assessed for both radiotracers and also correlated (Kappa). The influence of PSA and kinetics on both PET/CT (DR and miTNM) and predictive value of unfavourable kinetics on miTNM were determined. Cut-off PSA, PSAdt and PSAvel values able to predict PET/CT results were determined. Change in miTNM and treatment derived from [^{18}F]DCFPyL information compared with [^{18}F]F-choline were also evaluated. Results: We studied 138 patients. [^{18}F]DCFPyL showed a higher DR than [^{18}F]F-choline (64.5% versus 33.3%) with a fair agreement. [^{18}F]DCFPyL and [^{18}F]F-choline detected T in 33.3% versus 19.6%, N in 27.5% versus 13.8%, and M in 30.4% versus 8.7%. Both tracers' DR showed significant associations with PSA and PSAvel. Significant association was only found between miTNM and PSA on [^{18}F]F-choline-PET/CT ($p = 0.033$). For [^{18}F]F-choline and [^{18}F]DCFPyL-PET/CT, a PSAdt cut-off of 4.09 and 5.59 months, respectively, were able to predict M stage. [^{18}F]DCFPyL changed therapeutic management in 40/138 patients. Conclusions: [^{18}F]DCFPyL provides a higher DR and superior miTNM staging than [^{18}F]F-choline in restaging BCR, especially with high PSA and unfavourable PSA kinetics, showing a fair agreement to [^{18}F]F-choline.

Keywords: [^{18}F]DCFPyL; [^{18}F]F-choline; miTNM; PSA level; PSA kinetics; therapeutic impact

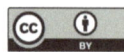

1. Introduction

Up to a half of pT2-3 node-negative prostate cancer (PCa) patients experience biochemical recurrence (BCR) after radical prostatectomy (RP) or radiotherapy [1]. Detection of responsible lesions in the context of a BCR constitutes a major challenge for conventional imaging modalities such as computed tomography (CT) and bone scan.

PET/CT with choline-based tracers has been the traditional imaging modality of choice in restaging patients following BCR [2]. However, multiple studies have shown low sensitivity and specificity, particularly at low prostate-specific antigen (PSA) levels, which can result in delays in salvage therapies [3,4]. For several years, and due to these limitations, the development of radionuclides that recognizes prostate-specific membrane antigen (PSMA) ligands has been proposed as an alternative, with higher sensitivity and specificity in BCR of PCa [5]. These "top diagnostic" radiotracers have increased the detection rate (DR) of oligometastatic disease that has driven recent advancements in metastasis-directed treatment strategies.

[^{18}F]DCFPyL[2-(3-(1-carboxy-5-[(6-[^{18}F]fluoro-pyridine-3-carbonyl)-amino]-pentyl)-ureido)-pentanedioic acid] is a radiofluorinated, small-molecule, high-affinity inhibitor of PSMA [6]. The current restrictions in its use in our environment explain the dual-tracer diagnostic approach in some cases of BCR, especially in those with a PSA level >2ng/mL and a previous negative or ambiguous PET/CT with choline-based tracers. Some studies have addressed utility of 68Ga-tracers PSMA-targeting radiopharmaceuticals and choline-based tracers in head-to-head comparison [7,8], although no previous reported experience exists using the newest developed [^{18}F]DCFPyL. On the other hand, if we only use DR to compare both radiotracers, the real diagnostic potential of PSMA-targeting radiopharmaceuticals compared with choline-based tracers may be limited. In addition, differences in therapeutic impact have been scarcely assessed [9].

The Prostate Cancer Molecular Imaging Standardized Evaluation (PROMISE) criteria summarize standards for study design and reporting of PCa molecular imaging. PROMISE criteria propose a molecular imaging TNM (miTNM) for the interpretation of PSMA-targeting radiopharmaceuticals PET/CT designed to organize findings in comprehensible categories and to promote the exchange of information among physicians and institutions [10].

The aim of our study was multiple: (i) to analyse the concordance between [^{18}F]DCFPyL and [^{18}F]F-choline, in head-to-head comparison, regarding DR and miTNM stage using PROMISE criteria, (ii) to address the predictive value of unfavourable PSA kinetics on miTNM, and (iii) to assess the therapeutic impact of [^{18}F]DCFPyL compared with [^{18}F]F-choline-PET/CT in patients with BCR of PCa.

2. Material and Methods

2.1. Patients

Patients with BCR of PCa after radical treatment (RP, radiotherapy or both) were recruited from different hospitals of our region for re-staging with [^{18}F]F-choline-PET/CT between August 2020 and December 2021. No patient was under androgen deprivation therapy (ADT). Patients with negative or ambiguous [^{18}F]F-choline-PET/CT, or with oligometastatic disease, underwent [^{18}F]DCFPyL-PET/CT and were included in a prospective dataset. We established as oligometastatic disease if there is a presence of ≤ 3 lesions affecting lymph node (pelvis and/or retroperitoneum) or bone.

[^{18}F]DCFPyL-PET/CT was performed within the context of compassionate use under the approval of the Spanish Agency of Medication and Health Care Products and after being approved by a multidisciplinary committee and after receiving patients' informed and signed consent. Database registry analysis of patients was approved by an Ethical Committee (internal code of 2022-53).

The inclusion criteria for the present analysis: (i) time window between both PET/CT within 2 months and (ii) minimum clinical follow-up of 6 months.

Patients were classified in groups taking into account: grade group (1 to 5) [11], European Association of Urology (EAU) classification adapted from D'Amico risk category (low/intermediate/high) [1], PSA value closest to PET/CTs (PSA ≤ 1 ng/mL, 1 < PSA ≤ 2 and PSA > 2), PSA doubling time (PSAdt)≤ or >6 months and PSA velocity (PSAvel)≥ or <0.2 ng/mL/month. The initial radical treatment and subsequent salvage treatment, if previous BCR, were obtained.

2.2. Acquisition Protocol

[^{18}F]F-choline and [^{18}F]DCFPyL PET/CTs were performed in a unique reference hospital and with the same hybrid PET/CT scanner (Discovery 5R/IQ, GE) in 3D acquisition mode for 2 min per bed position. Low dose CT (120 kV, 80 mA) without contrast was performed for attenuation correction and as an anatomical map. There was no fasting requirement and only a correct hydration previous to both radiotracer administrations was orally promoted.

The acquisition protocol of both PET/CTs included a standard study from skull to proximal legs 5–15 min and 100–120 min after [^{18}F]F-choline and [^{18}F]DCFPyL intravenous administration (activity of 2–4 MBq/Kg and 4–5 MBq/Kg, respectively). We also administrated diuretic medication before any tracer injection. A delayed study of the pelvis, in cases with significant urinary bladder retention or doubtful evaluation, was performed 30–60 min after [^{18}F]F-choline and [^{18}F]DCFPyL standard studies.

2.3. Image Analysis and Interpretation

The emission data was corrected for scatter, random coincidence events and system dead time using the provided software. All [^{18}F]F-choline and [^{18}F]DCFPyL scans were evaluated in the Advantage Workstation software version 4.7 (GE Healthcare) allowing review of PET, CT and fused imaging data. Two experienced nuclear medicine physicians evaluated both scans, and a third observer reviewed them in case of discordances. Any focal uptake higher than adjacent background, that did not correspond to physiological uptake, urinary excretion or benign conditions, was considered PET-positive and, thus, probably disease related.

Lesions identified with both tracers were classified in local recurrence (T), lymph nodes (N) and metastases (M), using miTNM stage defined by PROMISE criteria [10].

[^{18}F]F-choline or [^{18}F]DCFPyL avid lesions lacking histopathological verification were rated as malignant if there was a corresponding anatomical finding suspicious for malignancy on MRI or if it was considered clinically malignant in the follow-up by multidisciplinary committee (normalization of the PSA after targeted therapy). Otherwise, these uptakes were considered false positive. In addition, [^{18}F]F-choline avid lesions without any correspondence to [^{18}F]DCFPyL-PET/CT were considered false positive in some cases because of the false positive rate of [^{18}F]F-choline in inflammatory or infectious process demonstrated in the literature [12].

2.4. Therapeutic Management and Follow-Up

All diagnostic procedures and treatments undertaken, including biopsies, surgeries, radiotherapy and duration and type of systemic therapy were documented in the follow-up.

Different curative options for BCR are available depending on initial radical treatment. For patients who underwent RP, prostatic fossa radiotherapy is a possibility for either positive or negative prostatic fossa disease detection on PET/CT. Pelvic nodal recurrence can be treated with stereotactic body radiotherapy (SBRT) or surgery. On the other hand, patients who underwent radical prostate radiotherapy have more limitations for a new radiotherapy procedure, in case of prostatic radiotracer uptake on PET/CT, except for brachytherapy, needing a previous histologic confirmation of active disease. Polimetastatic disease (>3) with extension to the retroperitoneal territory and/or bones is treated with systemic therapy (ADT) with/without a combination of androgen receptor-axis-targeted therapies (ARAT) in cases of more extensive disease.

Changes in therapeutic management because of [^{18}F]DCFPyL, compared with [^{18}F]F-choline-PET/CT information, were assessed. We considered that changes in management happened when [^{18}F]DCFPyL-PET/CT modified treatment decision reached after [^{18}F]F-choline findings. Moreover, the added therapeutic impact of [^{18}F]DCFPyL-PET/CT over [^{18}F]F-choline-PET/CT (escalation vs. de-escalation) was assessed. Escalation was defined as locorregional radiotherapy/surgery or ARAT (Abiraterone, Apalutamide or Enzalutamide) in cases of regional or metastatic disease, respectively, only detected by [^{18}F]DCFPyL. De-escalation with only follow-up was decided in cases of a negative [^{18}F]DCFPyL and positive [^{18}F]F-choline, considering that the latter was false positive [12], or when PET/CT results were different and therapeutic decision after [^{18}F]F-choline was not performed, for example, more disease on [^{18}F]DCFPyL-PET/CT that allowed the standard treatment (ADT) instead of local treatment. No therapeutic impact was considered if (i) the results of both scans were concordant or whether different, no differences in treatment were reported compared with the information derived from [^{18}F]F-choline, and (ii) patients' clinical conditions did not allow the treatment change planned as a result of [^{18}F]DCFPyL-PET/CT.

In follow-up, all diagnostic procedures and treatments undertaken were documented. Serial PSA was obtained every 3 months after planned treatment. Initial treatment response was defined as a drop in PSA levels of greater than 50% from pre-treatment levels at least 6 months after treatment administration. For local curative treatments (surgery or radiotherapy) a minimum time window of 2 months with respect to [^{18}F]DCFPyL was considered reliable for assessing efficacy. Men with ADT as part of their treatment were not included in this analysis.

2.5. Statistical Analysis

Statistical analysis was performed using SPSS software (v. 28). Quantitative variables were represented by mean and standard deviation and qualitative variables by frequency and percentage. Relation between qualitative variables was studied using Chi-squared Pearson test. Kolmogorov–Smirnov test was used to study normality of the quantitative variables with result of non-normal variables, and the nonparametric tests Kruskal–Wallis and Mann–Whitney were used to compare the means of the quantitative variables. Overall, DR for [^{18}F]F-choline and [^{18}F]DCFPyL PET/CTs and concordance (Kappa, k) were assessed, classifying the results as poor (<0.20), weak (0.21–0.40), moderate (0.41–0.60), good (0.61–0.80) and very good (0.81–1.00). We also analysed DR of T, N and M recurrence for both tracers, and concordance.

We statistically analysed the correlation between patients' characteristics classified in groups (grade Gleason group, EAU classification, recurrence PSA and kinetics) and PET/CTs results, both DR and miTNM. In all cases, a p value < 0.05 was considered statistically significant. Based on the obtained results, a second assessment was focused on the search of strongest cut-off values of PSA, achieved by receiver operating characteristic (ROC) curve, for the prediction of metastatic disease in comparison with exclusively T and/or N disease.

2.6. Search Strategy and Study Selection for the Review

Two authors (LGZ and AMGV) performed a computer literature search on PubMed/MEDLINE databases to find relevant retrospective or prospective published articles on head-to-head comparison between choline-based tracers and PSMA-targeting radiopharmaceuticals in BCR PCa. The exclusion criteria were (i) articles not in English language, (ii) review articles, editorials or letters, comments, conference proceedings, case reports or small case series (<20) and (iii) no head-to-head comparison among these two imaging methods.

The researchers independently reviewed the titles and abstracts of the retrieved articles, applying the inclusion and exclusion criteria. After the selection, the full-text version of the remaining articles, to assess their eligibility for inclusion, were obtained resolving disagreements in a consensus meeting.

3. Results

One hundred and thirty-eight patients were enrolled. All the patients' characteristics are presented in Table 1.

Table 1. Baseline characteristics of 138 study subjects.

Characteristic	Value
Age (years)	
Mean ± SD	69.77 ± 7.54
Range	55–87
Grade group	
1	46 (33.3%)
2	39 (28.3%)
3	30 (21.7%)
4	12 (8.7%)
5	11 (8%)
EAU classification (D'Amico risk)	
Low	24 (17.4%)
Intermediate	38 (27.5%)
High	76 (55.1%)
Primary treatment	
Surgery	48 (34.8%)
Radiotherapy	60 (43.5%)
Both	30 (21.7%)
PSA closest to PET/CTs (ng/mL)	
Mean ± SD	2.80 ± 4.83
PSA ≤ 1	46 (33.4%)
1 < PSA ≤ 2	17 (12.3%)
PSA > 2	75 (54.3%)
PSAdt (month)	
Mean ± SD	7.34 ± 11.74
≤6	73 (52.9%)
>6	65 (47.1%)
PSAvel (ng/mL/month)	
Mean ± SD	0.26 ± 0.68
≥0.2	45 (32.6%)
<0.2	93 (67.4%)
Biochemical relapse	
First	100 (72.5%)
Second or further	38 (27.5%)

PSA: prostate-specific antigen; SD: standard deviation; PSAdt: PSA doubling time, PSAvel: PSA velocity; EAU: European Association of Urology.

3.1. Detection Rate and TNM Staging by [^{18}F]DCFPyL and [^{18}F]F-choline PET/CT

[^{18}F]DCFPyL showed a higher DR than [^{18}F]F-choline, 64.5% (89/138) and 33.3% (46/138), respectively. Both scans were negative in 44 patients (31.9%) and positive in 41 (29.7%). However, in 20/41 patients, [^{18}F]DCFPyL visualized additional lesions compared with [^{18}F]F-choline, which entailed miTNM stage change in 17 patients (Figure 1).

On the other hand, [^{18}F]DCFPyL was positive alone in 48/89 (53.9%) patients, being oligometastatic in 25 (Figure 2). Five patients were exclusively positive with [^{18}F]F-choline-PET/CT, and thus, [^{18}F]DCFPyL down-staged [^{18}F]F-choline results from positive to negative (3 follow-up, 1 biopsy (negative) and 1 ADT). [^{18}F]DCFPyL up-staged 5/21 patients with oligometastatic disease on [^{18}F]F-choline-PET/CT to polimetastatic disease after [^{18}F]DCFPyL.

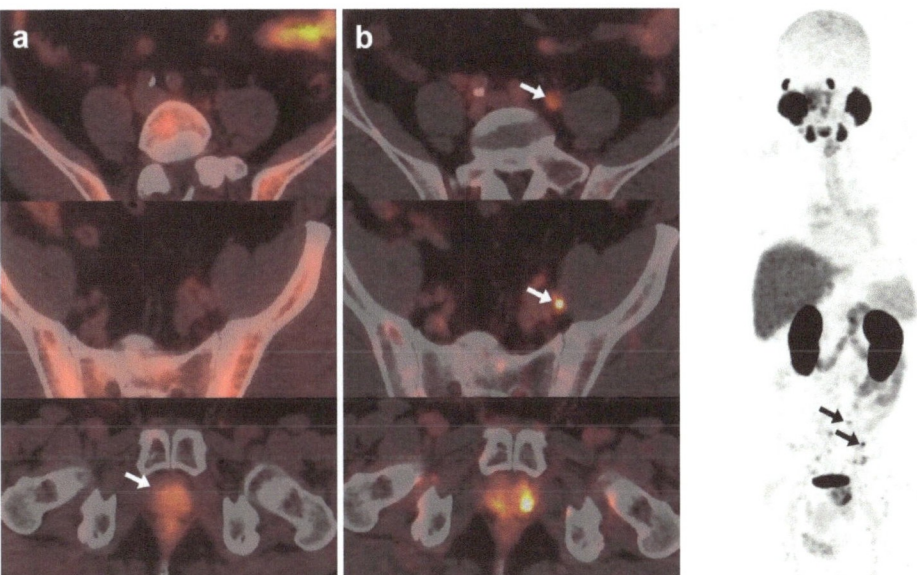

Figure 1. 59-year-old patient. Gleason 7 PCa treated with radiotherapy plus ADT. After ADT withdrawal BCR was detected (PSA 2.44 ng/mL, PSAdt 2.6 months, PSAvel 0.15 ng/mL/month). [^{18}F]F-choline (**a**) demonstrated only prostatic uptake (white arrow) and [^{18}F]DCFPyL-PET/CT (**b**) showed prostatic tracer uptake and lymph nodes metastases (white and black arrows). Time window of sixteen days between both scans. [^{18}F]DCFPyL changed therapeutic management allowing escalation (ADT + Apalutamide).

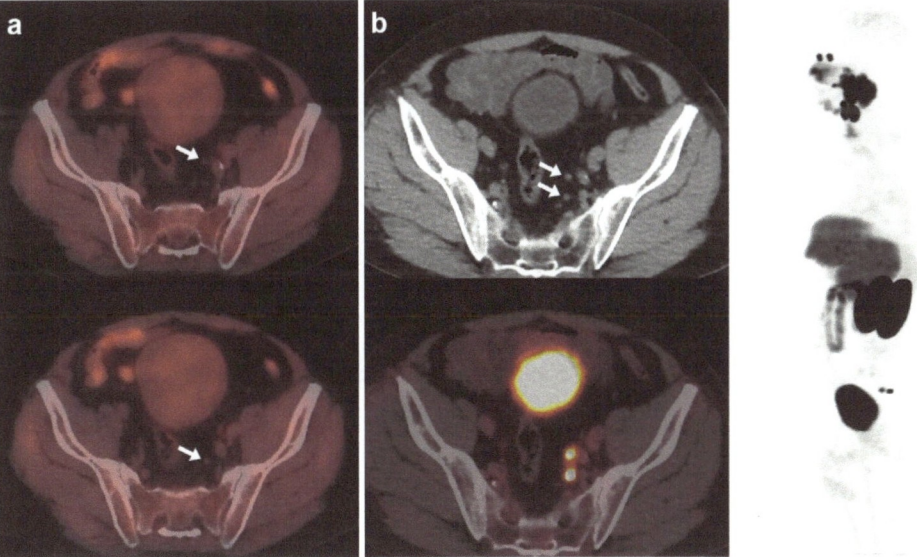

Figure 2. 67-year-old patient. Gleason 7 PCa treated with RP. First BCR treated with prostate fossa radiotherapy. Second BCR (PSA 0.63 ng/mL, PSAdt 8.6 months, PSAvel 0.04 ng/mL/month) scanned with [^{18}F]F-choline (**a**) and [^{18}F]DCFPyL PET/CT (**b**), time window of six days. Lymph nodes metastases (white arrows) were demonstrated only on [^{18}F]DCFPyL scan, changing therapeutic management (escalation). Patient underwent lymph nodes SBRT. PSA level decreased.

[^{18}F]DCFPyL and [^{18}F]F-choline PET/CTs T DR was 33.3% and 19.6%, respectively, with a moderate concordance. N DR was 27.5% and 13.8%, respectively. However, the most significant difference was found for M DR, 30.4% and 8.7%, for [^{18}F]DCFPyL and [^{18}F]F-choline, respectively (Table 2).

Table 2. Per patient miTNM obtained from [^{18}F]DCFPyL and [^{18}F]F-choline PET/CT, with concordance (kappa).

			[^{18}F]DCFPyL			
			(+)	(−)	Total	
T		(+)	20	7	27	
		(−)	26	85	111	
		Total	46	92	138	k = 0.403 (p < 0.001)
N1		(+)	4	8	12	
		(−)	15	111	126	
		Total	19	119	138	k = 0.143 (p = 0.086)
N2		(+)	4	2	6	
		(−)	14	118	132	
	[^{18}F]F-choline	Total	18	120	138	k = 0.287 (p < 0.001)
M1a		(+)	2	1	3	
		(−)	14	121	135	
		Total	16	122	138	k = 0.181 (p = 0.003)
M1b		(+)	5	2	7	
		(−)	16	115	131	
		Total	21	117	138	k = 0.304 (p < 0.001)
M1c		(+)	2	0	2	
		(−)	3	133	136	
		Total	5	133	138	k = 0.562 (p < 0.001)

T: local recurrence; N1: single lymph node region; N2: multiple lymph node regions (≥2); M1a: extrapelvic lymph nodes; M1b: bone involvement; M1c: other sites; k: kappa.

Regarding first to subsequent BCR, [^{18}F]F-choline DR was 35.6% and 27%, respectively, and [^{18}F]DCFPyL DR was 61.4% and 72.9%. No statistical differences were found in first to subsequent BCR DR in neither [^{18}F]F-choline or [^{18}F]DCFPyL ($p = 0.435$ and $p = 0.164$, respectively). We found weak (k = 0.378, $p < 0.001$) and poor (k = 0.079, $p < 0.467$) concordance in first to subsequent BCR DR between [^{18}F]F-choline and [^{18}F]DCFPyL.

3.2. Correlation between PET/CT Results and PSA Kinetics

Both [^{18}F]DCFPyL and [^{18}F]F-choline PET/CT DR showed significant associations with PSA groups and PSAvel. No significant association was found with PSAdt. [^{18}F]DCFPyL DR was 81.3% in patients with PSA > 2 ng/mL, higher than patients with $1 < \text{PSA} \leq 2$ (58.8%) and PSA ≤ 1 ng/mL (39.1%). It was also higher in patients with PSAvel > 0.2 ng/mL/month (90.5%) compared with those with PSAvel $\leq$ 0.2 ng/mL/month (53.7%). [^{18}F]F-choline DR was also higher in cases with PSA > 2 ng/mL (46.6%), being 35.3% and 13.04% in patients with $1 < \text{PSA} \leq 2$ and PSA ≤ 1 ng/mL, respectively, and 52.4% in cases with PSAvel > 0.2 ng/mL/month versus 26.3% with PSAvel $\leq$ 0.2 ng/mL/month. In addition, mean PSA was statistically different among patients with T and N recurrence on [^{18}F]F-choline-PET/CT ($p = 0.028$). Also, differences in mean PSA and PSAdt were found between N and M ($p = 0.034$) and T and M ($p = 0.031$) metabolic disease, respectively, on [^{18}F]DCFPyL-PET/CT (Table 3).

Using predefined cut-off values of PSA and PSA kinetics values, significant association was only found between miTNM and PSA groups on [^{18}F]F-choline-PET/CT ($p = 0.033$) and not for PSAdt or PSAvel. No statistical association was found between miTNM, PSA or PSA kinetics on [^{18}F]DCFPyL-PET/CT. In ROC analysis, only a PSAdt cut-off of 4.09 months showed significant association for the prediction of M stage with [^{18}F]F-choline-PET/CT (66.7% sensitivity, 73.8% specificity, 0.720 AUC, $p = 0.012$). For [^{18}F]DCFPyL-PET/CT, the obtained cut-offs in the prediction of M stage: PSA of 2.41 ng/mL (66.7% sensitivity, 64.4%

specificity, 0.675 AUC, $p = 0.002$), PSAdt of 5.59 months (61.1% sensitivity, 60.8% specificity, 0.679 AUC, $p = 0.001$) and PSAvel of 0.13 ng/mL/month (66.7% sensitivity, 61.4% specificity, 0.723 AUC, $p < 0.001$).

Table 3. PSA, PSAdt and PSAvel (mean ± SD) in miTNM comparison of [^{18}F]DCFPyL and [^{18}F]F-choline.

		[^{18}F]F-choline	[^{18}F]DCFPyL
PSA (ng/mL)	T	3.95 ± 1.92	3.17 ± 2.16
	N	2.68 ± 2.10	2.25 ± 2.14
	M	2.73 ± 1.86	4.63 ± 8.67
PSAdt (months)	T	5.07 ± 12.13	7.56 ± 10.83
	N	6.13 ± 4.23	5.87 ± 3.51
	M	9.32 ± 18.42	7.34 ± 11.20
PSAvel (ng/mL/month)	T	0.45 ± 0.79	0.23 ± 0.36
	N	0.28 ± 0.23	0.18 ± 0.15
	M	0.34 ± 0.44	0.56 ± 1.19

3.3. Therapeutic Impact and Follow-Up

As a result of [^{18}F]DCFPyL-PET/CT, therapeutic management was changed in 40/138 (29%) patients compared with [^{18}F]F-choline-PET/CT based planning treatment. Escalation was elected in 34 patients: 6 radiotherapy, 5 radiotherapy plus ADT, 6 surgery, 1 prostate cryoablation and 16 ARAT. De-escalation occurred in 6 patients: follow-up in 4 cases (3 [^{18}F]DCFPyL negative and 1 with prostatic uptake with both radiotracers and no malignant disease confirmed by biopsy) and ADT instead of local treatment in 2 cases. A potential therapeutic change, derived from [^{18}F]DCFPyL-PET/CT information, was not achieved because of patient comorbidities in 11 patients.

Derived from positive [^{18}F]DCFPyL-PET/CT, 19 patients underwent additional diagnostic procedures to confirm the results: 8 by imaging (3/8 was confirmed) and 11 by histological analysis (8/11 was confirmed) (Figures 3 and 4).

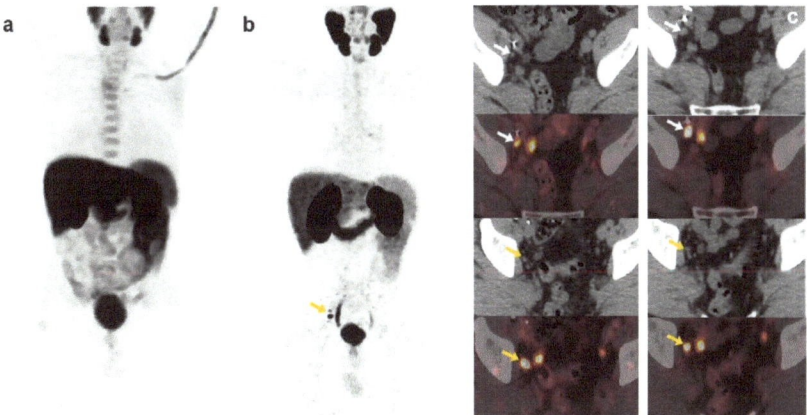

Figure 3. 55-year-old patient. Gleason 8 PCa treated with RP. First BCR treated with prostate fossa radiotherapy. Second BCR (PSA: 0.84 ng/mL, PSAdt 5.99 months, PSAvel 0.07 ng/mL/month). [^{18}F]F-choline-PET/CT negative (**a**). [^{18}F]DCFPyL-PET/CT (**b**), time window of twenty days, revealed two right external iliac lymph nodes metastases (white and yellow arrows). Lymphadenectomy was decided (escalation), without histopathological confirmation of malignancy. In follow-up, PSA progressed (2.07 ng/mL) and an additional [^{18}F]DCFPyL-PET/CT (**c**) showed exactly same lymph nodes (white and yellow arrows). SBRT was administered decreasing the PSA level, reclassifying [^{18}F]DCFPyL-PET/CT results as true positive.

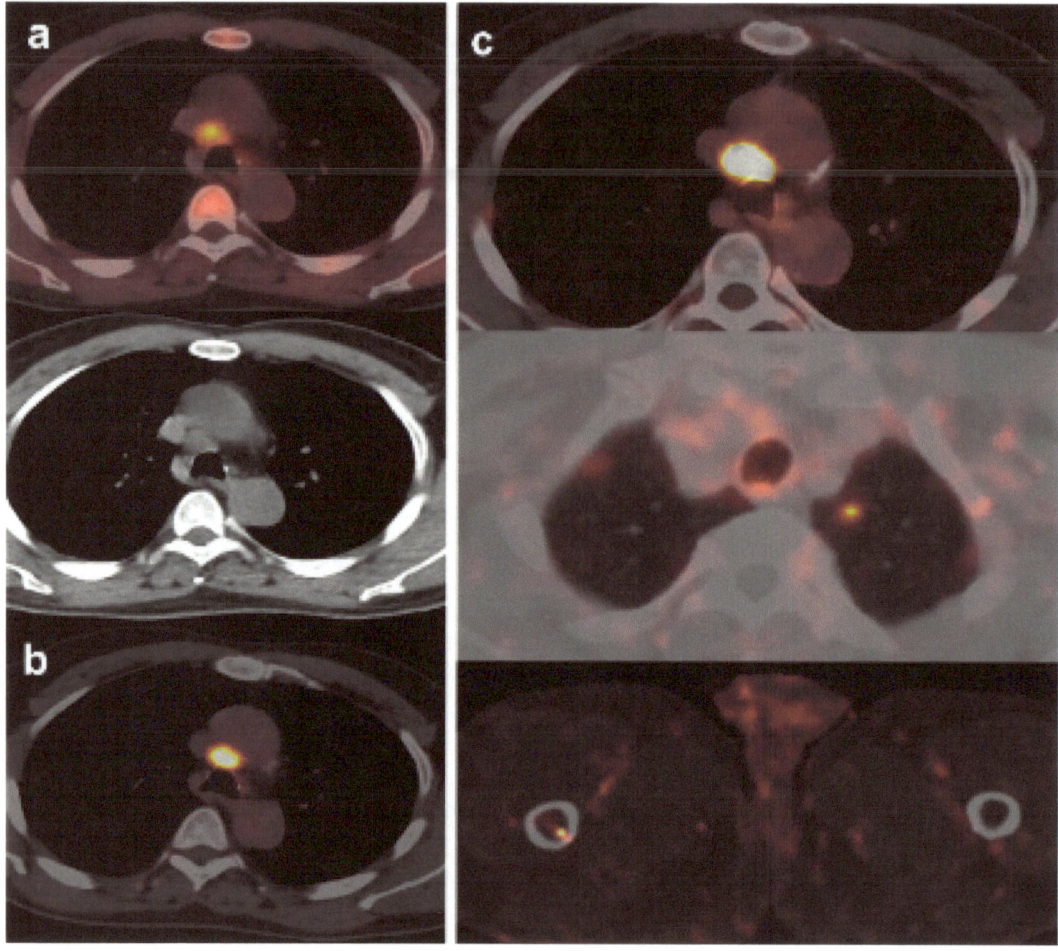

Figure 4. 70-year-old patient. Gleason 9 PCa, treated initially with RP and radiotherapy after his first BCR. Second BCR (PSA 0.7 ng/mL, PSAdt 5.6 months, PSAvel 0.05 ng/mL/month) with [^{18}F]F-choline (**a**) and [^{18}F]DCFPyL scans showing mediastinal lymph node tracer uptake (**b**) reported as inflammatory process. Follow-up was decided and PSA level continued increasing. A new [^{18}F]DCFPyL scan (**c**) was performed 3 months later, showing an increase in size and metabolism of mediastinal lymph node with additional microfoci of radiotracer uptake in lung and bone, suspicious of metastases. An endobronchial ultrasound-guided lymph node biopsy confirmed prostatic origin of metastasis. ADT + Apalutamide was initiated (escalation).

[^{18}F]DCFPyL-PET/CT was negative in 49/138 patients (7 low, 14 intermediate and 28 high risk). Follow-up without active treatment was adopted in 29 patients (4 positive [^{18}F]F-choline-PET/CT) and 20 intermediate/high risk patients underwent treatment (12 prostatic fossa radiotherapy, 8 ADT, 1/8 [^{18}F]F-choline-PET/CT positive). Regarding the false positive, six patients with positive [^{18}F]DCFPyL-PET/CT (2 prostate gland, 3 bone and 1 rectum) had a normal MRI (Figures 5 and 6). Ten patients were [^{18}F]F-choline-PET/CT positive and considered false positive (2 prostate gland, 5 lymph nodes, 2 bone, 1 pelvic mass) due to [^{18}F]DCFPyL-PET/CT result, biopsy or clinical follow-up.

For patients who benefited from a treatment change, local treatments were exclusively guided by [^{18}F]DCFPyL in eleven patients. Follow-up showed: PSA decreasing in 6 (4 radiotherapy, 1 cryoablation, 1 surgery), PSA increasing in 2 surgically treated patients (in one patient, an ulterior [^{18}F]DCFPyL-PET/CT revealed an incomplete surgical procedure, and in the other one, surgical procedure was performed almost 7 months after [^{18}F]DCFPyL-PET/CT), in 2 patients biochemical progression occurred before treatment decision and the remaining patient was missed.

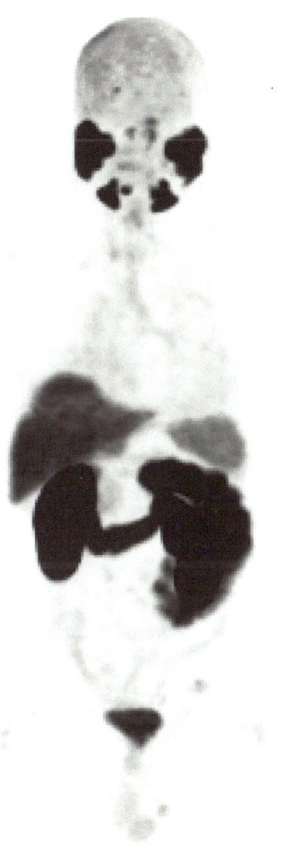
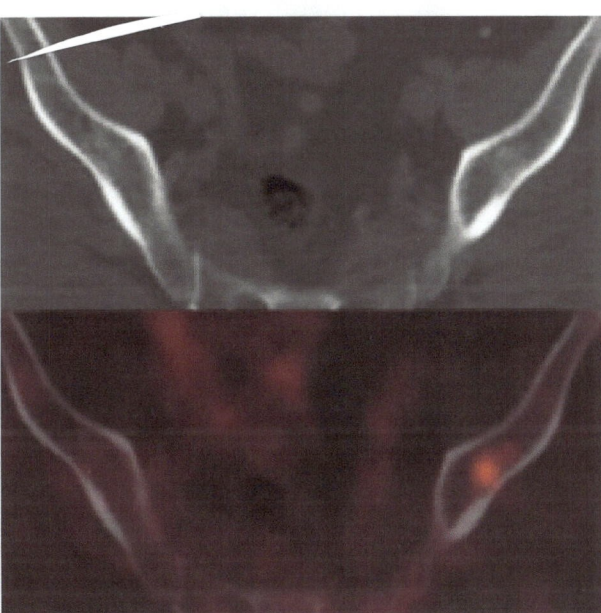

Figure 5. BCR in a 71-year-old patient (PSA: 0.26 ng/mL, PSAdt: 1.09 months, PSAvel: 0.2 ng/mL/month) after RP of PCa (Gleason 6, pT2c). [^{18}F]DCFPyL scan showed a slight uptake on left iliac bone with minimal sclerotic changes. Previous negative [^{18}F]F-choline scan (time window of one week). MRI did not confirm malignancy of PSMA uptake (false positive). Prostatic bed radiotherapy was given and PSA level decreased.

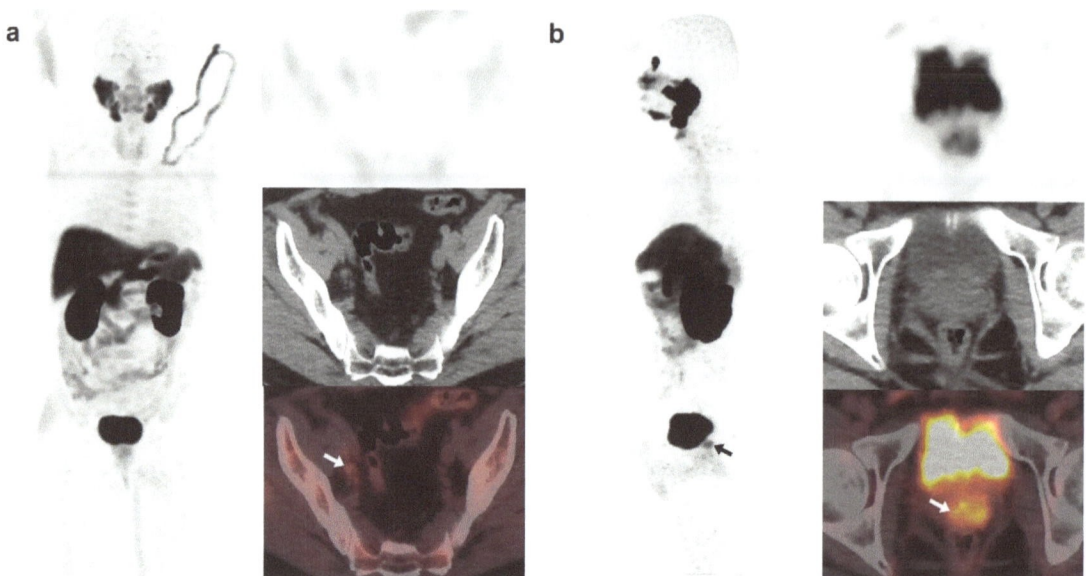

Figure 6. 56-year-old patient. PCa (Gleason 6) treated with braquitherapy. BCR (PSA: 5.4 ng/mL, PSAdt 6.17 months, PSAvel 0.55 ng/mL/month). [^{18}F]F-choline (**a**) showed prostate gland uptake and right external iliac lymph nodes metastasis (white arrow). One month later, the patient was also scanned with [^{18}F]DCFPyL (**b**) revealing only prostate gland pathological tracer uptake (white and black arrow). Prostate biopsy was negative (false positive). Follow-up was decided and PSA level keeps oscillating (4–5 ng/mL) with an additional negative [^{18}F]DCFPyL-PET/CT one year later.

3.4. Literature Review

Literature search results from PubMed/MEDLINE revealed 17 articles. Reviewing titles and abstracts, seven articles were excluded: four because they were not from the field of interest of this review and three as they were reviews. Ten articles were selected and retrieved in full-text version [7–9,13–19]. Data of 1868 patients with BCR PCa who underwent choline-based tracers and PSMA ligands PET/CT were eligible for the analysis (systematic review). Methodology and results of the selected papers are summarized on Table 4.

Table 4. Summary of studies comparing choline-labelled tracers and PSMA-targeting radiopharmaceuticals PET/CT in BR of PCa.

Author, Year, Study Type	n	Requirements for Requesting PET/CT with PSMA-Targeting Tracers. PSA Values (Median/Mean ± SD)	PET Radiotracers/Time Interval between Studies (Median/Mean ± SD/Range)	Diagnostic and Therapeutic Impact
Chevalme, 2021, R [7]	1084	Previous [18F]F-choline-PET/CT negative (924) or equivocal (160). Median PSA 1.7 ng/mL	[68Ga]Ga-PSMA-11 vs. [18F]F-choline/Median 42 days (4–100)	[68Ga]Ga-PSMA-11 was positive in 62% and in 82% of previous [18F]F-choline negative or equivocal, respectively. Overall DR of 68%. No therapeutic impact assessment.
Barbaud, 2019, R [8]	42	Previous [18F]F-choline-PET/CT negative (26) or doubtful. Mean PSA, PSAdt and PSAvel of 4.1 ± 5.1 ng/mL, 8.5 ± 7.4 months and 4 ± 4.8 ng/mL/y, respectively	[68Ga]Ga-PSMA-11 vs. [18F]F-choline/Median 41 days (14–243)	DR for [68Ga]Ga-PSMA-I: 80.9% (PB: 19 p, LN: 18p, M1b: 8p, M1c: 3p). Change in therapeutic management in 73.8%.
Witkowska-Patena, 2019, P [9]	40	None (90% negative or equivocal [18F]F-choline)/Mean PSA 0.77 ± 0.61 ng/mL	[18F]PSMA-1007 vs. [18F]F-choline/Mean 54 ± 21 days. Median 58 (12–105) d	DR for [18F]PSMA-1007 and [18F]F-choline of 60% and 5%, respectively. [18F]PSMA-1007 detected more lesions. In 70% of scans, [18F]PSMA-1007 upgrades [18F]F-choline result, from negative to positive. No therapeutic impact assessment.
Alonso, 2018, P [13]	36 (a)	None/Median PSA 3.3 ng/mL	[68Ga]Ga-PSMA-11 vs. [11C]-choline/1–2 weeks	DR for [68Ga]Ga-PSMA-11 and [11C]-choline of 75% and 53%, respectively. [68Ga]Ga-PSMA-11 detected more lesions.
Cantiello, 2018, R [14]	43	None/Median PSA, PSAdt and PSAvel of 0.8 ng/mL, 4 months and 2.6 ng/mL/y, respectively	[64Cu]PSMA-617 vs. [18F]F-choline/Median 2.2 weeks (1–3)	DR for [64Cu]PSMA-617 and [18F]F-choline of 74.4% and 44.2%, respectively. PB 30.2%, N1a ± PB: 9/43, M1b ± PB: 7/43. No therapeutic impact assessment.
Caroli, 2018, P [15]	314	Previous [18F]F-choline-PET/CT negative or dubious. Median PSA 0.83 ng/mL	[68Ga]Ga-PSMA-11 vs. [18F]F-choline/< 30 days	DR of 62.7% for [68Ga]Ga-PSMA-11 (67% in 88 patients with negative [18F]F-choline PET/CT). No therapeutic impact assessment.
Schwenck, 2017, R [16]	123 (b)	None. Median PSA and PSAdt of 2.7 ng/mL and 4 months, respectively	[68Ga]Ga-PSMA-11 vs. [11C]-choline/< 24 h	DR for [68Ga]Ga-PSMA-11 and [11C]-choline of 83% and 79%, respectively, in biochemical relapse (103 p). No therapeutic impact assessment.
Bluemel, 2016, R [17]	125 (c)	A previous [18F]F-choline-PET/CT negative in 41 patients. Mean PSA, PSAdt and PSAvel of 5.4 ± 12.73 ng/mL, 9.9 ± 10.6 months and 7 ± 25 ng/mL/y, respectively	[68Ga]Ga-PSMA-I&T vs. [18F]F-choline/Mean 19 ± 16 days	[68Ga]Ga-PSMA-I&T detected disease in 43.8% of patients with a previous negative [18F]F-choline. No therapeutic impact assessment.

Table 4. Cont.

Author, Year, Study Type	n	Requirements for Requesting PET/CT with PSMA-Targeting Tracers. PSA Values (Median/Mean ± SD)	PET Radiotracers/Time Interval between Studies (Median/Mean ± SD/Range)	Diagnostic and Therapeutic Impact
Morigi, 2015, P [18]	38	None/Mean PSA and PSAdt of 1.72 ± 2.54 ng/mL and 15.6 ± 22.1 months, respectively	[^{68}Ga]Ga-PSMA-11 vs. [^{18}F]F-choline/<30 days	DR for [^{68}Ga]Ga-PSMA-11 and [^{18}F]F-choline of 66% and 32%, respectively. [^{68}Ga]Ga-PSMA-11 detected more lesions. Change in therapeutic management in 63%.
Afshar-Oromieh, 2014, R [19]	37	None. Mean PSA 11.1 ± 24.1 ng/mL	[^{68}Ga]Ga-PSMA-11 vs. [^{18}F]F-choline/Mean 12.1 ± 8.4 days	DR for [^{68}Ga]Ga-PSMA-11 and [^{18}F]F-choline of 86.5% and 70.3%, respectively. PSMA detected more lesions. No therapeutic impact assessment.

n: number of patients, P: prospective, R: retrospective, PB: prostate bed, LN: lymph nodes, M1c: visceral metastases, p: patients, DR: detection rate, (^{a}) some nc specified patients with androgen deprivation therapy, (^{b}) primary and recurrent prostate cancer, (^{c}) only use PET/CT with PSMA-targeting tracers in patients with a previous negative [^{18}F]F-choline-PET/CT, PSAdt: PSA doubling time, PSAvel: PSA velocity, SD: standard deviation.

4. Discussion

In BCR, diagnostic impact of PSMA-targeting radiopharmaceuticals against choline-based tracers is significantly higher in patients with low PSA levels and previous negative/doubtful PET/CT with choline-based tracers in whom the detection of oligometastatic disease might enable metastasis-directed treatments [20,21]. In our study, patients with previous negative/oligometastatic [^{18}F]F-choline-PET/CT were referred to [^{18}F]DCFPyL expecting a benefit by the detection of more metastases. In fact, we found that 5/21 patients with oligometastatic disease in [^{18}F]F-choline-PET/CT were up-staged to polimetastatic after [^{18}F]DCFPyL, similar to previous reported results [16]. The absence of consensus about oligometastatic definition can limit diagnostic impact comparison of different radiotracers. In previous studies, oligometastatic disease was defined as M stage with ≤ 5 lesions [16,17], whereas other authors considered ≤ 3 as we did in this study [7]. Chevalme et al. found, using [^{68}Ga]Ga-PSMA-11, oligometastatic disease (1–3 foci) in 31% of the cases with previous negative/doubtful [^{18}F]F-choline [7]. In our sample, [^{18}F]DCFPyL-PET/CT detected oligometastatic disease in the 52.1% (25/48) of choline-negative cases. In a relevant number of cases, we detected positive lymph nodes and bone lesions that showed divergent findings with both tracers. The majority were only [^{18}F]DCFPyL-positive, probably due to higher lesion/background ratio and sensitivity compared with [^{18}F]F-choline that enables detection of smaller lesions.

Regarding the DR, our results are in accordance with previous works, with a [^{18}F]DCFPyL DR of 53.9% in patients with negative/equivocal [^{18}F]F-choline [7,8,15,17]. In addition, we did not observe differences in DR of first BCR with respect to the following, which is contrary to the study of Chevalme et al. [7] that reported a DR lower in first BCR versus previous (63 vs. 72%).

With respect to the influence of PSA kinetics, despite a PSAdt ≤ 6 months has been reported as a strong predictor of positivity of PET/CT with choline-based tracers [21], we did not find a significant association with DR or miTNM for any of the studied radiotracers with their counterparts. This absence of significant association with pre-defined unfavourable PSA kinetics promotes the interest in exploring other clinical, metabolic and laboratory parameters. In fact, we found that different cut-off values of PSA kinetics were able to predict M stage, especially for [^{18}F]DCFPyL-PET/CT, although with a moderate accuracy.

Regarding disease location on BCR PCa, [^{18}F]DCFPyL-PET/CT detected T in 33.3% of cases, similar to 26% reported by Chevalme et al. [7], but higher than 11% of Barbaud et al. [8], probably explained by higher rate of patients included with RP (76%). We observed higher T detection than [^{18}F]F-choline, although with a moderate concordance (k = 0.403, $p < 0.001$). Discrimination between benign and malignant intraprostatic tissue is hampered by low specificity of choline-based tracers based on high affinity of this radiotracer by benign hyperplasia [22,23]. Lymph node is the most prevalent disease location in BCR PCa, showing PSMA-targeting radiopharmaceuticals with a DR from 34% to 39% in patients with a previous choline-negative [7,8,16]. Our N disease detection using [^{18}F]DCFPyL was lower (27.5%), with a weak concordance with [^{18}F]F-choline. Previous authors found that 55% of the detected lymph nodes were identified with both tracers. Thus, using PSMA-ligands, increase in DR affecting both the number and locations of lymph nodes is a fact [16]. However, the most significant difference in our sample was M detection, 30.4% and 8.7% for [^{18}F]DCFPyL and [^{18}F]F-choline, respectively, in accordance with previous studies [7,16].

With respect to the discordances between both radiotracers, usually PSMA-targeting radiopharmaceuticals spot all choline-positive lesions, and discordances are mainly related to choline-negative/PSMA-positive findings [14,16]. The explanations of these discordances are contradictory and based on: (i) different metastasis environment with a loss of expression of PSMA that can occur in less than 10% of primary or metastatic prostate tumours [24]; (ii) tumour progression between scans in cases of a wide time interval [9]; and (iii) unspecific inflammation that promotes choline uptake in lymph nodes and can explain additionally choline-positive lymph nodes [25]. The higher PSMA-targeting radiopharmaceutical specificity with respect to choline-based tracers, explained by the overexpression of PSMA glycoprotein, seems more characteristic for PCa than up-regulation of choline kinase [26,27] and could support our consideration of PSMA-targeting tracer findings as standard, as previous authors did [16,18].

Prostatic fossa salvage radiation treatment (SRT) is the current standard of care in men with their first BCR after RP [28]. However, in patients with a previous radical radiotherapy, only brachytherapy is indicated if malignancy is histopathologically confirmed. On the other hand, a second BCR in patients that have undergone previous radiotherapy of prostatic fossa, with or without pelvic lymph nodes involved, reduces the potential local treatment options. Therefore, ADT becomes a real therapeutic option both in patients without located disease or with local disease but with no indication of an additional local treatment (SRT or surgery).

Therapeutic impact of PSMA-targeting radiopharmaceuticals compared with PET/CT with choline-based tracers has been scarcely analysed, ranging from 54% to 74% [8,18]. We observed an impact management in 29% of cases although it could be raised to 37% if patients with comorbidities limited the previously indicated treatment and could have been included. Escalation was considered when the treatment modification involved changing/adding radiotherapy fields or adding ARAT to the systemic ADT. Thus, men with a previous RP without disease or with disease confined to the prostatic fossa on PET/CT imaging were expected to proceed to SRT or a combination of radiotherapy and ADT if few lesions were defined on [^{18}F]DCFPyL-PET/CT or ADT plus ARAT in case of multiple locations (M stage) in patients with no chemotherapy indication. The therapeutic impact derived from [^{18}F]DCFPyL over [^{18}F]F-choline findings allowed treatment escalation in most of our patients (34/40). However, the assessment of therapeutic impact is challenging, being not only dependent of the accuracy of diagnostic techniques but on other factors as previously received treatments and the comorbidities/physical status of the patients, and although [^{18}F]DCFPyL-PET/CT result could have changed the therapeutic management of some patients, this decision was not carried out because of their clinical situation. Diagnostic escalation (additional diagnostic imaging vs. biopsy) to confirm [^{18}F]DCFPyL results is another relevant aspect to be assessed. In our sample, 19 patients underwent additional diagnostic procedures, only 11 by histological analysis, lower than the 24% reported by Morigi et al. [18].

Elective prostatic bed radiotherapy is a controversial issue. About half of men who experience BCR after RP and undergo SRT with the prostatic bed, even when there are no significant imaging findings, are currently cured [29], suggesting that SRT should still be considered despite a negative imaging result [30]. On the other hand, focused radiotherapy based on PET/CT with PSMA-targeting tracers exhibits higher response rates compared with the conventional procedure without metabolic guide, although cannot guarantee undetectable PSA in all the cases and that means PET/CT with PSMA-targeting tracers still underestimate the extent of the recurrent disease [8,30]. In the present analysis, 12 out of 49 patients with a negative [^{18}F]DCFPyL-PET/CT underwent prostatic fossa radiotherapy.

Thus, therapeutic implications derived from the use of PSMA-targeting radiopharmaceuticals can be significant. Target missed in BCR due to insufficient diagnostic work-up may lead to inadequate definition of local disease and to untreated microscopic or macroscopic disease distant from prostatic fossa (N1/M1). The expected result, derived from an earlier and more accurate diagnosis of PET/CT with PSMA-targeting radiopharmaceuticals, is the opportunity for focused therapies, with a reduction in the introduction of ADT and thus the time to ADT-resistance [31,32].

Regarding limitations, histopathological confirmation of our PET/CT results was not always feasible, although it is a controversial issue and probably neither indicated nor ethical. In addition, 2-month period used between both PET/CTs could limit a reliable comparison between both radiotracers in cases of a highly proliferative disease.

However, PCa usually presents with slow growth, and noticeable changes within this period are very unlikely.

With respect to the strengths, this is the first reported experience of the therapeutic impact of [^{18}F]DCFPyL in connection with [^{18}F]F-choline, in parallel comparison, in a significant sample of patients with BCR PCa.

5. Conclusions

[^{18}F]DCFPyL provided a higher DR than [^{18}F]F-choline in restaging of BCR, especially in patients with high PSA and unfavourable PSA kinetics, being superior in miTNM staging and showing a fair agreement to [^{18}F]F-choline-PET/CT. Information derived from [^{18}F]DCFPyL changed therapeutic management in a significant number of patients (29%) compared with [^{18}F]F-choline-PET/CT.

Author Contributions: Conceptualization, L.G.-Z. and A.M.G.-V.; methodology, L.G.-Z. and A.M.G.-V.; formal analysis, M.A.-S.; investigation, L.G.-Z. and A.M.G.-V.; writing—original draft preparation, L.G.-Z. and A.M.G.-V.; writing—review and editing, L.G.-Z. and A.M.G.-V.; visualization, L.G.-Z. and C.L. L.; supervision, Á.M.S.-C. All authors have read and agreed to the published version of the manuscript.

Funding: This research received no external funding.

Institutional Review Board Statement: The study was conducted in accordance with the Declaration of Helsinki and approved by the reference Ethical Committee (internal code of 2022-53; 24 May 2022) of GAI Albacete.

Informed Consent Statement: Informed consent was obtained from all subjects involved in the study.

Data Availability Statement: Data supporting reported results are only available for local investigators.

Conflicts of Interest: The authors have no relevant financial or non-financial interests to disclose.

References

1. Cornford, P.; Bellmunt, J.; Bolla, M.; Briers, E.; De Santis, M.; Gross, T.; Henry, A.M.; Joniau, S.; Lam, T.B.; Mason, M.D.; et al. EAU-ESTRO-SIOG guidelines on prostate cancer. Part II: Treatment of relapsing, metastatic, and castration-resistant prostate cancer. *Eur. Urol.* **2017**, *71*, 630–642. [CrossRef]
2. Fanti, S.; Minozzi, S.; Castellucci, P.; Balduzzi, S.; Herrmann, K.; Krause, B.J.; Oyen, W.; Chiti, A. PET/CT with ^{11}C-choline for evaluation of prostate cancer patients with biochemical recurrence: Meta-analysis and critical review of available data. *Eur. J. Nucl. Med. Mol. Imaging* **2016**, *43*, 55–69. [CrossRef]
3. Castellucci, P.; Fuccio, C.; Nanni, C.; Santi, I.; Rizzello, A.; Lodi, F.; Franceschelli, A.; Martorana, G.; Manferrari, F.; Fanti, S. Influence of trigger PSA and PSA kinetics on 11C-Choline PET/CT detection rate in patients with biochemical relapse after radical prostatectomy. *J. Nucl. Med.* **2009**, *50*, 1394–1400. [CrossRef]
4. Evangelista, L.; Briganti, A.; Fanti, S.; Joniau, S.; Reske, S.; Schiavina, R.; Stief, C.; Thalmann, G.N.; Picchio, M. New clinical indications for ^{18}F/^{11}C-choline, new tracers for positron emission tomography and a promising hybrid device for prostate cancer staging: A systematic review of the literature. *Eur. Urol.* **2016**, *70*, 161–175. [CrossRef]
5. Afshar-Oromieh, A.; Haberkorn, U.; Eder, M.; Eisenhut, M.; Zechmann, C.M. [^{68}Ga]Gallium-labelled PSMA ligand as superior PET tracer for the diagnosis of prostate cancer: Comparison with ^{18}F-FECH. *Eur. J. Nucl. Med. Mol. Imaging* **2012**, *39*, 1085–1086. [CrossRef]
6. Rowe, S.; Gorin, M.; Pienta, K.; Siegel, B.; Carroll, P.; Pouliot, F.; Probst, S.; Saperstein, L.; Preston, M.; Ajjai, A.; et al. Results from the OSPREY trial: A Prospective Phase 2/3 Multi-Center Study of ^{18}F-DCFPyL PET/CT imaging in patients with prostate cancer—Examination of diagnostic accuracy. *J. Nucl. Med.* **2019**, *60*, 586.
7. Chevalme, Y.M.; Boudali, L.; Gauthé, M.; Rousseau, C.; Skanjeti, A.; Merlin, C.; Robin, P.; Giraudet, A.L.; Janier, M.; Talbot, J.N. Survey by the French Medicine Agency (ANSM) of the imaging protocol, detection rate, and safety of ^{68}Ga-PSMA-11 PET/CT in the biochemical recurrence of prostate cancer in case of negative or equivocal ^{18}F-fluorocholine PET/CT: 1084 examinations. *Eur. J. Nucl. Med. Mol. Imaging* **2021**, *48*, 2935–2950. [CrossRef]
8. Barbaud, M.; Frindel, M.; Ferrer, L.; Le Thiec, M.; Rusu, D.; Rauscher, A.; Maucherat, B.; Baumgartner, P.; Fleury, V.; Colombié, M.; et al. ^{68}Ga-PSMA-11 PET-CT study in prostate cancer patients with biochemical recurrence and non-contributive ^{18}F-Choline PET-CT: Impact on therapeutic decision-making and biomarker changes. *Prostate* **2019**, *79*, 454–461. [CrossRef]
9. Witkowska-Patena, E.; Giżewska, A.; Dziuk, M.; Miśko, J.; Budzyńska, A.; Walęcka-Mazur, A. Head-to-Head Comparison of ^{18}F-Prostate-Specific Membrane Antigen-1007 and ^{18}F-Fluorocholine PET/CT in biochemically relapsed Prostate Cancer. *Clin. Nucl. Med.* **2019**, *44*, e629–e633. [CrossRef]

10. Eiber, M.; Herrmann, K.; Calais, J.; Hadaschik, B.; Giesel, F.L.; Hartenbach, M.; Hope, T.; Reiter, R.; Maurer, T.; Weber, W.A.; et al. Prostate Cancer Molecular Imaging Standardized Evaluation (PROMISE): Proposed miTNM Classification for the Interpretation of PSMA-Ligand PET/CT. *J. Nucl. Med.* **2018**, *59*, 469–478. [CrossRef]
11. van Leenders, G.J.L.H.; van der Kwast, T.H.; Grignon, D.J.; Evans, A.J.; Kristiansen, G.; Kweldam, C.F.; Litjens, G.; McKenney, J.K.; Melamed, J.; Mottet, N.; et al. The 2019 International Society of Urological Pathology (ISUP) Consensus Conference on Grading of Prostatic Carcinoma. *Am. J. Surg. Pathol.* **2020**, *44*, 87–99. [CrossRef]
12. Calabria, F.; Chiaravalloti, A.; Schillaci, O. ^{18}F-choline PET/CT pitfalls in image interpretation: An update on 300 examined patients with prostate cancer. *Clin. Nucl. Med.* **2014**, *39*, 122–130. [CrossRef]
13. Alonso, O.; Dos Santos, G.; García Fontes, M.; Balter, H.; Engler, H. ^{68}Ga-PSMA and ^{11}C-Choline comparison using a tri-modality PET/CT-MRI (3.0 T) system with a dedicated shuttle. *Eur. J. Hybrid Imaging* **2018**, *2*, 9. [CrossRef]
14. Cantiello, F.; Crocerossa, F.; Russo, G.I.; Gangemi, V.; Ferro, M.; Vartolomei, M.D.; Lucarelli, G.; Mirabelli, M.; Scafuro, C.; Ucciero, G.; et al. Comparison between ^{64}Cu-PSMA-617 PET/CT and ^{18}F-Choline PET/CT imaging in early diagnosis of prostate cancer biochemical recurrence. *Clin. Genitourin. Cancer* **2018**, *16*, 385–391. [CrossRef]
15. Caroli, P.; Sandler, I.; Matteucci, F.; De Giorgi, U.; Uccelli, L.; Celli, M.; Foca, F.; Barone, D.; Romeo, A.; Sarnelli, A.; et al. ^{68}Ga-PSMA PET/CT in patients with recurrent prostate cancer after radical treatment: Prospective results in 314 patients. *Eur. J. Nucl. Med. Mol. Imaging* **2018**, *45*, 2035–2044. [CrossRef]
16. Schwenck, J.; Rempp, H.; Reischl, G.; Kruck, S.; Stenzl, A.; Nikolaou, K.; Pfannenberg, C.; la Fougère, C. Comparison of ^{68}Ga-labelled PSMA-11 and ^{11}C-choline in the detection of prostate cancer metastases by PET/CT. *Eur. J. Nucl. Med. Mol. Imaging* **2017**, *44*, 92–101. [CrossRef]
17. Bluemel, C.; Krebs, M.; Polat, B.; Linke, F.; Eiber, M.; Samnick, S.; Lapa, C.; Lassmann, M.; Riedmiller, H.; Czernin, J.; et al. ^{68}Ga-PSMA-PET/CT in patients with biochemical prostate cancer recurrence and negative ^{18}F-Choline-PET/CT. *Clin. Nucl. Med.* **2016**, *41*, 515–521. [CrossRef]
18. Morigi, J.J.; Stricker, P.D.; van Leeuwen, P.J.; Tang, R.; Ho, B.; Nguyen, Q.; Hruby, G.; Fogarty, G.; Jagavkar, R.; Kneebone, A.; et al. Prospective comparison of ^{18}F-Fluoromethylcholine versus ^{68}Ga-PSMA PET/CT in prostate cancer patients who have rising PSA after curative treatment and are being considered for targeted therapy. *J. Nucl. Med.* **2015**, *56*, 1185–1190. [CrossRef]
19. Afshar-Oromieh, A.; Zechmann, C.M.; Malcher, A.; Eder, M.; Eisenhut, M.; Linhart, H.G.; Holland-Letz, T.; Hadaschik, B.A.; Giesel, F.L.; Debus, J.; et al. Comparison of PET imaging with a ^{68}Ga-labelled PSMA ligand and ^{18}F-choline-based PET/CT for the diagnosis of recurrent prostate cancer. *Eur. J. Nucl. Med. Mol. Imaging* **2014**, *41*, 11–20. [CrossRef]
20. Umbehr, M.H.; Müntener, M.; Hany, T.; Sulser, T.; Bachmann, L.M. The role of 11C-choline and ^{18}F-fluorocholine positron emission tomography (PET) and PET/CT in prostate cancer: A systematic review and meta-analysis. *Eur. Urol.* **2013**, *64*, 106–117. [CrossRef]
21. Treglia, G.; Ceriani, L.; Sadeghi, R.; Giovacchini, G.; Giovanella, L. Relationship between prostate-specific antigen kinetics and detection rate of radiolabelled choline PET/CT in restaging prostate cancer patients: A meta-analysis. *Clin. Chem. Lab. Med.* **2014**, *52*, 725–733. [CrossRef]
22. Souvatzoglou, M.; Weirich, G.; Schwarzenboeck, S.; Maurer, T.; Schuster, T.; Bundschuh, R.A.; Eiber, M.; Herrmann, K.; Kuebler, H.; Wester, H.J.; et al. The sensitivity of [^{11}C]choline PET/CT to localize prostate cancer depends on the tumor configuration. *Clin. Cancer Res.* **2011**, *17*, 3751–3759. [CrossRef]
23. Farsad, M.; Schiavina, R.; Castellucci, P.; Nanni, C.; Corti, B.; Martorana, G.; Canini, R.; Grigioni, W.; Boschi, S.; Marengo, M.; et al. Detection and localization of prostate cancer: Correlation of ^{11}C-choline PET/CT with histopathologic step-section analysis. *J. Nucl. Med.* **2005**, *46*, 1642–1649.
24. Mannweiler, S.; Amersdorfer, P.; Trajanoski, S.; Terrett, J.A.; King, D.; Mehes, G. Heterogeneity of prostate-specific membrane antigen (PSMA) expression in prostate carcinoma with distant metastasis. *Pathol. Oncol. Res.* **2009**, *15*, 167–172. [CrossRef]
25. van Waarde, A.; Jager, P.L.; Ishiwata, K.; Dierckx, R.A.; Elsinga, P.H. Comparison of sigma-ligands and metabolic PET tracers for differentiating tumor from inflammation. *J. Nucl. Med.* **2006**, *47*, 150–154.
26. Giesel, F.L.; Hadaschik, B.; Cardinale, J.; Radtke, J.; Vinsensia, M.; Lehnert, W.; Kesch, C.; Tolstov, Y.; Singer, S.; Grabe, N.; et al. F-18 labelled PSMA-1007: Biodistribution, radiation dosimetry and histopathological validation of tumor lesions in prostate cancer patients. *Eur. J. Nucl. Med. Mol. Imaging* **2017**, *44*, 678–688. [CrossRef]
27. Ghosh, A.; Heston, W.D. Tumor target prostate specific membrane antigen (PSMA) and its regulation in prostate cancer. *J. Cell. Biochem.* **2004**, *91*, 528–539. [CrossRef]
28. Carrie, C.; Hasbini, A.; de Laroche, G.; Richaud, P.; Guerif, S.; Latorzeff, I.; Supiot, S.; Bosset, M.; Lagrange, J.L.; Beckendorf, V.; et al. Salvage radiotherapy with or without short-term hormone therapy for rising prostate-specific antigen concentration after radical prostatectomy (GETUG-AFU 16): A randomised, multicentre, open-label phase 3 trial. *Lancet Oncol.* **2016**, *17*, 747–756. [CrossRef]
29. Stephenson, A.J.; Scardino, P.T.; Kattan, M.W.; Pisansky, T.M.; Slawin, K.M.; Klein, E.A.; Anscher, M.S.; Michalski, J.M.; Sandler, H.M.; Lin, D.W.; et al. Predicting the outcome of salvage radiation therapy for recurrent prostate cancer after radical prostatectomy. *J. Clin. Oncol.* **2007**, *25*, 2035–2041. [CrossRef]
30. Fendler, W.P.; Calais, J.; Eiber, M.; Flavell, R.R.; Mishoe, A.; Feng, F.Y.; Nguyen, H.G.; Reiter, R.E.; Rettig, M.B.; Okamoto, S.; et al. Assessment of ^{68}Ga-PSMA-11 PET accuracy in localizing recurrent prostate cancer: A prospective single-arm clinical trial. *JAMA Oncol.* **2019**, *5*, 856–863. [CrossRef]

31. Tosoian, J.J.; Gorin, M.A.; Ross, A.E.; Pienta, K.J.; Tran, P.T.; Schaeffer, E.M. Oligometastatic prostate cancer: Definitions, clinical outcomes and treatment considerations. *Nat. Rev. Urol.* **2017**, *14*, 15–25. [CrossRef]
32. Han, S.; Woo, S.; Kim, Y.J.; Suh, C.H. Impact of ^{68}Ga-PSMA PET on the management of patients with prostate cancer: A systematic review and meta-analysis. *Eur. Urol.* **2018**, *74*, 179–190. [CrossRef]

Disclaimer/Publisher's Note: The statements, opinions and data contained in all publications are solely those of the individual author(s) and contributor(s) and not of MDPI and/or the editor(s). MDPI and/or the editor(s) disclaim responsibility for any injury to people or property resulting from any ideas, methods, instructions or products referred to in the content.

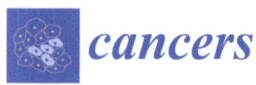

Article

'Stealth' Prostate Tumors

Vinayak G. Wagaskar [1], Osama Zaytoun [1,2], Swati Bhardwaj [3] and Ash Tewari [1,*]

[1] Department of Urology, Icahn School of Medicine at Mount Sinai Hospital, New York, NY 10029, USA
[2] Urology Department, Alexandria University, Alexandria 21113, Egypt
[3] Department of Pathology, Icahn School of Medicine at Mount Sinai Hospital, New York, NY 10029, USA
* Correspondence: ash.tewari@mountsinai.org; Tel.: +1-212-241-9955

Simple Summary: Efforts are ongoing to improve the diagnosis of prostate cancer. Novel blood and tissue-based biomarkers, advanced imaging modalities and image-guided biopsy techniques have further improved cancer detection rates. However, approximately 30–40% of cancers are still missed. Analysis of radical prostatectomy specimens is the only gold standard method for confirming the presence or absence of cancers. In this article, we aim to study those cancers that are missed by standard biopsy techniques and advanced imaging modalities, the so-called 'Stealth' prostate cancers. We focus on the lobe of the prostate where cancer is not detected on standard biopsy or by preoperative magnetic resonance imaging (MRI). This article helps to explain the significant false negative rates for current diagnostic modalities for prostate cancer. This will help future research to develop new strategies to improve the detection of these 'stealth' tumors.

Abstract: Background: The aim of this study was to determine the false negative rates of prebiopsy magnetic resonance imaging (MRI) and MRI–ultrasound (US) 12-core systematic prostate biopsy (PBx) by analyzing radical prostatectomy specimens. Methods: This retrospective study included 3600 prostate cancer (PCa) patients who underwent robot-assisted laparoscopic radical prostatectomy. Based on comparison of lobe-specific data on final pathology with preoperative biopsy and imaging data, the study population was subdivided into group I—contralateral (CL) benign PBx (n = 983), group II—CL and/or bilateral (BL) non-suspicious mpMRI (n = 2223) and group III—CL benign PBx + non-suspicious mpMRI (n = 688). This population was studied for the presence of PCa, clinically significant PCa (csPCa), extracapsular extension (ECE) (pathological stage pT3), positive frozen section and final positive surgical margin (PSM) in the CL lobe. Descriptive statistics were performed. Results: In subgroups I, II and III, PCa was respectively detected in 21.5%, 37.7% and 19.5% of cases, and csPCa in 11.3%, 16.3% and 10.3% of cases. CL pT3 disease was seen in 4.5%, 4% and 5.5%, and CL surgical margins and/or frozen section analysis were positive in 6%, 7% and 5% of cases in subgroups I, II and III, respectively. Conclusions: There are still significant rates of false negatives in the standard care diagnostics of PCa. Further strategies are required to improve the accuracy of diagnosis and determination of tumor location.

Keywords: prostate cancer; prostate biopsy; magnetic resonance imaging

Citation: Wagaskar, V.G.; Zaytoun, O.; Bhardwaj, S.; Tewari, A. 'Stealth' Prostate Tumors. *Cancers* 2023, 15, 3487. https://doi.org/10.3390/cancers15133487

Academic Editors: Ana Faustino, Paula A. Oliveira and Lúcio Lara Santos

Received: 25 February 2023
Revised: 21 April 2023
Accepted: 3 July 2023
Published: 4 July 2023

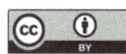

Copyright: © 2023 by the authors. Licensee MDPI, Basel, Switzerland. This article is an open access article distributed under the terms and conditions of the Creative Commons Attribution (CC BY) license (https:// creativecommons.org/licenses/by/ 4.0/).

1. Introduction

The widespread application of prostate-specific antigen (PSA) screening has led to more cases of prostate cancer (PCa) being diagnosed at an earlier clinical stage [1]. In this scenario, transrectal ultrasound-guided prostate biopsy (TRUS PBx) and subsequent pathological analysis are considered the gold standard for cancer diagnosis. Over the past two decades, the PBx scheme has witnessed numerous modifications to improve the biopsy yield [1–3]. Laterally directed extended PBx was found to significantly enhance the diagnosis of PCa compared with conventional sextant biopsy. However, the false negative rate remains substantial [4]. Serefoglou et al. performed repeat 12-core PBx on radical prostatectomy specimens, and surprisingly, the false negative rate of 12-core PBx in this series was 32.2% [5]. This relatively high false negative rate may be intuitively attributed to a limited amount of tissue sampled during PBx, the biopsy surgeon's experience, the lack of uniform and standardized biopsy techniques and the random nature of biopsy schemes with a resultant sampling error.

Multiparametric magnetic resonance imaging (mpMRI) has emerged as a promising tool for guiding PBx decision-making. The introduction of mpMRI-targeted PBx has increased the accuracy of clinically significant PCa (csPCa) detection [6–8]. Nevertheless, The American Urological Association raised concern regarding the risk of missing csPCa on negative mpMRI examinations [9]. We recently published our study on a series of 200 men with negative mpMRI, with 18% found to have PCa and 8% csPCa on the subsequent biopsy [9]. That study was performed with the reference standard as PBx. Our prior work on radical prostatectomy patients comparing suspicious vs. non-suspicious MRI demonstrated similar rates of csPCa, positive surgical margins and biochemical recurrence rates in both groups [10].

Here, we aimed to assess the accuracy of PBx and mpMRI in the diagnosis and localization of PCa and csPCa. This was performed by using lobe-specific final pathological data derived from radical prostatectomy specimens as a reference. We believe this will help to better understand the so-called 'stealth' PCa.

2. Materials and Methods

2.1. Study Design

The study was approved by the Institutional Review Board (GCO#14-0175) of the Icahn School of Medicine at Mount Sinai (New York, NY, USA). We retrospectively reviewed the data of 3600 men who underwent robotic-assessed laparoscopic radical prostatectomy (RALP) between 1 January 2014 and 31 December 2022. RALPs were performed by a single surgeon (A.T.) with more than 20 years of experience in the PCa field.

2.1.1. Inclusion and Exclusion Criteria

Patients who underwent RALP were included in the study if they had full preoperative PBx and mpMRI data. Exclusion criteria encompassed PBx schemes of fewer than 12 systemic cores, contraindications or unreadable mpMRI; prior hormonal or radiation manipulation; preoperative PSA > 20 ng/dL; absence of specific documentation on final pathology or missing information for clinical variables (Figure 1).

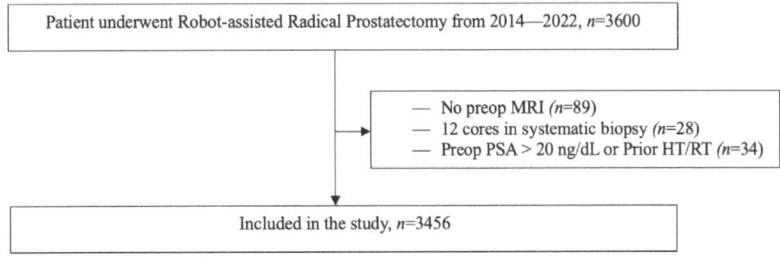

Figure 1. Flow chart depicting inclusion and exclusion criteria used to derive patient population used for data analysis. Abbreviations: MRI: magnetic resonance imaging, PSA: prostate-specific antigen, HT: Hormone therapy, RT: Radiation therapy.

2.1.2. MRI Protocol

Prostate evaluations were conducted using 3T MRI Siemens Skyra systems equipped with a phased-array coil. The following sequences were obtained: multiplanar high-resolution T2 fast spin echo (FSE); axial T1 FSE; axial diffusion-weighted imaging; axial T1 in and out of phase; and axial T1 perfusion before and after contrast injection (8 mL of Gadavist (gadobutrol) and 1 mg of glucagon via intramuscular injection). The mpMRI results were evaluated according to Prostate Imaging Reporting and Data System version

2 (PI-RADS v2) [11] by radiologists with more than 5 years of experience in mpMRI prostate imaging (>250 MRI scans per year). Non-suspicious MRI findings were defined as a PI-RADS v2 score of <3.

2.1.3. Biopsy Protocol and Technique

Indications for PBx were one or more of the following: PSA > 4 ng/mL, a 4K score (OPKO Diagnostics, Woburn, MA, USA) of >7%, PSA density of ≥ 0.15 ng/mL/cm^3 or suspicious digital rectal examination (DRE).

A transrectal ultrasound was performed. An amount of 5 cc of 1% Lidocaine was injected into each neurovascular bundle (a total of 10 cc was given). Care was taken to avoid intravascular injection. The prostate was then examined and measured using ellipsoid formula. For patients who had mpMRI suspicion (PI-RADS ≥ 3), the Artemis MRI/TRUS fusion device (Innomedicus, Cham, Switzerland) was attached to the ultrasound probe. Range of mobility of the arm was tested to ensure entire prostate from base to apex was reachable for the biopsy. After that, a repeat 360-degree scan was performed of the prostate. Semi-segmentation was performed in both transverse and sagittal views. After this, the MRI was loaded and fused with the ultrasound images.

The target/s on the MRI were identified on ultrasound and the biopsy targets were assigned to that zone. After this, motion artifact and recalibration were corrected under local anesthesia, and four targeted biopsies were taken; path of needle was documented on the Artemis. The targets biopsied were labeled as per location; e.g., Target Right Mid peripheral zone posteromedial. A systemic biopsy was then performed on all 12 quadrants. Systematic biopsies were labeled as Right Lateral Base, Right Medial Base, Right Lateral Mid, Right Medial Mid, Right Lateral Apex, Right Medial Apex, Left Lateral Base, Left Medial Base, Left Lateral Mid, Left Medial Mid, Left Lateral Apex and Left Medial Apex.

All biopsies were performed with a spring-loaded biopsy gun and 18-gauge needles with 12 mm average core length. Cores were placed on non-adherent gauze pad and, finally, in a bottle containing 10% formalin [12,13].

2.1.4. Pathological Assessment

An experienced genitourinary pathologist reviewed both PBx samples and RALP specimens (final pathology). Only H&E slides were reviewed for most cases. PIN-4 staining (including AMACR, high molecular weight cytokeratin and CK5/6) was performed on the few suspicious biopsy cases to confirm the diagnosis of cancer when not sufficiently evident based on morphology alone. The final pathology was comprehensively reviewed on a lobe-specific basis per the College of American Pathologists' (CAP) protocol for radical prostatectomy specimens [14]. This included comments on the presence of any PCa, Gleason score, grade group, presence of csPCa, presence of extracapsular extension (ECE) (pathological stage pT3), presence of positive neurosafe/frozen section margins and presence of positive surgical margins (PSM).

2.1.5. Outcome Definitions and Statistical Analysis

Gleason grading system was utilized as proposed by Epstein et al. [13], where Grade Group 1 = Gleason score ≤ 6, Grade Group 2 = Gleason score 3 + 4 = 7, Grade Group 3 = Gleason score 4 + 3 = 7, Grade Group 4 = Gleason score 4 + 4 = 8 and Grade Group 5 = Gleason scores 9 and 10. PCa is defined as Gleason Grade Group (GGG) 1 and above, while csPCa is defined as GGG ≥ 2 [15]. Based on comparison of lobe-specific data on final pathology with preoperative biopsy and imaging data, study population was further subdivided into three groups (Figure 2):

I. Contralateral (CL) benign PBx (n = 983).
II. CL and/or bilateral (BL) non-suspicious mpMRI (n = 2223).
III. CL benign PBx + non-suspicious mpMRI (n = 688).

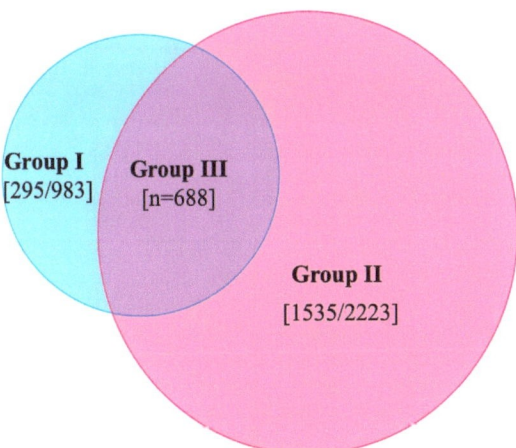

Figure 2. Venn diagram showing distribution of study population in each group. Group III population is an overlap between group I and group II.

This population was studied for presence of any PCa, csPCa, extra-capsular extension (pathological stage pT3), positive frozen section and positive surgical margins in CL lobe (Figure 3).

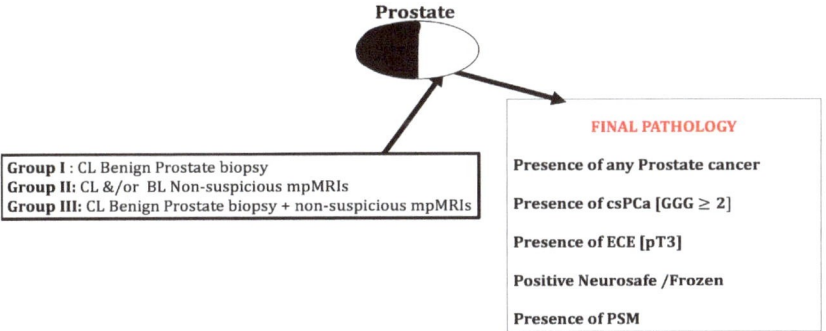

Figure 3. Schematic representation of methodology and study population classification. Patients with contralateral lobe benign prostate biopsy and/or non-suspicious MRI were studied for presence of cancer and other variables in radical prostatectomy specimens. Abbreviations: CL—contralateral, BL—bilateral, mpMRI—multiparametric magnetic resonance imaging, csPCa—clinically significant prostate cancer, ECE—extracapsular extension of cancer, PSM—positive surgical margins.

Descriptive statistics for the three groups were collected. Then, within each group, we compared patients with no CL cancer on final pathology (accurate) versus those with CL cancer (false negative). Results for continuous variables were reported as the median and interquartile range (IQR) and were compared using the Mann–Whitney U test. Results for categorical variables were reported as the frequency and proportion and were compared using a x2 test, as appropriate. All tests were two-tailed with a significance level of $p < 0.05$.

3. Results

PCa was detected in 21.5%, 37.7% and 19.5% of the three subgroups, respectively. Detection of csPCa was higher in group II (16.3%) than in the other two groups (11.3% and 10.3%, respectively). Other pathological findings were comparable between the study groups (Table 1).

Table 1. Comparative analysis between the three subgroups regarding the final pathological findings.

Final Pathology Parameters	Group I: n = 983 (%)	Group II: n = 2223 (%)	Group III: n = 688 (%)
Presence of any PCa, no (%)	212 (21.5)	825 (37.7)	134 (19.5)
Presence of csPCa, no (%)	111 (11.3)	362 (16.3)	71 (10.3)
Presence of ECE (pT3), no (%)	45 (4.5)	85 (3.8)	38 (5.5)
Positive frozen section analysis, no (%)	51 (5.2)	102 (4.5)	27 (4)
Presence of PSMs, no (%)	18 (1.8)	61 (2.7)	11 (1.5)

Abbreviations: PCa—prostate cancer, csPCa—clinically significant prostate cancer, ECE—extracapsular extension of cancer, PSM—positive surgical margins.

Table 2 depicts clinical characteristics for group I. Per final pathology, accurate concordance with biopsy results was shown in 78.5% (no CL cancer detected), while CL PCa was diagnosed in the rest, giving a false negative value of 21.5%. Both patient cohorts showed comparable age and median PSA at the time of diagnosis. Of note, the cohort with CL cancer on final pathology had statistically significant higher African American (AA) race, biopsy GGG, pathological T3 stage and PSM.

Table 2. Comparison between cohorts with accurate versus false negative results in group I.

Variable	Patients with No CL Cancer on Final Pathology: Accurate, n = 771 (78.5%)	Patient with CL Cancer on Final Pathology: False Negative, n = 212 (21.5%)	p Value
Median age in years	64	63	0.429
Race			
AA	80 (10.4)	37 (17.5)	<0.023 *
White	437 (56.7)	119 (56.1)	
Others	254 (32.9)	56 (26.4)	
BMI	26.9	27.1	0.362
Family history of PCa			
No	582 (75.5)	164 (77.4)	0.320
Yes	189 (24.5)	48 (22.6)	
Median PSA at diagnosis	6.1	6.3	0.258
Median prostate volume (cc)	40	39	0.381
Biopsy GGG			
1	101 (13.1)	21 (9.9)	
2	295 (38.3)	93 (43.9)	
3	201 (26.1)	51 (24.1)	0.019 *
4	122 (15.8)	22 (10.4)	
5	52 (6.7)	25 (11.8)	
MRI PI-RADS lesions			
1–2	105 (13.6)	23 (10.8)	
3	81 (10.5)	13 (6.1)	0.129
4	368 (47.7)	107 (50.5)	
5	217 (28.1)	69 (32.5)	
Final pathology GGG			
1	71 (9.2)	16 (7.5)	
2	412 (53.4)	103 (48.6)	
3	202 (26.2)	63 (29.7)	0.056
4	38 (4.9)	10 (4.7)	
5	48 (6.2)	20 (9.4)	

Table 2. Cont.

Variable	Patients with No CL Cancer on Final Pathology: Accurate, n = 771 (78.5%)	Patient with CL Cancer on Final Pathology: False Negative, n = 212 (21.5%)	p Value
Pathology T stage			<0.001 *
T2	660 (85.6)	133 (62.7)	
T3	111 (14.4)	79 (37.3)	
PSMs			<0.001 *
Absent	736 (95.5)	187 (88.2)	
Present	35 (4.5)	25 (11.8)	

Abbreviations: CL—contralateral, AA—African American race, PCa—prostate cancer, PSA—prostate specific antigen, GGG—Gleason Grade Group, MRI—magnetic resonance imaging, PI-RADS—Prostate Imaging Radiology And Data System, PSM—positive surgical margins. * p value < 0.05.

Regarding group II, accurate and false negative results were encountered in 62.3% and 37.7%, respectively. Patients with CL cancer on final pathology had non-suspicious MRI PI-RADS lesions in 40.2% compared to 1% in patients with no CL cancer cohort (p value < 0.001) (Table 3).

Table 3. Comparison between cohorts with accurate versus false negative results in group II.

Variable	Patients with No CL Cancer on Final Pathology: Accurate n = 1398 (62.3%)	Patient with CL Cancer on Final Pathology: False Negative n = 825 (37.7%)	p Value
Median age in years	64	63	0.429
Race			<0.001 *
AA	158 (11.3)	131 (15.9)	
White	855 (61.2)	497 (60.2)	
Others	385 (22.4)	197 (23.9)	
BMI	26.9	27.1	0.362
Family history of PCa			0.067
No	1072 (76.7)	656 (79.5)	
Yes	326 (23.3)	169 (20.5)	
Median PSA at diagnosis	6.0	6.0	0.258
Median prostate volume (cc)	39	39	0.381
Biopsy GGG			0.032 *
1	225 (16.1)	175 (21.2)	
2	553 (39.6)	323 (39.2)	
3	305 (21.8)	165 (20.0)	
4	196 (14.0)	98 (11.9)	
5	119 (8.5)	64 (7.8)	
MRI PI-RADS lesions			<0.001 *
1–2	13 (1)	332 (40.2)	
3	162 (11.6)	62 (7.5)	
4	716 (51.2)	252 (30.5)	
5	507 (36.3)	179 (21.7)	

Table 3. Cont.

Variable	Patients with No CL Cancer on Final Pathology: Accurate n = 1398 (62.3%)	Patient with CL Cancer on Final Pathology: False Negative n = 825 (37.7%)	p Value
Final pathology GGG			
1	127 (9.1)	98 (11.9)	
2	764 (54.6)	480 (58.2)	
3	344 (24.6)	174 (21.1)	0.017 *
4	60 (4.3)	24 (2.9)	
5	103 (7.4)	49 (5.9)	
Pathology T stage			
T2	1154 (82.5)	570 (69.1)	<0.001 *
T3	244 (17.5)	255 (30.9)	
PSMs			
Absent	1336 (95.6)	738 (89.5)	<0.001 *
Present	62 (4.4)	87 (10.5)	

Abbreviations: CL—contralateral, AA—African American race, PCa—prostate cancer, PSA—prostate-specific antigen, GGG—Gleason Grade Group, MRI—magnetic resonance imaging, PI-RADS—Prostate Imaging Radiology And Data System, PSM—positive surgical margins. * p value < 0.05.

False-negative results were encountered in 19.5% of patients in group III. This cohort showed statistically significant pathological T3 stage and PSMs in terms of cohort accurate correlation (Table 4). Figure 4 shows an example of GGG4 cancer that was missed on biopsy and prebiopsy MRI.

Table 4. Comparison between cohorts with accurate versus false negative results in group III.

Variable	Patients with No CL Cancer on Final Pathology: Accurate, n = 554 (81.5%)	Patient with CL Cancer on Final Pathology: False Negative, n = 134 (19.5%)	p Value
Median age in years	64	63	0.429
Race			
AA	53 (9.6)	19 (14.2)	
White	314 (56.7)	82 (61.2)	0.093
Others	187 (33.8)	33 (24.6)	
BMI	26.9	27.1	0.362
Family history of PCa			
No	416 (75.1)	103 (76.9)	0.320
Yes	138 (24.9)	31 (23.1)	
Median PSA at diagnosis	6.1	6.3	0.258
Median prostate volume (cc)	40	39	0.381
Biopsy GGG			
1	66 (11.9)	4 (3)	
2	210 (37.9)	57 (42.5)	
3	142 (25.6)	44 (32.8)	0.001 *
4	92 (16.6)	13 (9.7)	
5	44 (7.9)	16 (11.9)	

Table 4. Cont.

Variable	Patients with No CL Cancer on Final Pathology: Accurate, n = 554 (81.5%)	Patient with CL Cancer on Final Pathology: False Negative, n = 134 (19.5%)	p Value
MRI PI-RADS lesions			
1–2	5 (1)	2 (1)	
3	57 (10.3)	8 (6)	0.129
4	317 (57.2)	72 (53.7)	
5	175 (31.6)	52 (38.8)	
Final pathology GGG			
1	71 (9.2)	16 (7.5)	
2	412 (53.4)	103 (48.6)	
3	202 (26.2)	63 (29.7)	0.056
4	38 (4.9)	10 (4.7)	
5	48 (6.2)	20 (9.4)	
Pathology T stage			
T2	465 (83.9)	81 (60.4)	<0.001 *
T3	89 (16.1)	53 (39.6)	
PSMs			
Absent	532 (96)	118 (88.1)	<0.001 *
Present	22 (4)	16 (11.9)	

Abbreviations: CL—contralateral, AA—African American race, PCa—prostate cancer, PSA—prostate specific antigen, GGG—Gleason Grade Group, MRI—magnetic resonance imaging, PI-RADS—Prostate Imaging Radiology And Data System, PSM—positive surgical margins. * p value < 0.05.

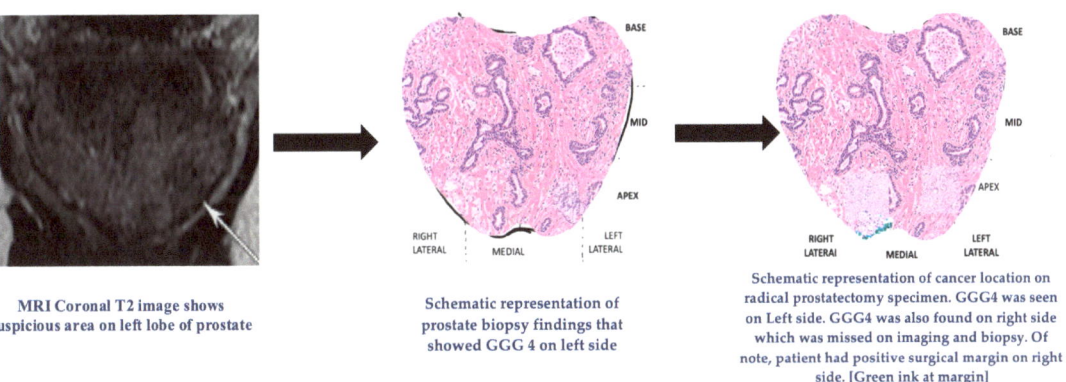

MRI Coronal T2 image shows suspicious area on left lobe of prostate

Schematic representation of prostate biopsy findings that showed GGG 4 on left side

Schematic representation of cancer location on radical prostatectomy specimen. GGG4 was seen on Left side. GGG4 was also found on right side which was missed on imaging and biopsy. Of note, patient had positive surgical margin on right side. [Green ink at margin]

Figure 4. Prebiopsy MRI followed by schematic representation of GGG4 cancer prostate biopsy and radical prostatectomy. Patient had cancer on right side that was missed on prebiopsy MRI and prostate biopsy. Abbreviations: MRI—magnetic resonance imaging, GGG—Gleason Grade Group.

4. Discussion

Diagnosis of PCa has primarily relied on laboratory tests and MRI followed by MRI-guided PBx. Efforts are ongoing to improve cancer diagnosis by involving biomarkers (4K score, select MDx, etc.) or using nomogram-derived calculators [16–18].

Military 'stealth' aircraft are designed with fascinating technology that makes their sonar or radar detection challenging. These aircraft are of similar size to other military aircraft but are made of special absorbent materials with unique shapes and contours that cannot be detected by radar [19]. In the current study, we introduce the term 'stealth PCa' to describe tumors that are missed on initial evaluation (systematic biopsy, mpMRI) and subsequently diagnosed via a prostatectomy specimen. We utilized lobe-specific final pathology of RALP specimens to assess the actual yield of current standard diagnostics for PCa.

Although the false negative rate of random biopsy protocols is well documented in the literature, we expect that the introduction of MRI and subsequent target biopsy will improve cancer detection and localization. However, counterintuitively, false negative results and, hence, 'stealth' tumors were still encountered. We still believe that we are far from precise tumor localization even with extensive expertise in the field of PCa similar to that of our surgeon.

Our study confers three key features: First, a significant number of csPCa cases are missed by mpMRI. It was shown that mpMRI improves the detection of csPCa as well as contributes to reducing the number of unnecessary PBx. Nevertheless, false negative rates of csPCa for non-suspicious MRI range from 2% to 18% [9,20]. We observed a 16% false negative rate in the diagnosis of csPCa in men with non-suspicious MRI, which is in concordance with published studies.

Second, non-suspicious mpMRI and systematic biopsy miss 11–16% of clinically significant 'stealth' PCa. The authors believe this is the most critical conclusion of our analysis and should be regarded with extreme caution. We still confirm that mpMRI and subsequent target biopsy have revolutionized the scope of PCa diagnosis. mpMRI provides anatomical and functional details as well as excellent positive predictive and negative predictive values.

In 2017, the PROMIS trial demonstrated that using mpMRI as an initial triage for men with an elevated PSA could allow 27% of patients to avoid a primary biopsy and diagnose 5% fewer clinically insignificant cancers. When compared to using a standard TRUS-guided PBx pathway, using mpMRI to guide biopsy can allow urologists to detect 18% more cases of significant cancers [21]. Hence, an MRI-guided biopsy followed by a systematic biopsy has been the gold standard in PCa diagnosis. Therefore, it is still an integral part of our own current practice that involves routine prebiopsy mpMRI. We believe that larger prospective studies are still needed to validate this critical conclusion.

Sampling error on needle PBx has been well demonstrated in the literature. It is due to a small amount of tissue (approximately 0.04% of the average gland volume) that is removed by thin-core needle biopsies [22]. Therefore, false negative rates are commonly encountered. Some authors confirmed a statement similar to our second conclusion. Kim et al. studied 730 radical prostatectomy specimens and compared them to combined systemic TRUS PBx of at least 12 cores and mpMRI. They concluded that this combination did not provide reliable accuracy in predicting the true unilaterality of PCa [23]. In another study by the same group, the sensitivity, specificity, positive predictive value and negative predictive value of mpMRI to predict csPCa were 74.3%, 45.5%, 95.5% and 10.2%, respectively [24].

We hypothesize that these challenges in accurate preoperative PCa localization may be attributed to the high heterogeneity and multifocality behavior of the disease itself. Additionally, this confirms that even with these marvelous advances in PCa diagnostics, we still lack the best tools for precise cancer detection and localization. We have initiated a trial on the wide application of micro-ultrasound to better localize PCa preoperatively; however, details of such trials are beyond the scope of this study.

Third, the presence of AA race and biopsy GGG $\geq$ 2 increases the possibilities of CL 'stealth' tumors. Molecular and genomic differences in the tumor biology of AA men have been widely studied to explain the aggressiveness and increased incidences of PCa compared with the non-Hispanic white population. Our prior work on AA men showed increased biopsy GGG upgrading and increased incidences of biochemical recurrence compared with other men. Herein, we found that AA men have increased incidences of 'stealth' tumors. The Gleason grading system is still a commanding predictor of PCa; the higher the grade, the worse the outcome. In our series, patients with GGG $\geq$ 2 have an increased incidence of CL stealth tumors. Surprisingly, our study also highlighted that there is no significance due to age, median PSA, family history of PCa or median prostate volume in determining the presence of CL 'stealth' tumors; i.e., we found no correlation of age, median PSA or prostate volume in men with vs. without CL 'stealth' tumors.

This study has its limitations. Firstly, it was retrospective in nature, where all the data were derived from our database. Second, the preoperative MRI/TRUS-guided 12-core PBxs were not performed by the same physician. Although there is no evidence to support any differences in the results of PBx between the performing urologists, we believe this factor may have influenced our data. Lastly, this study included only men with previously positive PBx that were recommended for and then underwent RALP and, therefore, excluded men with false negative initial biopsy, clinically insignificant prostate cancers not requiring RALP and others that underwent different treatment options (radiation, focal therapy, hormonal therapy, etc.). Therefore, the actual risk of a false negative biopsy may be much higher, and further studies are required to address this confounding factor.

5. Conclusions

The current standards of care for diagnostics for PCa (PSA, DRE, MRI and MRI–US-guided prostate biopsy or 12-core systematic biopsy) have significant false negative rates. Further strategies are required to improve the accuracy of diagnosis.

Author Contributions: Conceptualization, A.T. and V.G.W.; methodology, V.G.W., O.Z., S.B. and A.T.; software, V.G.W.; validation, V.G.W., O.Z., S.B. and A.T.; formal analysis, V.G.W., O.Z., S.B. and A.T.; investigation, V.G.W., O.Z., S.B. and A.T.; resources, V.G.W.; data curation, V.G.W.; writing—original draft preparation, V.G.W. and O.Z.; writing—review and editing, V.G.W., O.Z., S.B. and A.T.; visualization, V.G.W.; supervision, A.T.; project administration, A.T. All authors have read and agreed to the published version of the manuscript.

Funding: This research received no external funding.

Institutional Review Board Statement: This retrospective study was approved by the Institutional Review Board (GCO#14-0175) of the Icahn School of Medicine at Mount Sinai within the Mount Sinai Health System in New York City.

Informed Consent Statement: Informed consent was obtained from all subjects involved in the study.

Data Availability Statement: The data presented in this study are available on request from the corresponding author. The data are not publicly available due to ethical restrictions.

Conflicts of Interest: Dr. Ash Tewari has served as a site PI on pharma-/industry-sponsored clinical trials from Kite Pharma, Lumicell Inc., Dendreon and Oncovir Inc. His institution has received research funding (grants) from DOD, NIH, Axogen, Intuitive Surgical, AMBFF and other philanthropical organizations. Dr. A.K. Tewari has served as an unpaid consultant for Roivant Biosciences and advisor to Promaxo. He owns equity in Promaxo. The rest of the authors do not have conflict of interest.

References

1. Zaytoun, O.M.; Jones, J.S. Prostate cancer detection after a negative prostate biopsy: Lessons learnt in the Cleveland Clinic experience. *Int. J. Urol.* **2011**, *18*, 557–568. [CrossRef] [PubMed]
2. Heidenreich, A.; Aus, G.; Bolla, M.; Joniau, S.; Matveev, V.B.; Schmid, H.P.; Zattoni, F. EAU guidelines on prostate cancer. *Eur. Urol.* **2008**, *53*, 68–80. [CrossRef] [PubMed]
3. Scattoni, V.; Zlotta, A.; Montironi, R.; Schulman, C.; Rigatti, P.; Montorsi, F. Extended and saturation prostatic biopsy in the diagnosis and characterisation of prostate cancer: A critical analysis of the literature. *Eur. Urol.* **2007**, *52*, 1309–1322. [CrossRef]
4. Roehl, K.A.; Antenor, J.A.; Catalona, W.J. Serial biopsy results in prostate cancer screening study. *J. Urol.* **2002**, *167*, 2435–2439. [CrossRef] [PubMed]
5. Serefoglu, E.C.; Altinova, S.; Ugras, N.S.; Akincioglu, E.; Asil, E.; Balbay, M.D. How reliable is 12-core prostate biopsy procedure in the detection of prostate cancer? *Can. Urol. Assoc. J.* **2013**, *7*, E293–E298. [CrossRef]
6. Sonn, G.A.; Chang, E.; Natarajan, S.; Margolis, D.J.; Macairan, M.; Lieu, P.; Huang, J.; Dorey, F.J.; Reiter, R.E.; Marks, L.S. Value of targeted prostate biopsy using magnetic resonance-ultrasound fusion in men with prior negative biopsy and elevated prostate-specific antigen. *Eur. Urol.* **2014**, *65*, 809–815. [CrossRef]
7. Valerio, M.; Donaldson, I.; Emberton, M.; Ehdaie, B.; Hadaschik, B.A.; Marks, L.S.; Mozer, P.; Rastinehad, A.R.; Ahmed, H.U. Detection of Clinically Significant Prostate Cancer Using Magnetic Resonance Imaging-Ultrasound Fusion Targeted Biopsy: A Systematic Review. *Eur. Urol.* **2015**, *68*, 8–19. [CrossRef]

8. Tonttila, P.P.; Lantto, J.; Pääkkö, E.; Piippo, U.; Kauppila, S.; Lammentausta, E.; Ohtonen, P.; Vaarala, M.H. Prebiopsy Multiparametric Magnetic Resonance Imaging for Prostate Cancer Diagnosis in Biopsy-naive Men with Suspected Prostate Cancer Based on Elevated Prostate-specific Antigen Values: Results from a Randomized Prospective Blinded Controlled Trial. Eur. Urol. 2016, 69, 419–425. [CrossRef]
9. Wagaskar, V.G.; Levy, M.; Ratnani, P.; Moody, K.; Garcia, M.; Pedraza, A.M.; Parekh, S.; Pandav, K.; Shukla, B.; Prasad, S.; et al. Clinical Utility of Negative Multiparametric Magnetic Resonance Imaging in the Diagnosis of Prostate Cancer and Clinically Significant Prostate Cancer. Eur. Urol. Open Sci. 2021, 28, 9–16. [CrossRef]
10. Wagaskar, V.G.; Ratnani, P.; Levy, M.; Moody, K.; Garcia, M.; Pedraza, A.M.; Parekh, S.; Pandav, K.; Shukla, B.; Sobotka, S.; et al. Clinical characteristics and oncological outcomes in negative multiparametric MRI patients undergoing robot-assisted radical prostatectomy. Prostate 2021, 81, 772–777. [CrossRef]
11. Weinreb, J.C.; Barentsz, J.O.; Choyke, P.L.; Cornud, F.; Haider, M.A.; Macura, K.J.; Margolis, D.; Schnall, M.D.; Shtern, F.; Tempany, C.M.; et al. PI-RADS Prostate Imaging-Reporting and Data System: 2015, Version 2. Eur. Urol. 2016, 69, 16–40. [CrossRef] [PubMed]
12. Kanao, K.; Kajikawa, K.; Kobayashi, I.; Muramatsu, H.; Morinaga, S.; Nishikawa, G.; Kato, Y.; Watanabe, M.; Nakamura, K.; Sumitomo, M. Utility of a novel biopsy instrument with long side-notch needle in the selection of patients for active surveillance. J. Clin. Oncol. 2017, 35 (Suppl. 15), e16581. [CrossRef]
13. Wagaskar, V.G.; Zaytoun, O.; Kale, P.; Pedraza, A.; Haines, K., 3rd; Tewari, A. Robot-assisted simple prostatectomy for prostates greater than 100 g. World J. Urol. 2023, 41, 1169–1174. [CrossRef] [PubMed]
14. Protocol for the Examination of Radical Prostatectomy Specimens from Patients with Carcinoma of the Prostate Gland. Available online: https://documents.cap.org/protocols/Prostate_4.2.0.0.REL_CAPCP.pdf (accessed on 8 February 2023).
15. Epstein, J.I.; Zelefsky, M.J.; Sjoberg, D.D.; Nelson, J.B.; Egevad, L.; Magi-Galluzzi, C.; Vickers, A.J.; Parwani, A.V.; Reuter, V.E.; Fine, S.W.; et al. A Contemporary Prostate Cancer Grading System: A Validated Alternative to the Gleason Score. Eur. Urol. 2016, 69, 428–435. [CrossRef]
16. Wagaskar, V.G.; Sobotka, S.; Ratnani, P.; Young, J.; Lantz, A.; Parekh, S.; Falagario, U.G.; Li, L.; Lewis, S.; Haines, K., 3rd; et al. A 4K score/MRI-based nomogram for predicting prostate cancer, clinically significant prostate cancer, and unfavorable prostate cancer. Cancer Rep. 2021, 4, e1357. [CrossRef]
17. Wagaskar, V.G.; Levy, M.; Ratnani, P.; Sullimada, S.; Gerenia, M.; Schlussel, K.; Choudhury, S.; Gabriele, M.; Haas, I.; Haines, K., 3rd; et al. A SelectMDx/magnetic resonance imaging-based nomogram to diagnose prostate cancer. Cancer Rep. 2023, 6, e1668. [CrossRef]
18. Wagaskar, V.G.; Lantz, A.; Sobotka, S.; Ratnani, P.; Parekh, S.; Falagario, U.G.; Li, L.; Lewis, S.; Haines Iii, K.; Punnen, S.; et al. Development and External Validation of a Prediction Model to Identify Candidates for Prostate Biopsy. Urol. J. 2022, 19, 379–385. [PubMed]
19. Parker, M. Chapter 18-Radar Basics. In Digital Signal Processing 101, 2nd ed.; Parker, M., Ed.; Newnes: London, UK, 2017; pp. 231–240.
20. Oishi, M.; Shin, T.; Ohe, C.; Nassiri, N.; Palmer, S.L.; Aron, M.; Ashrafi, A.N.; Cacciamani, G.E.; Chen, F.; Duddalwar, V.; et al. Which Patients with Negative Magnetic Resonance Imaging Can Safely Avoid Biopsy for Prostate Cancer? J. Urol. 2019, 201, 268–276. [CrossRef]
21. Ahmed, H.U.; El-Shater Bosaily, A.; Brown, L.C.; Gabe, R.; Kaplan, R.; Parmar, M.K.; Collaco-Moraes, Y.; Ward, K.; Hindley, R.G.; Freeman, A.; et al. Diagnostic accuracy of multi-parametric MRI and TRUS biopsy in prostate cancer (PROMIS): A paired validating confirmatory study. Lancet 2017, 389, 815–822. [CrossRef]
22. Cheng, L.; Mazzucchelli, R.; Jones, T.D.; Lopez-Beltran, A.; Montironi, R. Chapter 3—The Pathology of Prostate Cancer. In Early Diagnosis and Treatment of Cancer Series: Prostate Cancer; Su, L.-M., Ed.; W.B. Saunders: Philadelphia, PA, USA, 2010; pp. 45–83.
23. Kim, J.J.; Kim, T.; Lee, H.; Byun, S.S.; Lee, S.E.; Choe, G.; Hong, S.K. Prediction of unilateral prostate cancer by the combination of transrectal ultrasonography-guided prostate biopsy and multi-parametric magnetic resonance imaging: A real-life experience. PLoS ONE 2018, 13, e0202872.
24. Kim, J.J.; Byun, S.-S.; Lee, S.E.; Lee, H.J.; Choe, G.; Hong, S.K. A negative multiparametric magnetic resonance imaging finding does not guarantee the absence of significant cancer among biopsy-proven prostate cancer patients: A real-life clinical experience. Int. Urol. Nephrol. 2018, 50, 1989–1997. [CrossRef] [PubMed]

Disclaimer/Publisher's Note: The statements, opinions and data contained in all publications are solely those of the individual author(s) and contributor(s) and not of MDPI and/or the editor(s). MDPI and/or the editor(s) disclaim responsibility for any injury to people or property resulting from any ideas, methods, instructions or products referred to in the content.

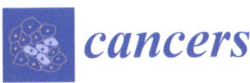

Article

Primary Total Prostate Cryoablation for Localized High-Risk Prostate Cancer: 10-Year Outcomes and Nomograms

Chung-Hsin Chen [1], Chung-You Tsai [2,3] and Yeong-Shiau Pu [1,*]

1. Department of Urology, National Taiwan University Hospital, Taipei 10002, Taiwan; chunghsinchen2@ntu.edu.tw
2. Division of Urology, Department of Surgery, Far Eastern Memorial Hospital, New Taipei City 22000, Taiwan; pgtsai@mail.femh.org.tw
3. Department of Electrical Engineering, Yuan Ze University, Taoyuan City 32003, Taiwan
* Correspondence: yspu@ntu.edu.tw; Tel.: +886-2-2312-3456 (ext. 65249); Fax: +886-2-2321-9145

Simple Summary: The role of prostate cryoablation was still uncertain for patients with high-risk prostate cancer (PC). This study was designed to investigate the 10-year outcomes and establish a nomogram for high-risk PC patients. We found prostate cryoablation to be an effective treatment option for selected men with high-risk PC. A preoperative nomogram that predicts biochemical recurrence would be useful for both patients and physicians to make clinical decisions when considering prostate cryoablation among other treatment modalities. A peri-operative nomogram that includes diagnostic PSA, PSA nadir, Gleason sum, and the number of cryoprobes deployed helps inform increased risk of biochemical recurrence, which would then justify early salvage treatments.

Abstract: The role of prostate cryoablation was still uncertain for patients with high-risk prostate cancer (PC). This study was designed to investigate 10-year disease-free survival and establish a nomogram in localized high-risk PC patients. Between October 2008 and December 2020, 191 patients with high-risk PC who received primary total prostate cryoablation (PTPC) were enrolled. The primary endpoint was biochemical recurrence (BCR), defined using Phoenix criteria. The performance of pre-operative and peri-operative nomograms was determined using the Harrell concordance index (C-index). Among the cohort, the median age and PSA levels at diagnosis were 71 years and 12.3 ng/mL, respectively. Gleason sum 8–10, stage ≥ T3a, and PSA > 20 ng/mL were noted in 27.2%, 74.4%, and 26.2% of patients, respectively. During the median follow-up duration of 120.4 months, BCR-free rates at 1, 3, 5, and 10 years were 92.6%, 76.6%, 66.7%, and 50.8%, respectively. The metastasis-free, cancer-specific, and overall survival rates were 89.5%, 97.4%, and 90.5% at 10 years, respectively. The variables in the pre-operative nomogram for BCR contained PSA at diagnosis, clinical stage, and Gleason score (C-index: 0.73, 95% CI, 0.67–0.79). The variables in the peri-operative nomogram for BCR included PSA at diagnosis, Gleason score, number of cryoprobes used, and PSA nadir (C-index: 0.83, 95% CI, 0.78–0.88). In conclusion, total prostate cryoablation appears to be an effective treatment option for selected men with high-risk PC. A pre-operative nomogram can help select patients suitable for cryoablation. A peri-operative nomogram signifies the importance of the ample use of cryoprobes and helps identify patients who may need early salvage treatment.

Keywords: cryotherapy; nomogram; outcome prediction; biochemical failure; prostate malignancy; recurrence

1. Introduction

Localized prostate cancer (PC) can be managed via several treatment options, including radical prostatectomy (RP), radiation therapy (RT), cryoablation, high-intensity focused ultrasound, and active surveillance/watchful waiting [1]. Among them, cryoablation is less recommended for patients with localized high-risk PC defined by at least one component

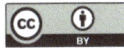

of prostate-specific antigen (PSA) > 20 ng/mL, Gleason grade group of 4 or 5, and clinical T stage of T2c or more [1,2]. However, its advantages of short hospital stay, minimal anesthesia, and rapid recovery due to the minimally invasive nature provide benefit to aged patients or those with multiple comorbidities [2–5]. Furthermore, focal cryoablation in highly select patients leads to few adverse events and preserves most functional outcomes [6,7]. In the aspect of oncological outcomes, a satisfactory 5-year biochemical recurrence (BCR)-free rate of 62.2% in patients with high-risk PC was reported by the Cryo On-Line Database (COLD) Registry, the largest database regarding prostate cryoablation in the world [3]. Although the treatment failure rate of primary total prostate cryoablation (PTPC) was significantly higher in patients with high-risk compared to intermediate- or low-risk PC [3], it was also high in high-risk PC treated with RP (5-year disease-free survival (DFS) rate, 38–65%) [8,9] or RT plus androgen deprivation therapy (ADT) (5-year DFS rate, 62–74%) [8,9]. PTPC may be still feasible for selected patients with high-risk PC. Until recently, long-term (10-year) oncological outcomes for high-risk PC patients and nomograms predicting recurrences were still lacking. To provide better clinical decision-making, we herein report the cohort of PTPC for patients with high-risk PC.

2. Materials and Methods

2.1. Patient Population

Between October 2008 and December 2020, consecutive patients with localized PC who received PTPC at National Taiwan University Hospital were prospectively collected. Bone scintigraphy and multi-parametric magnetic resonance imaging (MRI) were applied for the initial tumor staging in all patients. Among them, only patients with high-risk disease defined by EAU guidelines 2023 [2] were enrolled in the current study. (Flow diagram in Supplementary Figure S1) This study was reviewed and approved by Research Ethics Committee A of National Taiwan University Hospital (202204097RINA). We previously published the short-term results of our entire patient cohort, including non-high-risk disease [4].

2.2. Clinical Information Collection

Clinicopathological data regarding patient age, prostate size measured via transrectal ultrasound, pre-operative PSA, biopsy Gleason sum, clinical T stage, tumor location in MRI, neoadjuvant ADT, the amount of cryoprobes used intraoperatively, follow-up PSA values, time to BCR, recurrence patterns, and survival were prospectively collected. Clinical T stage was determined by means of either digital rectal examination or seminal vesicle biopsy prior to PTPC. Nine patients with clinical T3b disease were defined according to the result of seminal vesicle biopsy. Neoadjuvant ADT that usually took 4–12 weeks was mainly to reduce prostate size when the anterior–posterior diameter exceeded 35 mm to facilitate the cryoablation procedure. Twenty patients received adjuvant ADT under a clinical trial setting [10].

All cryoablation procedures were performed by the single surgical team, Drs. CH Chen and YS Pu. The detailed surgical procedures were described in the previous published article [11]. All patients were followed using the same protocol, including PSA every 3 months in the first year, every 6 months in the 2nd to 5th years, and then annually. The primary outcome was BCR, which was determined using the Phoenix criteria, i.e., PSA increase of ≥ 2 ng/mL above the nadir [12]. Upon BCR, we commended early restaging and early salvage therapy for these high-risk PC patients based on the consensus of the European Association of Urology Prostate Cancer Guidelines Panel [13]. Hence, we advised prostate and seminal biopsy, whole-body computed tomography/MRI imaging, and/or whole-body PET-CT scan (^{18}F-choline or ^{68}Ga-PSMA) to distinguish between local and distant failure. For patients with negative biopsy or unwilling to have a prostate biopsy, a whole-body PET-CT scan (^{18}F-choline or ^{68}Ga-PSMA) was conducted as an alternative. The primary outcome was BCR determined using the Phoenix criteria calculated from the serial follow-up PSA value.

2.3. Statistical Consideration

Contingency tables were constructed for comparisons using the Chi-square test. Non-parametric data were compared with the Mann–Whitney U rank-sum method to compare medians between groups. The log-rank test and Cox proportional hazards model were used to compare the BCR risk. All these analyses were conducted using R software, version 3.6.1 (http://www.r-project.org/, accessed on 1 September 2021). All tests were two-tailed with $p < 0.05$ indicating a significant difference.

The original patient cohort was randomly split into two cohorts: one (80% of patients) served as the training cohort for developing the predictive prognostic models, and the other (20%) as the validation cohort for external validation (Supplementary Table S1). Univariable and multivariable Cox proportional hazard models were applied to address the time to BCR after cryoablation. Multivariable Cox regression coefficients were used to generate prognostic nomograms. We intended to generate two prognostic nomograms: pre- and peri-operative predictive nomograms. Only pre-operative variables were incorporated into the pre-operative nomogram, while both pre- and peri-operative variables were used in the peri-operative nomogram. The final models were selected using a bidirectional stepwise regression process, which used the Akaike information criterion as a stopping rule [14]. The nomograms were constructed using the *survival* and *rms* packages in R [15].

The model performance for predicting the BCR-free survival was determined using the Harrell concordance index (C-index) [16]. To avoid the arbitrariness of cohort splitting, the bias-corrected C-index was further calculated using repeated five-fold cross-validation 20 times and 1000 bootstrapping methods for the entire cohort. Calibration plots were constructed to compare the nomogram-predicted probability of BCR-free survival at 1, 3, 5, and 7 years with the actual survival probability.

3. Results

3.1. Patient Demographics and Tumor Characteristics

A total of 233 consecutive PC patients who received PTPC were enrolled. Forty-two subjects were excluded because of low- or intermediate-risk disease. The median age of the remaining 191 high-risk PC patients was 71 years (range 48–88 years), and the median PSA value at diagnosis was 12.3 ng/mL (range 2–45.9 ng/mL; Table 1). The median time to BCR was 34.5 months and the 5-year BCR-free rate was 66.7%. There was PSA < 10, 10–20, and >20 ng/mL for 40.3%, 33.5%, and 26.2% of patients, respectively. About half of the patients had a Gleason sum $\geq 4 + 3$ (49.7%). Clinical T3a or above occurred in 74.4% of patients. Visible tumor lesions on MRI (PI-RADS 3–5) were noted in 83.3% of patients. Tumors located at the anterior apical prostate, which might be difficult to be treated [17], were identified in 29 (15.2%) patients. Neoadjuvant ADT for ≤ 3 and >3 months was applied in 94 (49.2%) and 9 (4.7%) patients, respectively. Twenty (10.5%) patients were given adjuvant ADT for 12 months under a prospective randomized study. Figure 1 shows that the higher the number of high-risk factors based on EAU guidelines 2023 (PSA, Gleason, and stage) that patients had, the faster the BCR occurred.

Table 1. Demographics of high-risk prostate cancer patients stratified by the status of biochemical failure.

Groups	All		No BCR		BCR		p Value
Patient number (n)	191	100.00%	111	58.1%	80	41.90%	
Median age (years, range)	71 (48–88)		72 (52–88)		69 (48–87)		0.014
Median PSA at diagnosis (ng/mL, range)	12.3 (2.0–45.9)		10.0 (2.0–45.9)		15.4 (4.5–44)		<0.001
PSA at diagnosis (ng/mL)							0.003
<10	77	40.31%	56	50.45%	21	26.25%	
10~20	64	33.51%	33	29.73%	31	38.75%	
>20	50	26.18%	22	19.82%	28	35.00%	

Table 1. Cont.

Groups	All		No BCR		BCR		p Value
Biopsy Gleason sum							0.004
≤6	35	18.32%	26	23.42%	9	11.25%	
3 + 4 = 7	61	31.94%	42	37.84%	19	23.75%	
4 + 3 = 7	43	22.51%	21	18.92%	22	27.50%	
8~10	52	27.23%	22	19.82%	30	37.50%	
Clinical T stage							0.006
T1c	8	4.19%	5	4.50%	3	3.75%	
T2a-2c	41	21.47%	29	26.13%	12	15.00%	
T3a	80	41.88%	52	46.85%	28	35.00%	
T3b	62	32.46%	25	22.52%	37	46.25%	
Visible lesions on MRI							0.084
No	32	16.75%	23	20.72%	9	11.25%	
Yes	159	83.25%	88	79.28%	71	88.75%	
Anterior apical tumor							0.449
No	162	84.82%	96	86.49%	66	82.50%	
Yes	29	15.18%	15	13.51%	14	17.50%	
Neoadjuvant hormonal therapy							0.153
No	88	46.07%	56	50.45%	32	40.00%	
Yes	103	53.93%	55	49.55%	48	60.00%	
Adjuvant hormonal therapy							0.437
No	171	89.53%	101	90.99%	70	87.50%	
Yes	20	10.47%	10	9.01%	10	12.50%	
Prostate volume (median in mL, range)	26.9 (11.9–81.9)		26.9 (11.9–81.9)		26.8 (12.6–64.0)		0.689
Cryoprobe number (median, range)	6 (5–9)		6 (5–8)		6 (5–9)		0.351
PSA nadir value (ng/mL)							<0.001
<0.01	87	45.55%	66	59.46%	21	26.25%	
0.01~<0.1	66	34.55%	35	31.53%	31	38.75%	
0.1~<0.5	27	14.14%	9	8.11%	18	22.50%	
0.5~	11	5.76%	1	0.90%	10	12.50%	
Time to PSA nadir (weeks)							0.084
<8	71	37.17%	34	28.57%	37	51.39%	
8~<12	76	39.79%	48	40.34%	28	38.89%	
12~	44	23.04%	29	24.37%	15	20.83%	

BCR = biochemical recurrence; PSA = prostate-specific antigen; CI = confidence interval; MRI = magnetic resonance imaging.

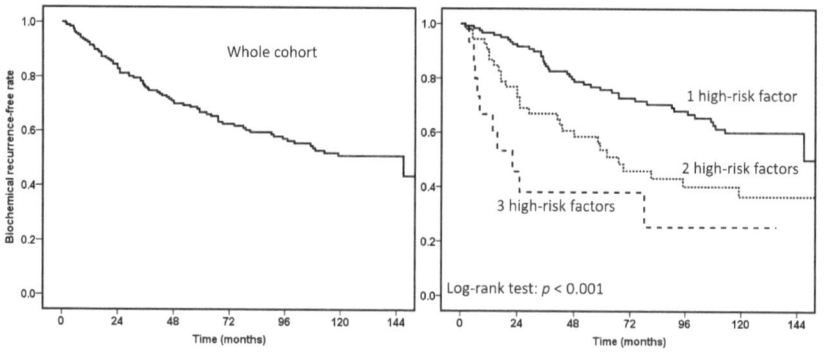

Figure 1. The Kaplan–Meier curve of biochemical failures in the high-risk prostate cancer patients receiving primary total prostate cryoablation. The high-risk factors were defined based on EAU guidelines 2023 and included Gleason sum of 8 or more, PSA value of 20 ng/mL or more, and clinical stage T3a or more.

3.2. Univariable and Multivariable Analyses Predicting BCR

Among the 191 patients, 111 (58.1%) remained BCR-free after a median follow-up duration of 120.4 months (IQR 63–137.7 months). Compared to patients without BCR, those with BCR (n = 80) tended to be younger (median 69 vs. 72 years, $p = 0.014$) and have higher PSA at diagnosis (median 15.4 vs. 10.0 ng/mL, $p < 0.001$), higher Gleason sum (8–10, 37.5% vs. 19.8%, $p = 0.004$), and higher clinical T stage ($\geq$T3b 46.3% vs. 22.5%, $p = 0.006$) (Table 1). There was no significant difference in prostate size, amount of cryoprobes used, the proportion of visible lesions on MRI, anterior apical tumors, or proportion of subjects receiving neoadjuvant ADT and adjuvant ADT between patients with and without BCR.

After PTPC, 77.0% of patients reached the PSA nadir within 3 months post-operatively. Eighty-seven (45.6%) patients had a PSA nadir value < 0.01 ng/mL. The PSA nadir values were significantly higher in men with subsequent BCR than those without ($p < 0.001$). For patients with a PSA nadir $\geq$ 0.5 ng/mL, up to 10 (91%) out 11 patients experienced BCR. In comparison, only 24.1% (21/87) of patients had BCR if the post-cryoablation PSA nadir was <0.01 ng/mL.

In the multivariable analysis of the pre-operative parameters, higher PSA, higher Gleason sum, and higher clinical T stage independently predicted BCR (Table 2). For the peri-operative predictive model, the multivariable analysis revealed that significant independent predictors for BCR included higher PSA, higher Gleason sum, fewer or inadequate number of cryoprobes used, and higher PSA nadir value (Table 2). More cryoprobes used appeared to lower the risk of BCR, suggesting that the effective coverage of cancer areas through adequately overlapping the cryoablation kill zone was crucial for treating high-risk PC. The PSA nadir value was the most powerful predictor in the peri-operative predictive model for BCR. Compared to patients with PSA nadir < 0.01 ng/mL, those with a nadir of 0.01 to <0.1 (hazard ratio (HR) = 2.98, 95% confidence interval (CI) 1.68–5.26), 0.1 to <0.5 (HR = 6.32, 95% CI 3.26–12.3), and $\geq$0.5 ng/mL (HR = 37.98, 95% CI 15.5–93.1) had significantly elevated risk of BCR. Although the time to PSA nadir was associated with BCR in the univariable analysis, it was a non-significant factor for BCR in the multivariable model because of the strong association with PSA nadir (Supplementary Table S2).

3.3. Predictive Nomograms and Calibration

To predict BCR-free survival probability, pre- and peri-operative nomograms (Figure 2) were constructed according to the multivariable predictive models. Three parameters were included in the pre-operative nomogram: PSA at diagnosis, biopsy Gleason sum, and clinical T stage. Four parameters were incorporated in the peri-operative nomogram: PSA at diagnosis, PSA nadir, biopsy Gleason sum, and number of cryoprobes used.

In the training cohort, the C-indexes for the pre- and peri-operative nomograms were 0.74 (95% CI 0.67–0.79) and 0.82 (95% CI 0.76–0.88), respectively. For the validation cohort, C-indexes were 0.76 (95% CI 0.61–0.91) and 0.84 (95% CI 0.69–0.99), respectively. Bias-corrected C-indexes for the two nomograms were 0.70 and 0.80, respectively. The calibration plots showed satisfactory agreement in the BCR-free survival probabilities calculated from either the nomograms or the actual survival data for both pre- and peri-operative nomograms (Figure 3).

Table 2. Univariable and multivariable analyses of biochemical recurrence in high-risk prostate cancer patients receiving primary total prostate cryoablation.

Variables	Case No.	Failure Events	Univariable Analysis			Multivariable Analysis					
						Preoperative Model			Peri-Operative Model		
			HR	Range	p Value	HR	Range	p Value	HR	Range	p Value
Pre-operative											
Age (year)	191	80	0.98	0.95–1.01	0.145	–	–	–	–	–	–
PSA at diagnosis (ng/mL)								0.001 *			<0.001 *
<10	77	21	1			1			1		
10–<20	64	31	2.01	1.15–3.50	0.014	1.93	1.10–3.38	0.022	2.48	1.38–4.46	0.002
20–<50	50	28	3.15	1.78–5.57	<0.001	2.75	1.54–4.91	0.001	3.68	1.91–7.09	<0.001
Biopsy Gleason sum								0.001 *			0.001
–6	35	9	1			1			1		
3 + 4 = 7	61	19	1.1	0.50–2.43	0.817	1.11	0.50–2.46	0.804	1.03	0.45–2.34	0.941
4 + 3 = 7	43	22	2.26	1.04–4.92	0.039	2.3	1.05–5.02	0.037	2.90	1.31–6.37	0.009
8–10	52	30	3.01	1.49–6.64	0.003	2.4	1.12–5.13	0.024	2.44	1.13–5.24	0.023
Clinical T stage								0.007			
T1c-2c	49	15	1			1			–	–	–
T3a	80	28	1.07	0.57–2.00	0.833	1.08	0.57–2.04	0.809	–	–	–
T3b	62	37	2.62	1.43–4.78	0.002	2.18	1.18–4.00	0.012	–	–	–
Visible lesions on MRI											
Yes	159	71	1			–	–	–	–	–	–
No	32	9	0.52	0.56–1.04	0.063	–	–	–	–	–	–
Anterior apical tumor											
No	162	66	1			–	–	–	–	–	–
Yes	29	14	1.31	0.74–2.33	0.361	–	–	–	–	–	–
Neoadjuvant hormonal therapy											
No	88	32	1			–	–	–	–	–	–
Yes	103	48	1.42	0.91–2.22	0.126	–	–	–	–	–	–
Prostate volume (mL)	191	80	1	0.98–1.02	0.908	–	–	–	–	–	–
Post-operative											
Cryoprobe number	191	80	0.87	0.70–1.10	0.239	–	–	–	0.69	0.53–0.92	0.002
Adjuvant hormonal therapy											
No	171	70	1			–	–	–	–	–	–
Yes	20	10	1.1	0.57–2.14	0.778	–	–	–	–	–	–
PSA nadir value (ng/mL)											<0.001 *
<0.01	87	21	1			–	–	–	1		
0.01–<0.1	66	31	2.37	1.36–4.14	0.002	–	–	–	2.98	1.68–5.26	<0.001
0.1–<0.5	27	18	6.56	3.46–12.5	<0.001	–	–	–	6.32	3.26–12.3	<0.001
0.5–	11	10	28.44	12.7–63.6	<0.001	–	–	–	37.98	15.5–93.1	<0.001
Time to PSA nadir (weeks)											
<8	71	37	1			–	–	–	–	–	–
8–<12	77	28	0.52	0.32–0.85	0.009	–	–	–	–	–	–
12–	43	15	0.48	0.27–0.89	0.019	–	–	–	–	–	–

PSA = prostate-specific antigen; HR = hazard ratio; MRI = magnetic resonance imaging; * p value of the variables which were considered to be ordered.

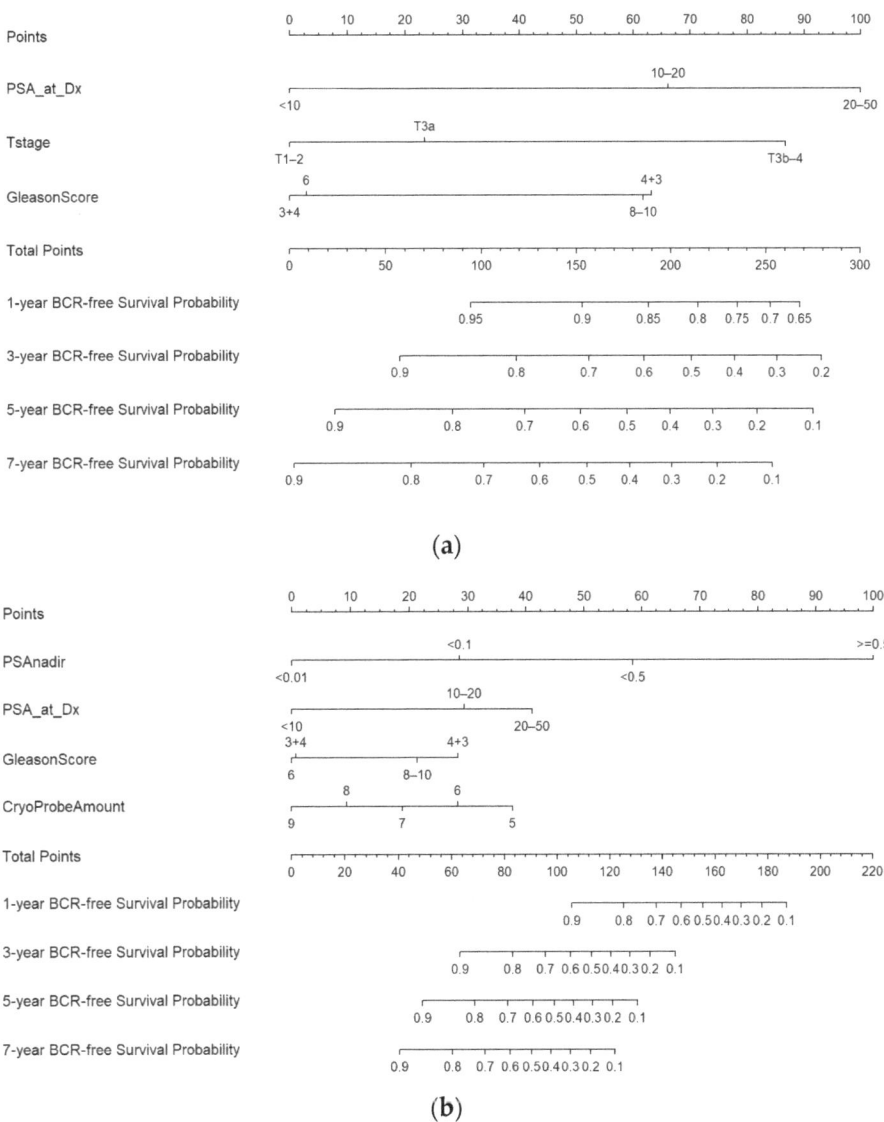

Figure 2. The nomograms for predicting biochemical recurrence in the high-risk or very high-risk prostate cancer patients: pre-operatively (**a**) and peri-operatively (**b**).

3.4. Pathological and Radiographic Evidence of Recurrence

The BCR-free rate at 1, 2, 3, 5, 7, and 10 years was 92.6%, 84.5%, 76.6%, 66.7%, 59.5%, and 50.8%, respectively (Figure 1). Among the 80 patients with BCR, 44 (55%) local recurrences were detected via either prostate biopsy ($n = 38$) or imaging studies ($n = 6$). Metastasis to the pelvic lymph node, bone, and both were found in 13 (16.3%), six (7.5%), and one (1.3%) patient, respectively. The remaining 16 (20.0%) patients who had BCR did not have any pathological or radiographic evidence of local recurrence or distant metastases. The estimated 10-year metastasis-free rate was 89.5% using Kaplan–Meier method. There was no visceral metastasis upon the identification of BCR. Two patients had lung metastases in 58 and 64 months after BCR. Three of the 191 patients had died of PC by the date of report preparation (January 2023). Eleven patients died of cardiovascular diseases, infection and other cancers. The estimated 10-year cancer-specific and overall survival rates were 97.4% and 90.5%.

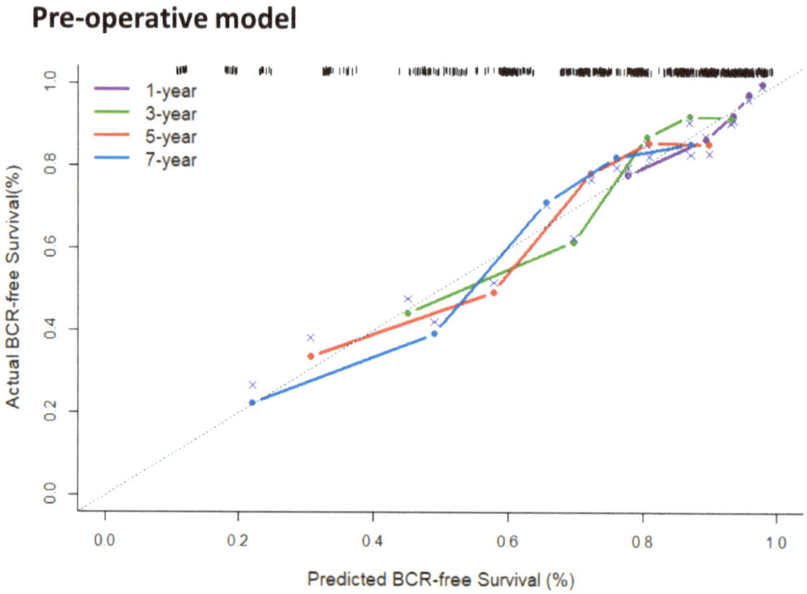

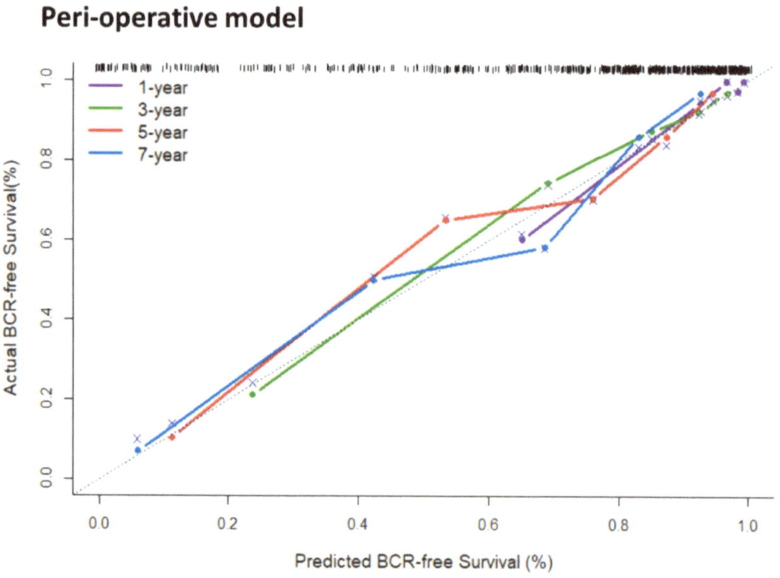

Figure 3. The calibration of the nomograms predicting biochemical failures: pre-operatively (**a**) and peri-operatively (**b**). BCR = biochemical recurrence. Remark "x": resampling optimism added.

3.5. Complications

A total of 44 (23.0%) patients had complications after PTPC in this cohort. The most common complication was bladder outlet obstruction ($n = 30$, 15.7%), which included bladder neck contracture ($n = 8$, 4.2%), urethral stricture ($n = 8$, 4.2%), urethral sloughing ($n = 10$, 5.2%), urethral stone ($n = 1$, 0.5%), and mixed type ($n = 3$, 1.6%). Eighteen (9.4%) patients had infection-related events, such as epididymitis ($n = 3$, 1.6%), prostatitis ($n = 8$, 4.2%), and urethrocystitis ($n = 7$, 3.7%). Among 81 patients with potency before PTPC, 9 (11.1%) recovered their erectile function with or without medication. No cryoprobe penetration wound infection was noted. Long-term urinary incontinence was observed in five (2.6%) patients. Transfusion was used for two (1.0%) patients. One patient encountered a suspected sigmoid injury which was handled with parenteral nutrition for 7 days and was discharged without any sequelae.

4. Discussion

Total prostate cryoablation is an alternative treatment option for localized PC, especially for low- and intermediate-risk disease [5,18]. Our data showed, in terms of BCR after a long-term follow-up duration, that PTPC provided adequate 10-year cancer control in 50.8% of patients with high-risk disease, which is generally comparable with historical control using other treatment modalities, such as RP [8,9] or RT [8,9]. The conventional pre-operative clinicopathological parameters, including PSA at diagnosis, Gleason sum, and clinical T stage helped predict BCR after PTPC. In the peri-operative setting, except for PSA at diagnosis and Gleason sum, PSA nadir and number of cryoprobes used comprised a powerful predictive model for BCR. The two models or nomograms provide valuable tools to inform clinical decision-making and prognostic information in PTPC. In addition, the peri-operative nomogram may help not only identify men at an increased risk of failure but also advise early salvage therapy.

Compared to lower risks, patients with high-risk disease have increased local recurrence and treatment failure rates regardless of treatment modality applied [1,8,9]. Therefore, the European Association of Urology guidelines suggested physicians offer multimodal therapy for the patients with high-risk localized PC [19]. Retrospective studies reported that the 5-year DFS rate with RP and RT was 38–65% and 62–74%, respectively [8,9]. In comparison, the COLD Registry and our series of PTPC demonstrated comparable outcomes of 62% and 66.7% for the 5-year BCR-free survival rate, respectively [3]. Although the definition of treatment failure differs between treatment modalities, that for RT and PTPC use the same Phoenix criteria. The BCR-free rates for high-risk disease between PTPC in our cohort and RT plus ADT [9] were similar at 5 (66.7% vs. 72%) and 10 years (46% vs. 53%), respectively. Since differences in demographics and tumor characteristics between patient populations may significantly affect clinical outcomes, it is inappropriate to compare these numbers directly. For example, clinical T3 disease was more frequent in our cohort (74%) than the RT cohort (14%). In contrast, the RT cohort had a higher proportion of PSA $\geq$ 20 ng/mL (36% vs. 26%) and Gleason score 8–10 (41% vs. 27%) compared with our PTPC cohort.

The addition of long-term adjuvant ADT to definitive RT has become a standard-of-care option for localized high-risk PC [20,21]. It was not clear whether adjuvant ADT would benefit patients receiving PTPC. In a small-scale ($n = 38$) prospective randomized study, adjuvant ADT for 12 months did not reduce BCR in patients with high-risk PC receiving PTPC [10]. The benefit of adjuvant ADT in PTPC may be minimal or uncertain and should be further investigated in large-scale studies. In our series, 103 (53.9%) had received neoadjuvant ADT to reduce prostate size before cryoablation. Only nine patients received neoadjuvant ADT for more than 3 months. However, our univariable analysis showed that neoadjuvant ADT did not significantly influence BCR-free survival ($p = 0.126$). In addition, we found no significant association between neoadjuvant ADT and PSA nadir after cryoablation (Supplementary Table S3).

The PSA nadir values have been identified as an important prognostic factor for clinical outcomes after PTPC. Tay et al. reported that patients with PSA nadir < 0.4 ng/mL in the COLD Registry had a significantly better 5-year DFS of about 70%, compared to those with PSA nadir ≥ 0.4 ng/mL where most patients failed within 5 years [22]. The multivariable analysis revealed that PSA nadir was a powerful prognosticator for BCR [22]. Many other Western reports [22,23] and our data on Asian men also showed consistent results in that PSA nadir values significantly predicted the treatment failures after PTPC. We also found that the earlier the PSA nadir was reached (<8 weeks), the higher the chance of BCR, suggesting that post-cryoablation residual cancer nests drove PSA recurrence and shortened the time to PSA nadir.

The number of cryoprobes used was a significant predictor of BCR in the multivariable peri-operative regression model. In general, the number of cryoprobes to be deployed in PTPC depends on several factors, including but not limited to prostate size, shape, and specific tumor locations [17]. Saturated prostate cryoablation via setting more cryoprobes and reducing the prostate volume to be covered per probe would improve cancer control [4]. A higher number of cryoprobes will reduce any possible inadequate ablation zone in the prostate and ensure that the overlapping ice balls in the prostate reach a substantially low killing temperature. These findings suggest that proactive and ample use of cryoprobes to cover as complete a prostate region as possible may reduce inadequate ablation zone and subsequent recurrence, especially when dealing with high-risk tumors.

Total prostate cryoablation had an acceptable rate of side effects in our patients with high-risk PC. Although infection-associated complications, such as epididymitis, prostatitis, and urethrocystitis, were up to 9.4%, all patients recovered well using the appropriate antibiotics. As a minimally invasive surgery [24], no infection at the penetration wound of the cryoprobes and thermoprobes was noted in our patients. The long-term continence rate, defined as 1 or less pad a day, was 97.4% and comparable to those of RP and RT series [25,26]. Bladder outlet obstruction resulting from bladder neck contracture, urethral stricture, and urethral sloughing was relatively higher in our high-risk PC patients than low- to intermediate-risk PC patients [3]. The possible reason was the intention to ablate as much of the prostate as possible and, subsequently, to break the protection zone of the urethral warming catheter in high-risk PC patients. Nevertheless, all these patients experienced improvement using endourological methods. In our high-risk cohort, we did not observe the most serious complication, namely, rectourethral fistula. A possible sigmoid injury was noted during prostate cryoablation in one patient, who was supported with total parenteral nutrition for one week and discharged without any sequelae. Considering high-risk PC patients, the complication rate of PTPC was acceptable and comparable to a non-nerve-sparing prostatectomy or radiation therapy plus androgen deprivation, which were considered as the preferred treatment options [1]. We did not identify significant clinical predictors for complications after PTPC in our series. The major reason was the patient selection bias. For example, we did not conduct PTPC in patients whose tumors were located near the urethra or who ever had transurethral resection of the prostate. To evaluate the possible predictors of complications from PTPC, a prospective cohort without significant selection criteria is warranted.

Several limitations exist in our study. First, the case number was not large enough for an extensive analysis of all clinical parameters in the multivariable model. However, the important demographic and tumor phenotype variables were all incorporated into the final model for establishing the predictive nomograms. Second, there was a lack of an independent cohort for external validation of the models or nomograms—this was well compensated using the bootstrap and cross-validation in our study. Third, this is a retrospective analysis that may have selection bias. However, the study enrolled all consecutive patients who received total prostate cryoablation, and all data variables were prospectively collected for all patients in a well-designed data entry file from the start of the study, which may significantly mitigate any selection bias or recall bias. Fourth, the current nomogram included only clinical parameters, but not molecular and detailed histological characters. Although this design made it convenient for the physician to use in clinical practice, the precision of outcome prediction may increase with more molecular/histological biomarkers, such as serine/arginine splicing factor 1 [27], microvessel density [27], insulin growth factor-1 [28], and so on.

5. Conclusions

Total prostate cryoablation appears to be an effective treatment option for men with high-risk PC. A pre-operative nomogram that predicts BCR would be useful for both patients and physicians to make clinical decisions when considering cryoablation among other treatment modalities. A peri-operative nomogram that includes diagnostic PSA, PSA nadir, Gleason sum, and the number of cryoprobes deployed may help inform increased risk of BCR, which would then justify early salvage treatments.

Supplementary Materials: The following are available online at https://www.mdpi.com/article/10.3390/cancers15153873/s1, Figure S1: Flow diagram of patient selection into the study cohort, Table S1: Demographics and characteristics of the training and validation cohorts, Table S2: The association of PSA nadir value and time to PSA nadir, Table S3: The association of PSA nadir value and neoadjuvant hormonal therapy.

Author Contributions: Conceptualization, C.-H.C. and Y.-S.P.; data curation, C.-H.C. and Y.-S.P., formal analysis, C.-H.C. and C.-Y.T.; investigation, C.-H.C.; methodology, C.-H.C. and C.-Y.T.; resources, Y.-S.P.; software, C.-Y.T.; supervision, Y.-S.P.; validation, C.-H.C.; writing—original draft, C.-H.C.; writing—review and editing, C.-Y.T. and Y.-S.P. All authors have read and agreed to the published version of the manuscript.

Funding: This research received no external funding.

Institutional Review Board Statement: This study was reviewed and approved by the Research Ethics Committee A of the National Taiwan University Hospital (202204097RINA).

Informed Consent Statement: Informed consent was waived based on the agreement of the Research Ethics Committee.

Data Availability Statement: Data are available on request due to restrictions of privacy consideration of our institutions. The data presented in this study are available on request from the corresponding author. The data are not publicly available due to the consideration of patients' privacy.

Acknowledgments: We thank all the participants and collaborators at the National Taiwan University.

Conflicts of Interest: The authors declare no potential conflict of interest.

Abbreviations

PC	prostate cancer
BCR	biochemical recurrence
COLD	Cryo On-Line Database
PSA	prostate-specific antigen
ADT	androgen deprivation therapy
PET	positron emission tomography
PTPC	primary total prostate cryoablation
MRI	magnetic resonance imaging

References

1. National Comprehensive Cancer Network. Prostate Cancer (Version 2.2022). Available online: https://www.nccn.org/professionals/physician_gls/pdf/prostate.pdf (accessed on 1 April 2022).
2. EAU. *EAU Guidelines. Edn. Presented at the EAU Annual Congress Milan 2023*; EAU Guidelines Office: Arnhem, The Netherlands, 2023.
3. Jones, J.S.; Rewcastle, J.C.; Donnelly, B.J.; Lugnani, F.M.; Pisters, L.L.; Katz, A.E. Whole gland primary prostate cryoablation: Initial results from the cryo on-line data registry. *J. Urol.* **2008**, *180*, 554–558. [CrossRef] [PubMed]
4. Chen, C.H.; Tai, Y.S.; Pu, Y.S. Prognostic value of saturated prostate cryoablation for localized prostate cancer. *World J. Urol.* **2015**, *33*, 1487–1494. [CrossRef] [PubMed]

5. Thompson, I.; Thrasher, J.B.; Aus, G.; Burnett, A.L.; Canby-Hagino, E.D.; Cookson, M.S.; D'Amico, A.V.; Dmochowski, R.R.; Eton, D.T.; Forman, J.D.; et al. Guideline for the management of clinically localized prostate cancer: 2007 update. *J. Urol.* **2007**, *177*, 2106–2131. [CrossRef] [PubMed]
6. Paladini, A.; Cochetti, G.; Colau, A.; Mouton, M.; Ciarletti, S.; Felici, G.; Maiolino, G.; Balzarini, F.; Sebe, P.; Mearini, E. The Challenges of Patient Selection for Prostate Cancer Focal Therapy: A Retrospective Observational Multicentre Study. *Curr. Oncol.* **2022**, *29*, 6826–6833. [CrossRef]
7. Kotamarti, S.; Polascik, T.J. Focal cryotherapy for prostate cancer: A contemporary literature review. *Ann. Transl. Med.* **2023**, *11*, 26. [CrossRef]
8. Aizer, A.A.; Yu, J.B.; Colberg, J.W.; McKeon, A.M.; Decker, R.H.; Peschel, R.E. Radical prostatectomy vs. intensity-modulated radiation therapy in the management of localized prostate adenocarcinoma. *Radiother. Oncol.* **2009**, *93*, 185–191. [CrossRef] [PubMed]
9. Ciezki, J.P.; Weller, M.; Reddy, C.A.; Kittel, J.; Singh, H.; Tendulkar, R.; Stephans, K.L.; Ulchaker, J.; Angermeier, K.; Stephenson, A.; et al. A Comparison Between Low-Dose-Rate Brachytherapy With or Without Androgen Deprivation, External Beam Radiation Therapy With or Without Androgen Deprivation, and Radical Prostatectomy With or Without Adjuvant or Salvage Radiation Therapy for High-Risk Prostate Cancer. *Int. J. Radiat. Oncol. Biol. Phys.* **2017**, *97*, 962–975. [CrossRef]
10. Chen, C.H.; Pu, Y.S. Adjuvant androgen-deprivation therapy following prostate total cryoablation in high-risk localized prostate cancer patients—Open-labeled randomized clinical trial. *Cryobiology* **2018**, *82*, 88–92. [CrossRef]
11. Chen, C.H.; Pu, Y.S. Proactive rectal warming during total-gland prostate cryoablation. *Cryobiology* **2014**, *68*, 431–435. [CrossRef] [PubMed]
12. Roach, M., 3rd; Hanks, G.; Thames, H., Jr.; Schellhammer, P.; Shipley, W.U.; Sokol, G.H.; Sandler, H. Defining biochemical failure following radiotherapy with or without hormonal therapy in men with clinically localized prostate cancer: Recommendations of the RTOG-ASTRO Phoenix Consensus Conference. *Int. J. Radiat. Oncol. Biol. Phys.* **2006**, *65*, 965–974. [CrossRef]
13. Van den Broeck, T.; van den Bergh, R.C.N.; Briers, E.; Cornford, P.; Cumberbatch, M.; Tilki, D.; De Santis, M.; Fanti, S.; Fossati, N.; Gillessen, S.; et al. Biochemical Recurrence in Prostate Cancer: The European Association of Urology Prostate Cancer Guidelines Panel Recommendations. *Eur. Urol. Focus* **2020**, *6*, 231–234. [CrossRef] [PubMed]
14. Harrell, F.E., Jr.; Lee, K.L.; Mark, D.B. Multivariable prognostic models: Issues in developing models, evaluating assumptions and adequacy, and measuring and reducing errors. *Stat. Med.* **1996**, *15*, 361–387. [CrossRef]
15. Harrell, F.E., Jr. Rms: Regression Modeling Strategies. R Package Version 6.2-0. Available online: https://cran.r-project.org/web/packages/rms/rms.pdf (accessed on 15 April 2021).
16. Harrell, F.E., Jr.; Califf, R.M.; Pryor, D.B.; Lee, K.L.; Rosati, R.A. Evaluating the yield of medical tests. *JAMA* **1982**, *247*, 2543–2546. [CrossRef] [PubMed]
17. Chen, C.H.; Chen, Y.C.; Pu, Y.S. Tumor location on MRI determines outcomes of patients with prostate cancer after total prostate cryoablation. *Cryobiology* **2021**, *98*, 39–45. [CrossRef]
18. Sanda, M.G.; Cadeddu, J.A.; Kirkby, E.; Chen, R.C.; Crispino, T.; Fontanarosa, J.; Freedland, S.J.; Greene, K.; Klotz, L.H.; Makarov, D.V.; et al. Clinically Localized Prostate Cancer: AUA/ASTRO/SUO Guideline. Part I: Risk Stratification, Shared Decision Making, and Care Options. *J. Urol.* **2018**, *199*, 683–690. [CrossRef]
19. Mottet, N.; van den Bergh, R.C.N.; Briers, E.; Van den Broeck, T.; Cumberbatch, M.G.; De Santis, M.; Fanti, S.; Fossati, N.; Gandaglia, G.; Gillessen, S.; et al. EAU-EANM-ESTRO-ESUR-SIOG Guidelines on Prostate Cancer-2020 Update. Part 1: Screening, Diagnosis, and Local Treatment with Curative Intent. *Eur. Urol.* **2021**, *79*, 243–262. [CrossRef]
20. Pilepich, M.V.; Winter, K.; Lawton, C.A.; Krisch, R.E.; Wolkov, H.B.; Movsas, B.; Hug, E.B.; Asbell, S.O.; Grignon, D. Androgen suppression adjuvant to definitive radiotherapy in prostate carcinoma--long-term results of phase III RTOG 85-31. *Int. J. Radiat. Oncol. Biol. Phys.* **2005**, *61*, 1285–1290. [CrossRef]
21. Bolla, M.; Van Tienhoven, G.; Warde, P.; Dubois, J.B.; Mirimanoff, R.O.; Storme, G.; Bernier, J.; Kuten, A.; Sternberg, C.; Billiet, I.; et al. External irradiation with or without long-term androgen suppression for prostate cancer with high metastatic risk: 10-Year results of an EORTC randomised study. *Lancet Oncol.* **2010**, *11*, 1066–1073. [CrossRef]
22. Tay, K.J.; Polascik, T.J.; Elshafei, A.; Cher, M.L.; Given, R.W.; Mouraviev, V.; Ross, A.E.; Jones, J.S. Primary Cryotherapy for High-Grade Clinically Localized Prostate Cancer: Oncologic and Functional Outcomes from the COLD Registry. *J. Endourol.* **2016**, *30*, 43–48. [CrossRef]
23. Mercader, C.; Musquera, M.; Franco, A.; Alcaraz, A.; Ribal, M.J. Primary cryotherapy for localized prostate cancer treatment. *Aging Male* **2020**, *23*, 1460–1466. [CrossRef]
24. de Vermandois, J.A.R.; Cochetti, G.; Zingaro, M.D.; Santoro, A.; Panciarola, M.; Boni, A.; Marsico, M.; Gaudio, G.; Paladini, A.; Guiggi, P.; et al. Evaluation of Surgical Site Infection in Mini-invasive Urological Surgery. *Open Med.* **2019**, *14*, 711–718. [CrossRef] [PubMed]
25. Ataman, F.; Zurlo, A.; Artignan, X.; van Tienhoven, G.; Blank, L.E.; Warde, P.; Dubois, J.B.; Jeanneret, W.; Keuppens, F.; Bernier, J.; et al. Late toxicity following conventional radiotherapy for prostate cancer: Analysis of the EORTC trial 22863. *Eur. J. Cancer* **2004**, *40*, 1674–1681. [CrossRef]
26. Ficarra, V.; Novara, G.; Rosen, R.C.; Artibani, W.; Carroll, P.R.; Costello, A.; Menon, M.; Montorsi, F.; Patel, V.R.; Stolzenburg, J.U.; et al. Systematic review and meta-analysis of studies reporting urinary continence recovery after robot-assisted radical prostatectomy. *Eur. Urol.* **2012**, *62*, 405–417. [CrossRef] [PubMed]

27. Broggi, G.; Lo Giudice, A.; Di Mauro, M.; Asmundo, M.G.; Pricoco, E.; Piombino, E.; Caltabiano, R.; Morgia, G.; Russo, G.I. SRSF-1 and microvessel density immunohistochemical analysis by semi-automated tissue microarray in prostate cancer patients with diabetes (DIAMOND study). *Prostate* **2021**, *81*, 882–892. [CrossRef] [PubMed]
28. Heni, M.; Hennenlotter, J.; Scharpf, M.; Lutz, S.Z.; Schwentner, C.; Todenhofer, T.; Schilling, D.; Kuhs, U.; Gerber, V.; Machicao, F.; et al. Insulin receptor isoforms A and B as well as insulin receptor substrates-1 and -2 are differentially expressed in prostate cancer. *PLoS ONE* **2012**, *7*, e50953. [CrossRef]

Disclaimer/Publisher's Note: The statements, opinions and data contained in all publications are solely those of the individual author(s) and contributor(s) and not of MDPI and/or the editor(s). MDPI and/or the editor(s) disclaim responsibility for any injury to people or property resulting from any ideas, methods, instructions or products referred to in the content.

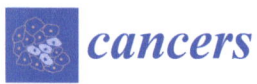 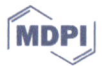

Systematic Review

Malignancy Associated with Low-Risk HPV6 and HPV11: A Systematic Review and Implications for Cancer Prevention

Leandro Lima da Silva [1], Amanda Mara Teles [1,2], Joana M. O. Santos [3], Marcelo Souza de Andrade [1], Rui Medeiros [3], Ana I. Faustino-Rocha [4,5], Paula A. Oliveira [4,5], Ana Paula Azevedo dos Santos [1,6], Fernanda Ferreira Lopes [7], Geraldo Braz [8], Haissa O. Brito [1] and Rui M. Gil da Costa [1,3,4,5,9,10,*]

[1] Post-Graduate Program in Adult Health (PPGSAD), Federal University of Maranhão (UFMA), São Luís 65080-805, MA, Brazil; ana.azevedo@ufma.br (A.P.A.d.S.); haissa.brito@ufma.br (H.O.B.)
[2] Post-Graduate Program in Animal Health, State University of Maranhão, São Luís 65099-110, MA, Brazil
[3] Molecular Oncology and Viral Pathology Group, Portuguese Institute of Oncology of Porto Research Center (CI-IPOP)/RISE@CI-IPOP (Health Research Network), Portuguese Institute of Oncology of Porto (IPO-Porto)/Porto Comprehensive Cancer Center (Porto.CCC), 4200-072 Porto, Portugal
[4] Centre for the Research and Technology of Agro-Environmental and Biological Sciences (CITAB), University of Trás-os-Montes and Alto Douro, 5000-801 Vila Real, Portugal; anafaustino.faustino@sapo.pt (A.I.F.-R.)
[5] Inov4Agro—Institute for Innovation, Capacity Building and Sustainability of Agri-Food Production, University of Trás-os-Montes and Alto Douro, 5000-801 Vila Real, Portugal
[6] Post-Graduate Program in Health Sciences, Federal University of Maranhão (UFMA), São Luís 65080-805, MA, Brazil
[7] Post-Graduate Program in Odontology, Federal University of Maranhão (UFMA), São Luís 65080-805, MA, Brazil; fernanda.ferreira@ufma.br
[8] Post-Graduate Program in Computing Sciences, Federal University of Maranhão (UFMA), São Luís 65080-805, MA, Brazil; geraldo.braz@ufma.br
[9] Laboratory for Process Engineering, Environment, Biotechnology and Energy (LEPABE), Faculty of Engineering, University of Porto, 4200-465 Porto, Portugal
[10] Associate Laboratory in Chemical Engineering (ALiCE), Faculty of Engineering, University of Porto, 4200-465 Porto, Portugal
* Correspondence: rui.costa@ufma.br

Citation: Silva, L.L.d.; Teles, A.M.; Santos, J.M.O.; Souza de Andrade, M.; Medeiros, R.; Faustino-Rocha, A.I.; Oliveira, P.A.; dos Santos, A.P.A.; Ferreira Lopes, F.; Braz, G.; et al. Malignancy Associated with Low-Risk HPV6 and HPV11: A Systematic Review and Implications for Cancer Prevention. *Cancers* 2023, 15, 4068. https://doi.org/10.3390/cancers15164068

Academic Editor: Brian Gabrielli

Received: 30 June 2023
Revised: 28 July 2023
Accepted: 8 August 2023
Published: 11 August 2023

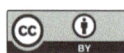

Copyright: © 2023 by the authors. Licensee MDPI, Basel, Switzerland. This article is an open access article distributed under the terms and conditions of the Creative Commons Attribution (CC BY) license (https://creativecommons.org/licenses/by/4.0/).

Simple Summary: Vaccination against human papillomavirus (HPV) helps prevent cancer caused by this virus. Determining which viral genotypes should be included is key for developing successful vaccination strategies. Low-risk genotypes, especially HPV6 and HPV11, are associated with benign warts. However, some studies also report their presence in cancers. We reviewed the scientific literature to estimate the proportion of cancers that bear single or dual HPV6/11 infections. HPV6 and HPV11 have been reported in up to 5.5% of penile and 87.5% of laryngeal cancers; however, they have not been reported in vulvar, vaginal or oral cancers. Next, we compared the HPV6/11 genomes with HPV16, the most common high-risk HPV genotype, and observed that the similarities mainly involved the *E7* gene, suggesting a limited ability to interfere with the differentiation of the host cells. These findings support the use of HPV vaccines that cover HPV6/11 not only for preventing genital warts but also for preventing specific types of cancers.

Abstract: High-risk human papillomavirus (HPV) is etiologically related to cervical cancer, other anogenital cancers and oropharyngeal carcinomas. Low-risk HPV, especially HPV6 and HPV11, cause genital warts and laryngeal papillomas. However, the accumulating data suggests that HPV6 and HPV11 may cause malignant lesions at non-cervical anatomic sites. This review aims to estimate the proportions of single and dual HPV6/11 infections in multiple cancers reported in the last 10 years in the Cochrane, Embasa and PubMed databases. Secondly, the genomes of HPV6/11 were compared with the most common high-risk genotype, HPV16, to determine the similarities and differences. A total of 11 articles were selected, including between one and 334 HPV+ cancer patients. The frequencies of single or dual HPV6/11 infections ranged between 0–5.5% for penile and 0–87.5% for laryngeal cancers and were null for vulvar, vaginal and oral cancers. The genomic similarities between HPV6/11 and HPV16 mainly involved the *E7* gene, indicating a limited ability to block cell differentiation. The presence of single or dual HPV6/11 infections in variable proportions of penile and laryngeal cancers support the vaccination strategies that cover these genotypes, not only for preventing genital warts but also for cancer prevention. Other risk factors and co-carcinogens are likely to participate in epithelial carcinogenesis associated with low-risk HPV.

Keywords: vaccine; squamous cell carcinoma; papillomavirus; retinoblastoma protein; low-risk HPV

1. Introduction

Human papillomaviruses are host species-specific, double-stranded DNA viruses that exhibit a conserved icosahedral morphology, ranging between 50–55 nm in diameter with a molecular weight of 5×10^6 Da [1,2]. Infection through tissue microdamage allows the virus to gain access to basal keratinocytes in the epidermis and keratinized mucosae [3,4]. The HPV genome contains a set of genes that are expressed early in the viral cycle upon cell entry, designated the "early" (E) genes, and two "late" (L) genes, L1 and L2, which are expressed later in the viral cycle and encode the structural capsid proteins as well as the regulatory regions [5]. Based on their nucleotide sequence of the L1 gene, HPVs are divided into types which are grouped in five genera (alpha, beta, gamma, mu and nu), where alpha is the main genus, comprising the HPV types associated with the development of cervical cancer known as high-risk (HR) HPVs (e.g., HPV16 and HPV18) and the types associated with genital warts, termed low-risk (LR) HPVs (e.g., HPV6 and HPV11) [6–10]. The HPV types are defined based on a 10% variation in their L1 nucleotide sequence and may be further subdivided into variants with different biological properties based on smaller differences [11–14]. The HPV types may also be divided according to their target epithelial site, i.e., cutaneous versus mucocutaneous [15]. Quadrivalent and nonavalent HPV vaccines are protective against HPV6 and HPV11 infections along with infections by HR-HPVs, while the bivalent vaccine only targets HPV16 and HPV18 [16]. Low-risk genital types are often responsible for benign lesions, such as condyloma acuminata, and may also cause low-grade cervical dysplasia. However, the risk of developing invasive cervical carcinoma is low [17]. HPV6 and HPV11 are most frequently found in genital warts [18] and are also involved in respiratory papillomas [19,20]. In contrast, HR-HPVs are able to establish persistent infections; interfere with cell proliferation, differentiation and survival; and are the etiologic agents of cervical cancer [5]. However, in contrast with cervical cancer, a limited number of studies have found single infections caused by LR-HPV, specifically HPV6 and HPV11, in small proportions of some non-cervical anogenital cancers, such as vulvar [21] and penile [22] cancers. Such observations suggest the hypothesis that these two HPV types may exert a more significant oncogenic effect on those specific anatomic sites than in the uterine cervix. If this is the case, the knowledge of the proportion of cancers potentially associated with HPV6/11 would help tailor vaccination strategies, especially in world regions where such cancers are more common. The present work adopted two complementary approaches to study this hypothesis. First, we performed a systematic review of the scientific literature from the last 10 years to determine the prevalence of single or dual HPV6 and HPV11 infections in the sites of HPV-associated cancers. Secondly, the genomic organization of these viruses was comparatively studied against HPV16, the most common high-risk HPV genotype, to identify meaningful similarities and differences. Finally, based on the results from both these studies, the factors that may contribute to a possible oncogenic role for HPV6 and HPV11 were discussed.

2. Materials and Methods

2.1. Systematic Review of HPV6 and HPV11 in Cancer

The systematic review was performed in accordance with the preferred reporting items for systematic reviews and meta-analyses (PRISMA) guidelines [23], according to the following parameters. Population: HNSCCs, anal, cervical, penile, vaginal and vulvar cancer patients. Intervention: the frequency of HPV6 and HPV11 single infections. The search strategy contemplated three standard databases on biomedicine: PubMed, Embase and Cochrane, accessed in March and April 2022. The keywords "cancer AND HPV6" or "cancer AND HPV11" were applied. A total of 541 articles were retrieved from PubMed, 695 articles from Embase and 29 articles from Cochrane. Duplicated records were excluded based on the article's bibliographic reference. The following inclusion criteria were established concerning the type of study (case series and case–control studies in humans), tumor sample type (formalin-fixed paraffin-embedded and fresh tissue biopsies), tumor location (head and neck, uterine cervix, anorectum, penis, prepuce, vulva and vagina), histological diagnosis (squamous cell carcinoma), HPV detection methodology performed (PCR-based or sequencing techniques) and the type of agents identified (the frequency of single or dual HPV6 and HPV11 infections reported with or without a report of the infections by other LR-HPV types). The exclusion criteria were a lack of histological confirmation of cancer, a lack of identification of single/dual HPV6 or HPV11 infections, case reports, review articles and meta-analyses. The abstracts and, when necessary, the materials and methods were analyzed to apply the inclusion and exclusion criteria.

2.2. Comparative Genomic Analysis of HPV6, HPV11 and HPV16

The HPV6 and HPV11 genomes were compared with HPV16, the most commonly identified high-risk HPV in cancer, to identify the similarities and differences in the key genes involved in the cell transformation. The complete genomes of HPV16 (NC_001526.4) and HPV6 (NC_001355.1) were retrieved from the RefSeq database, available at NCBI. The RefSeq database was unavailable for HPV11. Therefore, its complete genome was retrieved from the GeneBank database, available at NCBI (MW404328.1). Then, the complete genomes of HPV16, HPV6 and HVP11 were uploaded to the Proksee/CGView Server online tool, which is a system for genome assembly, annotation and visualization [24]. In this tool, BLAST (blastn) was used to identify the regions of similarity between the genomic sequences. The amino acid sequences of the early proteins E6, E7, E5A and E5B from HPV16 and HPV6 were retrieved from the RefSeq database, available at NCBI, and the proteins from HPV11 were retrieved from the GenePept database, available at NCBI. The blastp tool from NCBI was used to evaluate the similarities between the early protein sequences.

3. Results

3.1. Systematic Review of HPV6 and HPV11 in Cancer

Most of the initially screened publications were excluded since they dealt with benign lesions instead of cancer, which was in line with the known role of HPV6 and HPV11 in warts. Overall, after applying the inclusion and exclusion criteria, 11 articles were selected for further analysis (Figure 1). A total of three articles were analyzed for cervical cancer [25–27], six for HNSCCs [28–33], none for anal cancer, three for penile cancer [28,34,35], one for vaginal cancer [28] and one for vulvar cancer [28]. The characteristics of all 11 publications that were selected for further analysis are summarized in Table 1.

The selected publications (Table 1) spanned the period between 2012 and 2021 and dealt with patient cohorts varying in size between eight and 1010 total patients. HPV detection was primarily performed using PCR-based methods, except for Aldersley et al. (2021) who used previously obtained whole exome data. The proportion of HPV-positive cases ranged between 1/85 [30] and 142/142 [25]. Seven studies used formalin-fixed paraffin-embedded (FFPE) material [28–32,34,35]; however, one used fresh biopsies [33] and another used tissue stored in RNAlater [26]. HPV genotyping was performed using a variety of commercial and custom methods. Three studies addressed the frequency of HPV6/11 infections in cervical cancer [25–27] (Table 2).

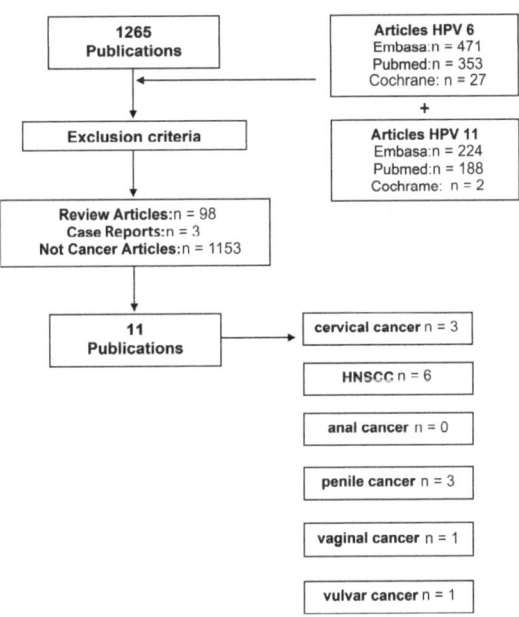

Figure 1. Systematic review of HPV6 and HPV11 in cancer and the resulting publications selected for analysis.

Table 1. Characteristics of the 11 articles included in the HPV6 and HPV11 systematic review.

References	Type of Sample	Detection Method	Genotyping Method	Total Sample and (HPV + Sample)
Tao et al., 2017 [25]	Cervical scrappings	PCR/Luminex 200 (Tellgen, Shanghai, China)	PCR/Luminex 200 (Tellgen, China)	142 (142)
Das et al., 2013 [26]	Tissue biopsy in RNAlater (Qiagen, Hilden, Germany)	Nested PCR	Digene HPV Hybrid Capture II Test (Qiagen, Germany)	107 (105)
Aldersley et al., 2021 [27]	Whole exome data from previous publications	SureSelect Exon Capture (Agilent, Santa Clara, CA, USA) and HiSeq sequencing (Illumina, San Diego, CA, USA)	SureSelect Exon Capture (Agilent) and HiSeq sequencing (Illumina, USA)	72 (62)
Barzon et al., 2014 [34]	FFPE	PCR (Inno-LiPa, Tokyo, Japan)	Real-time PCR	59 (18)
Alemany et al., 2016 [35]	FFPE	SPF-10/DEIA/LIPA25 (Laboratory Biomedical Products, Rijswijk, The Netherlands)	LIPA25 (Laboratory Biomedical Products, The Netherlands) and Sanger sequencing	1010 (334)
Vietía et al., 2014 [33]	Fresh biopsies	PCR (Inno-LiPa, Japan)	PCR (Inno-LiPa, Japan)	71 (48)
Taberna et al., 2016 [29]	FFPE	PCR (Inno-LiPa, Japan)	Real-Time PCR	404 (54)
Lam et al., 2018 [30]	FFPE	Nested PCR	Sanger sequncing	85 (1)

Table 1. Cont.

References	Type of Sample	Detection Method	Genotyping Method	Total Sample and (HPV + Sample)
Weiss et al., 2015 [31]	FFPE	Real-Time PCR GP5+/6+ and In Situ Hybridization	Real-Time PCR	8 (6)
Sun et al., 2012 [32]	FFPE	PCR for HPV 6/11 and HPV 16/18	PCR for HPV 6/11 and HPV 16/18	83 (42)
Magaña-León et al., 2015 [28]	FFPE	SPF-10/DEIA/LIPA25 (Laboratory Biomedical Products, The Netherlands)	PCR (Inno-LiPa, Japan)	35 (10)

These studies generally identified an extremely low prevalence of single HPV6/11 infections or infections with HPV6/11 in the context of other LR-HPV in cervical cancer. A single case of HPV11 mono-infection was reported by [25], which also had the largest caseload of the three. Three studies addressed penile cancer [28,34,35]. Alemany et al. (2016) presented the largest caseload of the three and reported that 3.6% and 1.2% of HPV-positive cases carried HPV6 and HPV11 mono-infections, respectively. Barzon et al. (2014) reported a case showing HPV11 mono-infection and Magaña-León et al. (2015) reported none. In the larynx, the proportions of single infections varied between 0% and 75% cases for HPV6 and between 0% and 12.5% cases for HPV11. No studies observed single HPV6/11 infections in oral, vaginal or vulvar SCCs.

Table 2. Prevalence of HPV6 and HPV11 single infections in different types of HPV-associated cancers.

Anatomic Location		HPV6 % (n/N)	HPV11 % (n/N)	Multiple Low-Risk% (n/N)	Geographical Location	References
Uterine cervix		0/142	1/142	1/142	China	Tao et al., 2017 [25]
		0/105	0/105	0/105	India	Das et al., 2013 [26]
		1.4% (1/62)	0/62	1/62	Republic of Korea/United States/France	Aldersley et al., 2021 [27]
Penis		0/18	5.5% (1/18)	1/18	Italy	Barzon et al., 2014 [34]
		3.6% (12/334)	1.2% (4/334)	4.8% (16/334)	25 Countries	Alemany et al., 2016 [35]
		0/8	0/8	0/8	Mexico	Magaña-León et al., 2015 [28]
Head and neck	Oral cavity	0/9	0/9	0/9	Mexico	Magaña-León et al., 2015 [28]
	Larynx	3.7% (2/54)	3.7% (2/54)	4/54	United States	Taberna et al., 2016 [29]
		1.2% (1/85)	0/85	1/85	China	Lam et al., 2018 [30]
		75.0% (6/8)	12.5% (1/8)	7/8	Germany	Weiss et al., 2015 [31]
		Not tested	Not tested	9.6% (8/42)	China	Sun et al., 2012 [32]
		0/9	0/9	0/9	Mexico	Magaña-León et al., 2015 [28]
	Mixed locations	12.5% (6/48)	0% (0/48)	16.67% (8/48)	Venezuela	Vietía et al., 2014 [33]
Vagina		0/7	0/7	1/7 *	Mexico	Magaña-León et al., 2015 [28]
Vulva		0/1	0/1	0/1	Mexico	Magaña-León et al., 2015 [28]

* One single HPV54 infection among seven vaginal SCC cases in the Magaña-Leon et al. (2015) study, which included 35 SCCs from multiple locations.

The HPV surrogate marker p16^{INK4a} was studied using immunohistochemistry in five articles. Two studies found that most penile cancers harboring HR-HPV were p16^{INK4a}-positive [34,35]. However, the larger Alemany et al. [35] study found that only a small proportion of cancers with LR-HPV were p16^{INK4a}-positive. Three studies described p16^{INK4a} immunostaining in laryngeal cancers [29–31] and reported a poor correlation with the presence of HPV DNA. Weiss et al. found two positive LR-HPV cases [31].

3.2. HPV6/11/16 Comparative Genomic Analysis

HPV16 had a circular dsDNA with a total of 7906 bp and eight coding sequences (Figure 2). When performing a blastn analysis at Proksee/CGView to compare both the HPV16/HPV6 and HPV16/HPV11 genomes, it was possible to observe that the majority of the similarities between the genomic sequences were located in the E1, E2, L2, L1 and E7 coding regions. No similarities between the genomic sequences at the E6 and E5 regions were found using these tools. The early proteins from HPV16 and HPV6/11 were then evaluated regarding the similarity of their amino acid sequence (Supplementary Table S1) using blastp. The identities, positives and expected values are presented in Tables 3 and 4, where the identity describes the similarities of the sequences (the number of identical amino acids) and positives correspond to the number of amino acids that were either identical or had similar chemical properties.

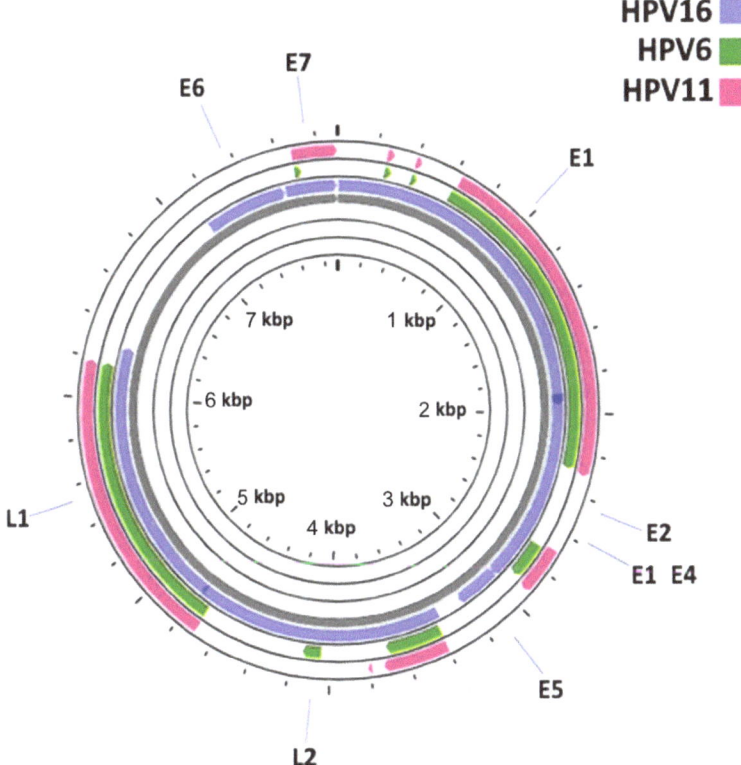

Figure 2. Comparative genomic organization of HPV6, HV11 and HPV16.

According to the data obtained, the protein with highest similarity between HPV16 and HPV6 was E7, while E5 was the protein with lowest similarity. Similar results were obtained for HPV16 and HPV11.

Table 3. A comparative analysis of the HPV6 and HPV16 E6, E7 and E5 oncoproteins.

		HPV6			
		E6 (NP_040296.1)	E7 (NP_040297.1)	E5A (NP_040301.1)	E5B (NP_040302.1)
HPV16	E6 (NP_041325.1)	Identities: 39%; Positives: 60%; Expect: 2×10^{-41}			
	E7 (NP_041326.1)		Identities: 57%; Positives: 69%; Expect: 3×10^{-34}		
	E5 (NP_041330.2)			Identities: 24%; Positives: 58%; Expect: 0.018	No significant similarity found.

Table 4. A comparative analysis of the HPV11 and HPV16 E6, E7 and E5 oncoproteins.

		HPV11			
		E6 (QXM18822.1)	E7 (QXM18823.1)	E5A (QXM18827.1)	E5B (QXM18828.1)
HPV16	E6 (NP_041325.1)	Identities: 37%; Positives: 61%; Expect: 2×10^{-40}			
	E7 (NP_041326.1)		Identities: 55%; Positives: 70%; Expect: 1×10^{-33}		
	E5 (NP_041330.2)			No significant similarity found.	No significant similarity found.

4. Discussion

High-risk (HR)-HPVs, particularly HPV16, have been identified as the etiologic agents of multiple anogenital and oropharyngeal cancers, as shown by numerous observational and experimental studies [36–41]. LR-HPVs mostly cause benign lesions, such as condylomas, but have also been suggested to be involved in subsets of malignant non-cervical lesions [42,43]. The present work provided a systematic analysis of the data published in the last 10 years to determine the frequencies of HPV6 and HPV11 as single infections in anogenital and head and neck cancers. The 11 selected articles showed significant geographic diversity, including works from four continents, as well as a large international penile cancer study by Alemany et al. (2016). While some studies showed a low HPV-positive caseload for specific sites, such as the Weiss et al. (2015) and Magaña-Leon et al. (2015) reports, others were much larger and included dozens or hundreds of patients, such as the Taberna et al. (2016) or Alemany et al. (2016) articles. These heterogeneous results recommended caution when interpreting the findings from our systematic review. Smaller studies may highlight locally important phenomena, such as a higher HPV6/11 infection rate, while larger studies may dilute those observations and provide a more general picture. One study from Venezuela [33] reported data from multiple head and neck locations. However, it was impossible to ascribe specific HPV genotypes to each anatomical site. We chose to include this study because it provided data on the frequencies of LR-HPVs in head and neck SCCs in general. However, it could not replace the detailed reports ascribing HPV6 and HPV11 to more specific anatomic sites. We began by analyzing the studies focused on cervical cancer. Approx. 95% of women with cervical cancer were infected with one or more HR-HPV subtype, with HPV16 and 18 being the most common [44,45]. LR-HPV was associated with benign neoplasia and scientific data accumulated over decades does not support its involvement in cervical SCCs [46,47]. In line with such observations, our systematic review showed considerably low frequencies for HPV6 and HPV11 mono-infections in cervical cancer. Quadrivalent and nonavalent HPV vaccines conferred protection against these LR-HPV types and their associated lesions [16]. Advanced cervical cancer had dramatic consequences for patients due to cancer invasion and metastasis, but also due to psychological issues and paraneoplastic syndromes [48–50]. Even intraepithelial lesions were associated with significant morbidity, which could recur after surgical excision [51,52]. HPV-associated head and neck cancers were most frequently located in the oropharynx, where HPV16 was responsible for approximately 95% of the HPV-related cases [13,36,53]. The head and neck studies in our systematic review mostly reported data from the larynx, which likely reflected the known role of HPV6 and HPV11 in respiratory papillomas in this anatomic area [17]. HPV6 and HPV11 were the main causative agents of laryngeal papillomas, the most frequent benign tumors in the lower respiratory tract [17]. Respiratory lesions associated with the HPV11 type are suggested to be more aggressive compared to those associated with HPV6 [54]. Our systematic review showed that laryngeal SCCs carried HPV6 and HPV11 in varying proportions. While large studies from China and the USA showed frequencies ranging between 1% and 4%, a smaller German study showed much higher figures, with up to 75% of cases showing HPV11 mono-infections. It is likely that these widely varying figures reflected different geographical realities, but the results supported the involvement of HPV6 and HPV11 in a significant proportion of laryngeal SCCs. Other studies showed similar results [55]. The association between HPV6, HPV11 and this anatomic area may reflect local microenvironmental factors and an exposure to chemical carcinogens, as well as immunological impairment. These factors were not screened in this systematic review. Minimal data were available concerning other head and neck locations, with one study indicating null figures for oral SCCs [28] and the [33] study reporting figures for mixed locations. LR-HPV, such as HPV6 and HPV11, were associated with penile condylomas [56]. While it is possible that some penile condylomas may progress to SCCs [57], there is still insufficient data to support this hypothesis. Our systematic review showed that HPV6 and HPV11 infections were found in a significant proportion of penile SCCs, in agreement with the previous reports on penile cancer and penile intraepithelial neoplasia by multiple teams [58,59], including a meta-analysis by [22]. While the Magaña-Leon study with only eight cases did not identify any HPV6 orHPV11 single infections, larger studies such as those of Barzon et al. (2014) and especially Alemany et al. (2016), indicated that HPV6 and HPV11 mono-infections were found in approximately 5% of penile SCCs. Multiple LR-HPV infections were also found in 4% of other cases, according to Alemany et al. (2016). Taken together, these observations support the involvement of the LR-HPV types in a significant proportion of penile SCCs, suggesting that the penis and prepuce are anatomical sites with a particular susceptibility to carcinogenesis induced by these agents. Vaccines covering HPV6 and HPV11 may be more adequate for preventing penile neoplasia than bivalent vaccines targeting only HPV16 and HPV18. In the vulva and vagina, HPV6 and HPV11 were commonly associated with benign neoplasia, most often condylomas [47,60,61]. In our systematic review, a single study [28] addressed the frequency of HPV6 and HPV11 mono-infections in the vagina and vulva, limiting our ability to draw conclusions. This study suggested that a low frequency of infection caused by these LR-HPV types could be associated with vaginal SCCs. However, no cases of vulva SCCs with HPV6/11 were identified. These results were in agreement with the previous reports [62]. In our 10-year study period, no studies focused on anal cancer fulfilled the inclusion criteria, and we could not conclude the involvement of HPV6 and HPV11 mono-infections in this type of cancer. This was regrettable, as other studies identified the presence of a small proportion of anal SCCs associated with those LR-HPV types, especially in the context of immunosuppression induced by HIV [63–66].

It is possible that genomic similarities with high-risk HPV allow for HPV6 and HPV11 to interact with important cellular targets, conferring a limited carcinogenic potential. The HPV early proteins had regulatory functions and could be found in both high- and low-risk HPVs [67–72]. Among these, the E5, E6 and E7 oncoproteins were believed to be the main transforming proteins of HR-HPV [5]. While E5 may have a low transforming activity when expressed alone in a cell culture, it could play important roles in carcinogenesis induced by high-risk HPV [73,74]. The E6 protein was able to inactivate the p53 tumor suppressor protein and also perform p53-independent functions, thus playing a major role in the HPV-induced cell transformation [75,76]. The E7 protein played several major roles in carcinogenesis, especially by driving the degradation of the retinoblastoma protein (pRb) and thereby promoting cell proliferation [77,78]. It has been previously suggested that low-risk HPV types do not use their E6 and E7 gene products to drive extensive cell proliferation in the basal and parabasal cell layers, thereby drastically reducing their ability to induce cancer [79]. Indeed, our genomic analysis showed that the HPV6/11 and HPV16 genomes shared important differences concerning the E5, E6 and E7 oncogenes. However, they also exhibited some similarities. The E7 coding region was most conserved among all three viruses, while no similarities were found between the genomic sequences at the E6 and E5 regions. This suggests that the lower oncogenic potential of HPV6 and HPV11 compared with HPV16 was at least partly related to the differences on their E5 and E6 oncogenes. Conversely, the similarities observed in the E7 oncogene could help explain why HPV6 and HPV11 seemed to show some carcinogenic potential towards non-cervical tissues. Indeed, the HPV6 and HPV11 E7 proteins interacted with the pRb family member p130, inducing its proteasomal degradation. This mechanism could contribute to deregulating cell differentiation and proliferation in the suprabasal epithelial layers [80–82]. Classically, the accumulation of the p16INK4a protein was assessed immunohistochemically in squamous cell carcinomas as a surrogate marker for pRb downregulation to confirm viral activity [83]. Two of the studies included in this review [34,35] reported results for p16INK4a immunostaining in penile cancer, suggesting that only a minority of cases with LR-HPV were positive for this marker, which was in line with their limited ability to induce the degradation of pRb family proteins. Three studies of laryngeal cancer [29–31] reported that p16INK4a immunostaining had a poor correlation with the HPV DNA status in this type of cancer and, as observed for penile cancer, some LR-HPV-positive cases were p16INK4a-positive [29,31].

5. Conclusions

Overall, the present review combined and analyzed the data concerning the frequency of HPV6 and HPV11 mono-infections across multiple types of cancer. This analysis was limited by the small caseload of some studies and also by the absence of data concerning possible carcinogenic co-factors that could synergize with HPV6 and HPV11 to promote their tumorigenic potential. HPV6 and HPV11 mono-infections were mostly associated with SCCs of the larynx and penis. SCCs of the cervix, vagina, vulva and the head and neck (apart from the pharynx) showed the lowest frequencies of HPV6 and HPV11 mono-infections. It is plausible that factors such as immune suppression and specific changes to the local microbiome may contribute to the enhancement of viral persistence, while chemical agents may also act as co-carcinogens in the pharyngeal and penile mucosae. Establishing the etiologic role of these LR-HPVs in the penis and pharynx and the contributions of other co-factors will require additional studies and experimental demonstrations.

Supplementary Materials: The following supporting information can be downloaded at: https://www.mdpi.com/article/10.3390/cancers15164068/s1, Table S1: HPV6, HPV11 and HPV16 E5, E6 and E7 protein sequences.

Author Contributions: Conceptualization, M.S.d.A., H.O.B. and R.M.G.d.C.; methodology, M.S.d.A., G.B., R.M. and J.M.O.S.; validation, F.F.L. and A.P.A.d.S.; investigation, L.L.d.S. and A.M.T.; resources, P.A.O., R.M. and R.M.G.d.C.; data curation, A.I.F.-R., P.A.O. and R.M.G.d.C.; writing—original draft preparation, A.M.T. and R.M.G.d.C.; writing—review and editing, L.L.d.S., J.M.O.S., M.S.d.A., R.M., A.I.F.-R., P.A.O., A.P.A.d.S., F.F.L., G.B. and H.O.B.; supervision, R.M., R.M.G.d.C. and H.O.B.; project administration, R.M.G.d.C. and R.M.; funding acquisition, R.M., P.A.O. and R.M.G.d.C. All authors have read and agreed to the published version of the manuscript.

Funding: This research was funded by the following institutions: CAPES (finance code 001 and grant 13/2020), PDPG Amazônia Legal 0810/2020/88881.510244/2020-01 (grants IECT-FAPEMA-05796/18 and FAPEMA IECT 30/2018), IECT Saúde (grant PPSUS-02160/20 financed by FAPEMA, CNPq and the Brazilian Ministry of Health), the Research Center of the Portuguese Oncology Institute of Porto (project no. PI86-CI-IPOP-66-2017), the European Investment Fund, the FEDER/COMPETE/POCI—Operational Competitiveness and Internationalization Program, and national funds from the FCT—Portuguese Foundation for Science and Technology under projects UID/AGR/04033/2020 and UIDB/CVT/00772/2020. This work was also supported by LA/P/0045/2020 (ALiCE), UIDB/00511/2020 and UIDP/00511/2020 (LEPABE), funded by national funds through FCT/MCTES (PIDDAC) and 2SMART (NORTE-01-0145-FEDER-000054) and supported by the Norte Portugal Regional Operational Programme (NORTE 2020) under the PORTUGAL 2020 Partnership Agreement through the European Regional Development Fund (ERDF). Rui Gil da Costa received a FAPEMA postdoctoral grant (BPD-01343/23). Leando Lima da Silva and Amanda Teles were supported by CAPES research grants under the project PDPG Amazônia Legal 0810/2020/88881.510244/2020-01.

Institutional Review Board Statement: Not applicable.

Informed Consent Statement: Not applicable.

Data Availability Statement: The data produced in this study are available in this article and in Supplementary Table S1.

Conflicts of Interest: The authors declare no conflict of interest. The funders had no role in the design of the study; in the collection, analyses, or interpretation of the data; in the writing of the manuscript; or in the decision to publish the results.

References

1. Tommasino, M. The human papillomavirus family and its role in carcinogenesis. *Semin. Cancer Biol.* **2014**, *26*, 13–21. [CrossRef] [PubMed]
2. Vashisht, S.; Mishra, H.; Mishra, P.K.; Ekielski, A.; Talegaonkar, S. Structure, genome, infection cycle and clinical manifestations associated with human papillomavirus. *Curr. Pharm. Biotechnol.* **2019**, *20*, 1260–1280. [CrossRef] [PubMed]
3. Liu, Y.; Baleja, J. Structure and function of the papillomavirus E6 protein and its interacting proteins. *Front. Biosci.* **2008**, *1*, 121–134. [CrossRef]
4. De Sanjose, S.; Brotons, M.; Pavon, M.A. The natural history of human papillomavirus infection. *Best Pract. Res. Clin. Obstet. Gynaecol.* **2018**, *47*, 2–13. [CrossRef]
5. Estêvão, D.; Costa, N.R.; da Costa RM, G.; Medeiros, R. Hallmarks of HPV carcinogenesis: The role of E6, E7 and E5 oncoproteins in cellular malignancy. *Biochim. Biophys. Acta-Gene Regul. Mech.* **2019**, *1862*, 153–162. [CrossRef]
6. Zur Hausen, H. Papillomaviruses and cancer: From basic studies to clinical application. *Nat. Rev. Cancer* **2002**, *2*, 342–350. [CrossRef]
7. Zur Hausen, H. Papillomavirus infections: A major cause of human cancers. In *Infections Causing Human Cancer*; Zur Hausen, H., Ed.; Wiley–VCH: Weinheim, Germany, 2006; pp. 145–243.
8. Bernard, H.U.; Burk, R.D.; Chen, Z.; van Doorslaer, K.; Zur Hausen, H.; de Villiers, E.M. Classification of papillomaviruses (PVs) based on 189 PV types and proposal of taxonomic amendments. *Virology* **2010**, *401*, 70–79. [CrossRef]
9. De Villiers, E.M.; Fauquet, C.; Broker, T.R.; Bernard, H.U.; Zur Hausen, H. Classification of papillomaviruses. *Virology* **2004**, *324*, 17–27. [CrossRef]
10. Muñoz, N.; Bosch, F.X.; De Sanjosé, S.; Herrero, R.; Castellsagué, X.; Shah, K.V.; Snijders, P.J.F.; Meijer, C.J.L.M. Epidemiologic classifcation of human papillomavirus types associated with cervical cancer. *N. Engl. J. Med.* **2003**, *348*, 518–527. [CrossRef]
11. Salgado, A.H.; Martín-Gámez, D.C.; Moreno, P.; Murillo, R.; Bravo, M.M.; Villa, L.; Molano, M. E6 molecular variants of human papillomavirus (HPV) type 16: An updated and unified criterion for clustering and nomenclature. *Virology* **2011**, *410*, 201–215. [CrossRef]
12. Sichero, L.; Sobrinho, J.S.; Villa, L.L. Oncogenic potential diverge among human papillomavirus type 16 natural variants. *Virology* **2012**, *432*, 127–132. [CrossRef]
13. Cochicho, D.; da Costa, R.G.; Felix, A. Exploring the roles of HPV16 variants in head and neck squamous cell carcinoma: Current challenges and opportunities. *Virol. J.* **2021**, *18*, 217. [CrossRef]
14. Leto, M.D.G.P.; Santos Júnior, G.F.D.; Porro, A.M.; Tomimori, J. Human papillomavirus infection: Etiopathogenesis, molecular biology and clinical manifestations. *An. Bras. Dermatol.* **2011**, *86*, 306–317. [CrossRef] [PubMed]
15. Kroupis, C.; Vourlidis, N. Human papilloma virus (HPV) molecular diagnostics. *Clin. Chem. Lab. Med.* **2011**, *49*, 1783–1799. [CrossRef] [PubMed]
16. Hampson, I.N. Effects of the prophylactic HPV vaccines on HPV type prevalence and cervical pathology. *Viruses* **2022**, *14*, 757. [CrossRef] [PubMed]

17. Handisurya, A.; Schellenbacher, C.; Kirnbauer, R. Diseases caused by human papillomaviruses (HPV). *J. Dtsch. Dermatol. Ges.* **2009**, *7*, 453–666, quiz 466, 467. [CrossRef] [PubMed]
18. Forman, D.; de Martel, C.; Lacey, C.J.; Soerjomataram, I.; Lortet-Tieulent, J.; Bruni, L.; Vignat, J.; Ferlay, J.; Bray, F.; Plummer, M.; et al. Global burden of human papillomavirus and related diseases. *Vaccine* **2012**, *30*, F12–F23. [CrossRef]
19. Yuan, H.; Zhou, D.; Wang, J.; Schlegel, R. Divergent human papillomavirus associated with recurrent respiratory papillomatosis with lung involvement. *Genome Announc.* **2013**, *1*, 10. [CrossRef]
20. Donne, A.; Hampson, L.; Homer, J.; Hampson, I. The role of HPV type in recurrent respiratory papillomatosis. *Int. J. Pediatr. Otorhinolaryngol.* **2010**, *74*, 7–14. [CrossRef]
21. Faber, M.T.; Sand, F.L.; Albieri, V.; Norrild, B.; Kjær, S.K.; Verdoodt, F. Prevalence and type distribution of human papillomavirus in squamous cell carcinoma and intraepithelial neoplasia of the vulva. *Int. J. Cancer* **2017**, *141*, 1161–1169. [CrossRef]
22. Olesen, T.B.; Sand, F.L.; Rasmussen, C.L.; Albieri, V.; Toft, B.G.; Norrild, B.; Munk, C.; Kjær, S.K. Prevalence of human papillomavirus DNA and p16INK4a in penile cancer and penile intraepithelial neoplasia: A systematic review and meta-analysis. *Lancet Oncol.* **2019**, *20*, 145–158. [CrossRef]
23. Page, M.J.; McKenzie, J.E.; Bossuyt, P.M.; Boutron, I.; Hoffmann, T.C.; Mulrow, C.D.; Shamseer, L.; Tetzlaff, J.M.; Akl, E.A.; Brennan, S.E.; et al. The PRISMA 2020 statement: An updated guideline for reporting systematic reviews. *Int. J. Surg.* **2021**, *88*, 105906. [CrossRef]
24. Grant, J.R.; Stothard, P. The CGView server: A comparative genomics tool for circular genomes. *Nucleic Acids Res.* **2008**, *36*, W181–W184. [CrossRef] [PubMed]
25. Tao, G.; Yaling, G.; Zhan, G.; Pu, L.; Miao, H. Human papillomavirus genotype distribution among HPV-positive women in Sichuan province, Southwest China. *Arch. Virol.* **2017**, *163*, 65–72. [CrossRef]
26. Das, D.; Rai, A.K.; Kataki, A.C.; Barmon, D.; Deka, P.; Sharma, J.D.; Sarma, A.; Shrivastava, S.; Bhattacharyya, M.; Kalita, A.K.; et al. Nested multiplex PCR based detection of human papillomavirus in cervical carcinoma patients of North-East India. *Asian Pac. J. Cancer Prev.* **2013**, *14*, 785–790. [CrossRef] [PubMed]
27. Aldersley, J.; Lorenz, D.R.; Mouw, K.W.; D'Andrea, A.D.; Gabuzda, D. Genomic landscape of primary and recurrent anal squamous cell carcinomas in relation to HPV integration, copy-number variation, and DNA damage response genes. *Mol. Cancer Res.* **2021**, *19*, 1308–1321. [CrossRef]
28. Magaña-León, C.; Oros, C.; López-Revilla, R. Human papillomavirus types in non-cervical high-grade intraepithelial neoplasias and invasive carcinomas from San Luis Potosí, Mexico: A retrospective cross-sectional study. *Infect. Agents Cancer* **2015**, *10*, 33. [CrossRef] [PubMed]
29. Taberna, M.; Resteghini, C.; Swanson, B.; Pickard, R.K.; Jiang, B.; Xiao, W.; Mena, M.; Kreinbrink, P.; Chio, E.; Gillison, M.L. Low etiologic fraction for human papillomavirus in larynx squamous cell carcinoma. *Oral. Oncol.* **2016**, *61*, 55–61. [CrossRef]
30. Lam, E.W.H.; Chan, M.M.H.; Wai, C.K.C.; Ngai, C.M.; Chen, Z.; Wong, M.C.S.; Yeung, A.C.M.; Tong, J.H.M.; Chan, A.B.W.; To, K.F.; et al. The role of human papillomavirus in laryngeal cancer in Southern China. *J. Med. Virol.* **2018**, *90*, 1150–1159. [CrossRef] [PubMed]
31. Weiss, D.; Heinkele, T.; Rudack, C. Reliable detection of human papillomavirus in recurrent laryngeal papillomatosis and associated carcinoma of archival tissue. *J. Med. Virol.* **2015**, *87*, 860–870. [CrossRef]
32. Sun, J.; Xiong, J.; Zhen, Y.; Chen, Z.L.; Zhang, H. P53 and PCNA is positively correlated with HPV infection in laryngeal epitheliopapillomatous lesions in patiets with different ethnic backgrounds in Xinjiang. *Asian Pac. J. Cancer Prev.* **2012**, *13*, 5439–5444. [CrossRef]
33. Vietía, D.; Liuzzi, J.; Avila, M.; De Guglielmo, Z.; Prado, Y.; Correnti, M. Human papillomavirus detection in head and neck squamous cell carcinoma. *Ecancermedicalscience* **2014**, *8*, 475. [CrossRef]
34. Barzon, L.; Cappellesso, R.; Peta, E.; Militello, V.; Sinigaglia, A.; Fassan, M.; Simonato, F.; Guzzardo, V.; Ventura, L.; Blandamura, S.; et al. Profiling of expression of human papillomavirus-related cancer miRNAs in penile squamous cell carcinomas. *Am. J. Pathol.* **2014**, *184*, 3376–3383. [CrossRef]
35. Alemany, L.; Cubilla, A.; Halec, G.; Kasamatsu, E.; Quirós, B.; Masferrer, E.; Tous, S.; Lloveras, B.; Hernández-Suarez, G.; Lonsdale, R.; et al. Role of human papillomavirus in penile carcinomas worldwide. *Eur. Urol.* **2016**, *69*, 953–961. [CrossRef]
36. Lechner, M.; Liu, J.; Masterson, L.; Fenton, T.R. HPV-associated oropharyngeal cancer: Epidemiology, molecular biology and clinical mangement. *Nat. Rev. Clin. Oncol.* **2022**, *19*, 306–327. [CrossRef]
37. Serrano, B.; Brotons, M.; Bosch, F.X.; Bruni, L. Epidemiology and burden of HPV-related disease. *Clin. Obstet. Gynaecol.* **2018**, *47*, 14–26. [CrossRef]
38. Mestre, V.F.; Medeiros-Fonseca, B.; Estêvão, D.; Casaca, F.; Silva, S.; Félix, A.; Silva, F.; Colaço, B.; Seixas, F.; Bastos, M.M.; et al. HPV16 is sufficient to induce squamous cell carcinoma specifically in the tongue base in transgenic mice. *J. Pathol.* **2020**, *251*, 4–11. [CrossRef]
39. Medeiros-Fonseca, B.; Mestre, V.F.; Estêvão, D.; Sánchez, D.F.; Cañete-Portillo, S.; Fernández-Nestosa, M.J.; Casaca, F.; Silva, S.; Brito, H.; Félix, A.; et al. HPV16 induces penile intraepithelial neoplasia and squamous cell carcinoma in transgenic mice: First mpouse model for HPV-related penile cancer. *J. Pathol.* **2020**, *251*, 411–419. [CrossRef]
40. Stelzer, M.K.; Pitot, H.C.; Liem, A.; Schweizer, J.; Mahoney, C.; Lambert, P.F. A mouse model for human anal cancer. *Cancer Prev. Res.* **2010**, *3*, 1534–1541. [CrossRef]

41. Cochicho, D.; Nunes, A.; Gomes, J.P.; Martins, L.; Cunha, M.; Medeiros-Fonseca, B.; Oliveira, P.; Bastos, M.M.S.M.; Medeiros, R.; Mendonça, J.; et al. Characterization of the human papillomavirus 16 oncogenes in K14HPV16 mice: Sublineage A1 drives multi-organ carcinogenesis. *Int. J. Mol. Sci.* **2022**, *23*, 12371. [CrossRef]
42. Trottier, H.; Franco, E.L. The epidemiology of genital human papillomavirus infection. *Vaccine* **2006**, *24*, S4–S15. [CrossRef]
43. Garbuglia, A.R.; Gentile, M.; Del Nonno, F.; Lorenzini, P.; Lapa, D.; Lupi, F.; Pinnetti, C.; Baiocchini, A.; Libertone, R.; Cicalini, S.; et al. An anal cancer screening program for MSM in Italy: Prevalence of multiple HPV types and vaccine-targeted infections. *J. Clin. Virol.* **2015**, *72*, 49–54. [CrossRef]
44. Jain, M.A.; Limaiem, F. *Cervical Intraepithelial Squamous Cell Lesion*; StatPearls Publishing: Treasure Island, FL, USA, 2021.
45. Cohen, P.A.; Jhingran, A.; Oaknin, A.; Denny, L. Cervical cancer. *Lancet* **2019**, *393*, 169–182. [CrossRef]
46. Li, N.; Franceschi, S.; Howell-Jones, R.; Snijders, P.J.; Clifford, G.M. Human papillomavirus type distribution in 30,848 invasive cervical cancers worldwide: Variation by geographical region, histological type and year of publication. *Int. J. Cancer* **2011**, *128*, 927–935. [CrossRef]
47. Manyere, N.R.; Dube Mandishora, R.S.; Magwali, T.; Mtisi, F.; Mataruka, K.; Mtede, B.; Palefsky, J.M.; Chirenje, Z.M. Human papillomavirus genotype distribution in genital warts among women in Harare-Zimbabwe. *J. Obstet. Gynaecol.* **2020**, *40*, 830–836. [CrossRef]
48. Viau, M.; Renaud, M.C.; Grégoire, J.; Sebastianelli, A.; Plante, M. Paraneoplastic syndromes associated with gynecological cancers: A systematic review. *Gynecol. Oncol.* **2017**, *146*, P661–P671. [CrossRef]
49. Pang, S.S.; Murphy, M.; Markham, M.J. Current management of locally advanced and metastatic cervical cancer in the United States. *JCO Oncol. Pract.* **2022**, *18*, 417–422. [CrossRef]
50. Peixoto da Silva, S.; Santos, J.M.; Costa e Silva, M.P.; Gil da Costa, R.M.; Medeiros, R. Cancer cachexia and its pathophysiology: Links with sarcopenia, anorexia and asthenia. *J. Cachexia Sarcopenia Muscle* **2020**, *11*, 619–635. [CrossRef]
51. Monti, M.; D'Aniello, D.; Scopelliti, A.; Tibaldi, V.; Santangelo, G.; Colagiovanni, V.; Giannini, A.; DI Donato, V.; Palaia, I.; Perniola, G.; et al. Relationship between cervical excisional treatment for cervical intraepithelial neoplasia and obstetrical outcome. *Minerva Obstet. Gynecol.* **2020**, *73*, 233–246.
52. Giannini, A.; Di Donato, V.; Sopracordevole, F.; Ciavattini, A.; Ghelardi, A.; Vizza, E.; D'Oria, O.; Simoncini, T.; Plotti, F.; Casarin, J.; et al. Outcomes of high-grade cervical dysplasia with positive margins anf HPV persistence after cervical conization. *Vaccines* **2022**, *11*, 698. [CrossRef]
53. Cochicho, D.; Esteves, S.; Rito, M.; Silva, F.; Martins, L.; Montalvão, P.; Cunha, M.; Magalhães, M.; Gil da Costa, R.M.; Felix, A. PIK3CA gene mutations in HNSCC: Systematic review and correlations with HPV status and patient survival. *Cancers* **2022**, *14*, 1286. [CrossRef]
54. Rabah, R.; Lancaster, W.D.; Thomas, R.; Gregoire, L. Human papillomavirus-11-associated recurrent respiratory papillomatosis is more aggressive than human papillomavirus-6-associated disease. *Pediatr. Dev. Pathol.* **2001**, *4*, 68–72. [CrossRef]
55. Lee, L.-A.; Cheng, A.-J.; Fang, T.-J.; Huang, C.-G.; Liao, C.-T.; Chang, J.T.-C.; Li, H.-Y. High incidence of malignant transformation of laryngeal papilloma in Taiwan. *Laryngoscope* **2008**, *118*, 50–55. [CrossRef]
56. Wieland, U.; Kreuter, A. HPV-induced anal lesions. *Hautarzt* **2015**, *66*, 439–445. [CrossRef]
57. Zaouak, A.; Ebdelli, W.; Bacha, T.; Koubaa, W.; Hammami, H.; Fenniche, S. Verrucous carcinoma arising in an extended giant condyloma acuminatum. *Skinmed* **2023**, *21*, 53–54.
58. De Sousa, I.D.B.; Vidal, F.C.B.; Vidal, J.P.C.B.; de Mello, G.C.F.; Nascimento, M.D.D.S.B.; Brito, L.M.O. Prevalence of human papillomavirus in penile malignant tumors: Viral genotyping and clinical aspects. *BMC Urol.* **2015**, *15*, 13. [CrossRef]
59. Fernández-Nestosa, M.J.; Guimerà, N.; Sanchez, D.F.; Cañete-Portillo, S.; Velazquez, E.F.; Jenkins, D.; Quint, W.; Cubilla, A.L. Human papillomavirus (HPV) genotypes in condylomas, intraepithelial neoplasia, and invasive carcinoma of the penis using laser capture microdissection (LCM)-PCR: A study of 191 lesions in 43 patients. *Am. J. Surg. Pathol.* **2017**, *41*, 820–832. [CrossRef]
60. Srodon, M.; Stoler, M.H.; Baber, G.B.; Kurman, R.J. The distribution of low and high-risk HPV types in vulvar and vaginal intraepithelial neoplasia (VIN and VaIN). *Am. J. Surg. Pathol.* **2006**, *30*, 1513–1518. [CrossRef]
61. Facio, F.N., Jr.; Facio, M.F.W.; Spessoto, A.C.N.; Godoy, M.; Tessaro, H.; Campos, R.; Zanatto, D.; Calmon, M.; Rahal, P.; Fava, L.C.; et al. Clinical and molecular profile of patients with condyloma acuminatum treated in the Brazilian public healthcare system. *Cureus* **2022**, *14*, e21961. [CrossRef]
62. Horn, L.C.; Klostermann, K.; Hautmann, S.; Höhn, A.K.; Beckmann, M.W.; Mehlhorn, G. HPV-associated alterations of the vulva and vagina. Morphology and molecular pathology. *Pathologe* **2011**, *32*, 467–475. [CrossRef]
63. Cornall, A.M.; Roberts, J.M.; Garland, S.M.; Hillman, R.J.; Grulich, A.E.; Tabrizi, S.N. Anal and perianal squamous carcinomas and high-grade intraepithelial lesions exclusively associated with "low-risk" HPV genotypes 6 and 11. *Int. J. Cancer* **2013**, *133*, 2253–2258. [CrossRef]
64. de Pokomandy, A.; Rouleau, D.; Ghattas, G.; Vézina, S.; Coté, P.; Macleod, J.; Allaire, G.; Franco, E.L.; HIPVIRG Study Group. Prevalence, clearance, and incidence of anal human papillomavirus infection in HIV-infected men: The HIPVIRG Cohort Study. *J. Infect. Dis.* **2009**, *199*, 965–973. [CrossRef]
65. Goldstone, S.; Palefsky, J.M.; Giuliano, A.R.; Moreira, E.D.; Aranda, C.; Jessen, H.; Hillman, R.J.; Ferris, D.G.; Coutlee, F.; Liaw, K.-L.; et al. Prevalence of and risk factors for human papillomavirus (HPV) infection among HIV-seronegative men who have sex with men. *J. Infect. Dis.* **2011**, *203*, 66–74. [CrossRef]

66. Alexandrou, A.; Dimitriou, N.; Levidou, G.; Griniatsos, J.; Sougioultzis, S.; Korkolopoulou, P.; Felekouras, E.; Pikoulis, E.; Diamantis, T.; Tsigris, C.; et al. The incidence of HPV infection in anal cancer patients in Greece. *Acta Gastroenterol. Belg.* **2014**, *77*, 213–216. [PubMed]
67. Egawa, N.; Nakahara, T.; Ohno, S.; Narisawa-Saito, M.; Yugawa, T.; Fujita, M.; Yamato, K.; Natori, Y.; Kiyono, T. The E1 protein of human papillomavirus type 16 is dispensable for maintenance replication of the viral genome. *J. Virol.* **2012**, *86*, 3276–3283. [CrossRef] [PubMed]
68. Hughes, F.J.; Romanos, M.A. E1 protein of human papillomavirus is a DNA helicase/ATPase. *Nucleic Acids Res.* **1993**, *21*, 5817–5823. [CrossRef] [PubMed]
69. Doorbar, J.; Egawa, N.; Griffin, H.; Kranjec, C.; Murakami, I. Human papillomavirus molecular biology and disease association. *Rev. Med. Virol.* **2015**, *25* (Suppl. S1), 2–23. [CrossRef]
70. Sanders, C.M.; Stenlund, A. Transcription factor-dependent loading of the E1 initiator reveals modular assembly of the papillomavirus origin melting complex. *J. Biol. Chem.* **2000**, *275*, 3522–3534. [CrossRef]
71. Võsa, L.; Sudakov, A.; Remm, M.; Ustav, M.; Kurg, R. Identification and analysis of papillomavirus E2 protein binding sites in the human genome. *J. Virol.* **2012**, *86*, 348–357. [CrossRef]
72. Wang, X.; Meyers, C.; Wang, H.-K.; Chow, L.T.; Zheng, Z.-M. Construction of a full transcription map of human papillomavirus type 18 during productive viral infection. *J. Virol.* **2011**, *85*, 8080–8092. [CrossRef]
73. Müller, M.; Prescott, E.L.; Wasson, C.W.; Macdonald, A. Human papillomavirus E5 oncoprotein: Function and potential target for antiviral therapeutics. *Future Virol.* **2015**, *10*, 27–39. [CrossRef]
74. DiMaio, D.; Petti, L.M. The E5 proteins. *Virology* **2013**, *445*, 99–114. [CrossRef] [PubMed]
75. Filippova, M.; Johnson, M.M.; Bautista, M.; Filippov, V.; Fodor, N.; Tungteakkhun, S.S.; Williams, K.; Duerksen-Hughes, P.J. The large and small isoforms of human papillomavirus type 16 E6 bind to and differentially affect procaspase 8 stability and activity. *J. Virol.* **2007**, *81*, 4116–4129. [CrossRef]
76. Genther Williams, S.M.; Disbrow, G.L.; Schlegel, R.; Lee, D.; Threadgill, D.W.; Lambert, P.F. Requirement of epidermal growth factor receptor for hyperplasia induced by E5, a high-risk human papillomavirus oncogene. *Cancer Res.* **2005**, *65*, 6534–6542. [CrossRef] [PubMed]
77. Roman, A.; Munger, K. The papillomavirus E7 proteins. *Virology* **2013**, *445*, 138–168. [CrossRef] [PubMed]
78. McLaughlin-Drubin, M.E.; Bromberg-White, J.L.; Meyers, C. The role of the human papillomavirus type 18 E7 oncoprotein during the complete viral life cycle. *Virology* **2005**, *338*, 61–68. [CrossRef]
79. Egawa, N.; Doorbar, J. The low-risk papillomaviruses. *Virus Res.* **2017**, *231*, 119–127. [CrossRef]
80. Barrow-Laing, L.; Chen, W.; Romão, A. Low- and high-risk human papillomavirusE7 proteins regulate p130 differently. *Virology* **2010**, *400*, 233–239. [CrossRef]
81. Zhang, B.; Chen, W.; Roman, A. The E7 proteins of low- and high-risk human papillomaviruses share the ability to target the pRB family member p130 for degradation. *Proc. Natl. Acad. Sci. USA* **2006**, *103*, 437–442. [CrossRef]
82. Genovese, N.J.; Broker, T.R.; Chow, L.T. Nonconserved lysine residues attenuate the biological function of the low-risk human papillomavirus E7 protein. *J. Virol.* **2011**, *85*, 5546–5554. [CrossRef]
83. Singhi, A.D.; Westra, W.H. Comparison of human papillomavirus in situ hybridization and p16 immunohistochemistry in the detection of human papillomavirus-associated head and neck cancer based on a prospective clinical experience. *Cancer* **2010**, *116*, 2166–2173. [CrossRef] [PubMed]

Disclaimer/Publisher's Note: The statements, opinions and data contained in all publications are solely those of the individual author(s) and contributor(s) and not of MDPI and/or the editor(s). MDPI and/or the editor(s) disclaim responsibility for any injury to people or property resulting from any ideas, methods, instructions or products referred to in the content.

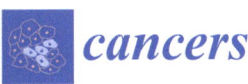

Article

Planning CT Identifies Patients at Risk of High Prostate Intrafraction Motion

Hendrik Ballhausen *, Minglun Li, Elia Lombardo, Guillaume Landry and Claus Belka

Department of Radiation Oncology, LMU University Hospital, LMU Munich, 81377 Munich, Germany
* Correspondence: hendrik.ballhausen@med.uni-muenchen.de

Simple Summary: Motion of the prostate may adversely affect the outcome of radiotherapy. Online tracking of the prostate during irradiation is technologically feasible but only available at select institutions. It would be beneficial to be able to identify patients at risk of particularly high prostate intrafraction motion with simpler technology. In this paper, we present a larger inner diameter of the lesser pelvis as an anatomical predictor for high prostate intrafraction motion. It can be measured with a single planning CT, which should always be available. Risk patients identified in this way could then be selected for more rigorous online motion management or benefit from increased safety margins.

Abstract: Prostate motion (standard deviation, range of motion, and diffusion coefficient) was calculated from 4D ultrasound data of 1791 fractions of radiation therapy in N = 100 patients. The inner diameter of the lesser pelvis was obtained from transversal slices through the pubic symphysis in planning CTs. On the lateral and craniocaudal axes, motility increases significantly (t-test, $p < 0.005$) with the inner diameter of the lesser pelvis. A diameter of >106 mm (ca. 6th decile) is a good predictor for high prostate intrafraction motion (ca. 9th decile). The corresponding area under the receiver operator curve (AUROC) is 80% in the lateral direction, 68% to 80% in the craniocaudal direction, and 62% to 70% in the vertical direction. On the lateral x-axis, the proposed test is 100% sensitive and has a 100% negative predictive value for all three characteristics (standard deviation, range of motion, and diffusion coefficient). On the craniocaudal z-axis, the proposed test is 79% to 100% sensitive and reaches 95% to 100% negative predictive value. On the vertical axis, the proposed test still delivers 98% negative predictive value but is not particularly sensitive. Overall, the proposed predictor is able to help identify patients at risk of high prostate motion based on a single planning CT.

Keywords: radiation oncology; external beam radiotherapy; prostate carcinoma; intrafraction motion; motion management; risk management; planning CT

1. Introduction

External beam radiotherapy (EBRT) is used in the treatment of prostate carcinoma [1–3]. The intrafraction motion of the prostate can significantly impact delivery to the prostate gland. The prostate gland is a mobile organ, and larger movements during treatment could result in irradiation of healthy tissue or underdosing of the tumor target volume, adversely affecting tumor control [4,5]. Conversely, patients with higher intrafraction motion might benefit from continuous tracking and intrabeam adjustments through smaller required safety margins [6,7].

Several studies have investigated the effects of intrafraction motion on EBRT of the prostate, and the results have demonstrated the need for motion management strategies to optimize treatment outcomes. For example, an early study found a maximal range of motion of 6.8 mm anterior and 4.6 mm posterior [8].

While intrafraction motion may be insignificant in one patient or fraction, it may be substantial in another. A study in 184 patients found a "large variation in typical shifts between" ranging from 1 to 6 mm radially [9].

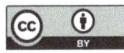

Citation: Ballhausen, H.; Li, M.; Lombardo, E.; Landry, G.; Belka, C. Planning CT Identifies Patients at Risk of High Prostate Intrafraction Motion. *Cancers* **2023**, *15*, 4103. https://doi.org/10.3390/cancers15164103

Academic Editor: Hideya Yamazaki

Received: 25 July 2023
Revised: 11 August 2023
Accepted: 12 August 2023
Published: 15 August 2023

Copyright: © 2023 by the authors. Licensee MDPI, Basel, Switzerland. This article is an open access article distributed under the terms and conditions of the Creative Commons Attribution (CC BY) license (https://creativecommons.org/licenses/by/4.0/).

Typically, the effect of prostate bed motion requires safety margins of 3 to 5 mm during image-guided radiation therapy [10].

In image guided therapy, several modalities have been available to pinpoint the location of the prostate and track its motion between fractions ("inter-fraction"). Examples include cone-beam computed tomography (CBCT), electronic portal imaging (EPI) with or without fiducial markers, stereotactic three-dimensional (3D) ultrasound and full 3D computed tomography [11,12]. The same or similar modalities are available to track the prostate's motion during a fraction ("intra-fraction").

One strategy is to limit intra-fraction motion by determining optimal levels of bladder filling [13] or restricting motion via endorectal balloons [14–16]. A more modern and generally advantageous approach is to reduce treatment times, limiting the opportunity for the prostate to wander off-beam [17].

Another approach is to use real-time tracking and beam adaptation, such as the Calypso 4D localization system, which allows for continuous monitoring and correction of the target position during treatment [18].

Similarly, four-dimensional (4D) ultrasound is a non-invasive technique used to visualize and track the motion of internal organs, including the prostate gland, during radiation therapy [19–21]. This method is not widely available in clinical practice, and its use is limited to specialized centers with the necessary equipment and expertise.

On the other hand, planning CT scans are routinely used in the treatment planning process for prostate cancer patients. This imaging modality provides high-quality images of the prostate gland and surrounding structures, which are used to generate a treatment plan that optimizes tumor coverage and minimizes the dose to nearby healthy tissues.

Because 4D ultrasound is not widely available, a planning CT would be particularly useful to identify patients at risk of high prostate intrafraction motion. In this paper, a CT-based anatomical criterion is derived and assessed. It may serve as a univariate predictor and identify patients at risk of high prostate intrafraction motion.

2. Materials and Methods

Infra-fraction motion of the prostate was recorded at our institution during 2.385 fractions of image-guided radiotherapy (IGRT) in 126 patients. The raw data is publicly available (see the data availability statement below) and has been described in detail at [22,23].

For this paper, those fractions were selected for which ultrasound recordings of at least 2 min were available. Of each fraction, the central one-minute time window was selected for analysis; see Figure 1. The rationale was to work with recordings of standardized length and to exclude possible motion artefacts at the beginning or end of the recordings.

For each of the clipped recordings, the standard deviation σ of the prostate position, the range of motion ρ, and the diffusion coefficient δ of the random walk model [24,25] were calculated for each of the three axes. In the case of the lateral x-axis:

$$\sigma_x = \sqrt{\frac{1}{N}\sum(x_i - \bar{x})^2} \tag{1}$$

$$\rho_x = \max(x) - \min(x) \tag{2}$$

$$\delta_x = \frac{(\Delta x)^2}{\Delta T} \tag{3}$$

σ and ρ are measured in mm. To be comparable across fractions and patients, they require a static time window of fixed duration (here: one minute). The diffusion coefficient δ is measured in mm^2 per minute and describes a linearly increasing variance over time.

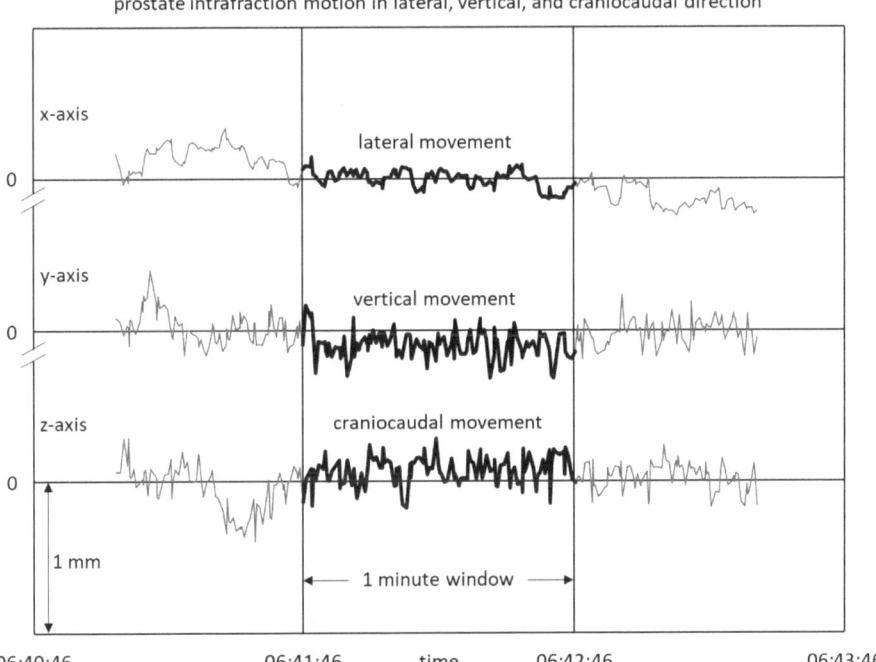

Figure 1. One minute of prostate tracking is evaluated per fraction.

Planning CTs were available for all patients. Transversal slices had been stored as DICOM images of 512 by 512 pixels with a pixel size of (1.074 mm)^2 in 97 out of 102 cases, (1.367 mm)^2 in 4 cases, and (1.073 mm)^2 in 1 case. Using these pixel pitches, all measurements were converted to mm for further analysis.

Planning CTs were manually evaluated by a physicist. The inner diameter D of the lesser pelvis was measured; see Figure 2.

Raw data processing: For each patient, their inner diameter D of the lesser pelvis was tabulated together with their average standard deviation σ, range of motion ρ, and diffusion coefficient δ along each of the three axes (for a total of 10 data points per patient).

Calculation of aggregate statistics: Across all patients, the average ± standard deviation, the minimum, the median, the maximum, and the other two quartiles of the ten quantities were tabulated. Histograms of the ten quantities were plotted.

Exploratory statistics: Scatter plots of the patient-average standard deviation σ, range of motion ρ, and diffusion coefficient δ in relation to the inner diameter D of the lesser pelvis were drawn.

Receiver Operator Characteristics: Sensitivity against specificity was plotted, and the area under the receiver operator curve (AUROC) was measured.

Explaining variable: Any inner diameter of the lesser pelvis below the 6th decile is considered "low D", while any diameter at or above the 6th decile is considered "high D". The threshold was informed by receiver operator curves and selected to maximize sensitivity while still providing at least some specificity.

Graphical Analysis: Box plots of the patient-average standard deviation σ, range of motion ρ, and diffusion coefficient δ were drawn comparing patients with "low D" vs. "high D".

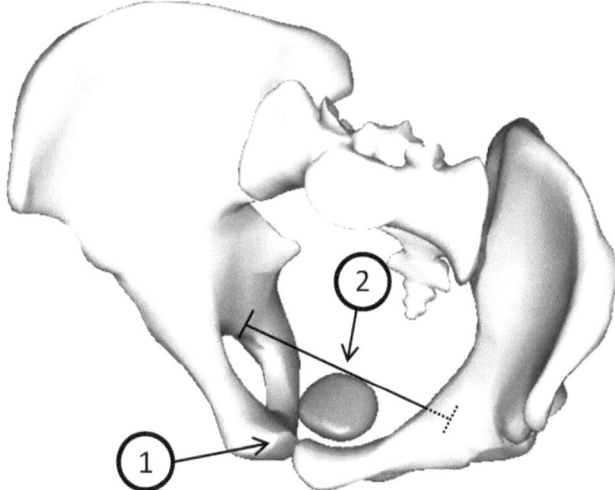

Figure 2. The inner diameter of the lesser pelvis is measured by identifying the most cranial slice of the planning CT that features the symphysis and then measuring the lateral distance between the two pubic bones. The 3D model shows the location of the prostate (1) in relation to the measured diameter (2) of the lesser pelvis.

Statistical Tests: Patient-average standard deviations σ, patient-average ranges of motion ρ, and patient-average diffusion coefficients δ above the 9th decile are considered "high". The test predicts "high" prostate motility if and only if the inner diameter D of the lesser pelvis is "high". Two-by-two contingency tables were drawn for each of the nine qualities, and the p-value was calculated by Fisher's two-sided exact test. Sensitivity, specificity, negative predictive value (NPV), and positive predictive value (PPV) were calculated.

3. Results

3.1. Available Data

One patient had to be excluded from the analysis because their ultrasound recordings contained outlier data. Another patient had to be excluded from the analysis because the relevant transversal slice was not assessable because multiple metal implants cast shadows on the symphysis ("metal artefacts"). This reduced the number of available patients to N = 100 and the number of available fractions to 1791. Table 1 shows the format of the input data for all the following analyses.

Table 1. Sample of N = 100 patients of the inner diameter of the lesser pelvis (D) and patient-average prostate motion characteristics (σ, ρ, δ).

Patient	D [mm]	σ_x [mm]	σ_y [mm]	σ_z [mm]	ρ_x [mm]	ρ_y [mm]	ρ_z [mm]	δ_x [mm²/s]	δ_y [mm²/s]	δ_z [mm²/s]
1	102.0	0.143	0.086	0.155	0.549	0.455	0.633	0.181	0.034	0.223
2	99.9	0.169	0.125	0.148	0.615	0.579	0.661	0.084	0.181	0.099
3	97.7	0.467	0.300	0.688	1.668	1.219	2.484	2.140	0.493	5.739
4	109.5	0.427	0.154	0.866	1.344	0.694	2.869	1.688	0.067	5.759
5	109.5	0.103	0.110	0.178	0.444	0.596	0.810	0.057	0.013	0.132
...	...	...	...	...	...	...	...	...	...	...
100	101.0	0.300	0.181	0.487	1.183	0.887	1.782	1.678	0.098	3.107

3.2. Inner Diameter of the Lesser Pelvis

In the sample of N = 100 patients, the inner diameter D of the lesser pelvis ranged from 89 mm to 115 mm. The average diameter was 103 mm plus or minus 6 mm of standard deviation, and the median diameter was 104 mm. See Table 2. Note that these numbers are significantly lower than what is often reported as the transverse diameter of the pelvic inlet. The latter is commonly measured in females and in the superior pelvis.

Table 2. Distribution of the inner diameter of the lesser pelvis (D) and patient-average prostate motion characteristics (σ, ρ, δ).

N = 100	D [mm]	σ_x [mm]	σ_y [mm]	σ_z [mm]	ρ_x [mm]	ρ_y [mm]	ρ_z [mm]	δ_x [mm²/s]	δ_y [mm²/s]	δ_z [mm²/s]
average	103.3	0.25	0.19	0.32	0.90	0.84	1.22	1.46	0.75	1.91
std. dev.	5.9	0.26	0.12	0.29	0.72	0.39	0.85	4.16	2.32	4.59
minimum	89.1	0.05	0.08	0.08	0.19	0.34	0.38	0.01	0.01	0.02
1st quartile	99.9	0.12	0.12	0.17	0.51	0.61	0.76	0.09	0.05	0.18
median	104.2	0.16	0.16	0.22	0.65	0.71	0.89	0.20	0.12	0.42
3rd quartile	108.5	0.26	0.19	0.34	0.98	0.94	1.38	0.61	0.28	1.16
maximum	114.9	1.98	0.76	2.15	5.01	2.26	5.65	29.70	20.08	29.30

Figure 3 shows a histogram of D. In the following, D ≥ 106 mm is considered "high D" and D < 106 mm is labeled "low D". Using this cutoff at the 6th decile, N = 61 or 61% of the patients were "low D", and N = 39 or 39% were "high D".

3.3. Prostate Motility

The patient-average standard deviation of the prostate position σ ranged from <0.1 mm to ca. 2.0 mm in the lateral and craniocaudal axes and 0.8 mm in the vertical axes. The average values were 0.25 mm (x-axis), 0.19 mm (y-axis), and 0.32 mm (z-axis), respectively. See Table 2 for further details. A joint histogram of all three axes is shown in Figure 4a. A joint cutoff of 0.5 mm corresponds roughly to the 9th decile.

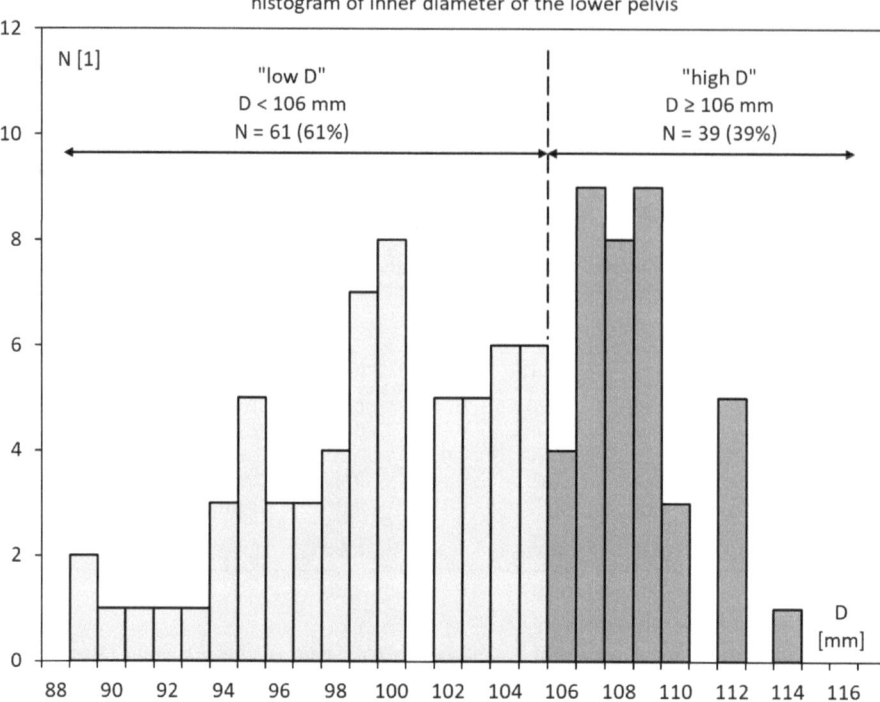

Figure 3. Histogram of the inner diameter of the lesser pelvis in the patient sample (D).

Similarly, the patient-average range of motion of the prostate ρ ranged from <0.4 mm to ca. 2 mm on the y-axis and >5 mm on the x- and z-axes. The average values were 0.90 mm (x-axis), 0.84 mm (y-axis), and 1.22 mm (z-axis), respectively. See Table 2 for further details. A joint histogram of all three axes is shown in Figure 4b. A joint cutoff of 2.0 mm corresponds roughly to the 9th decile.

Finally, the patient-average diffusion coefficient of prostate motion ranged from close to zero to almost 30 mm^2/s in some cases. High-motility cases pushed the averages to 1.46, 0.75, and 1.91 mm^2/s in the three axes. However, medians were much more moderate at 0.20, 0.12, and 0.42 mm^2, respectively. See Table 2 for further details. A joint histogram of all three axes is shown in Figure 4c. A joint cutoff of 7.5 mm is above the 9th decile, as the distribution is quite centered on zero.

In general, prostate motion was lower in the vertical direction than in the lateral and craniocaudal directions. This was true for all the tree measures σ, ρ and δ.

3.4. Prostate Motility vs. Inner Diameter of the Lesser Pelvis

The three scatter plots in Figure 5a–c show each 100 patients × 3 axes = 300 data points. The three plots show the patient-average standard deviation σ, patient-average range of motion ρ, and patient-average diffusion coefficient δ, respectively. The axes intersections are chosen such that they split each plot into four quadrants.

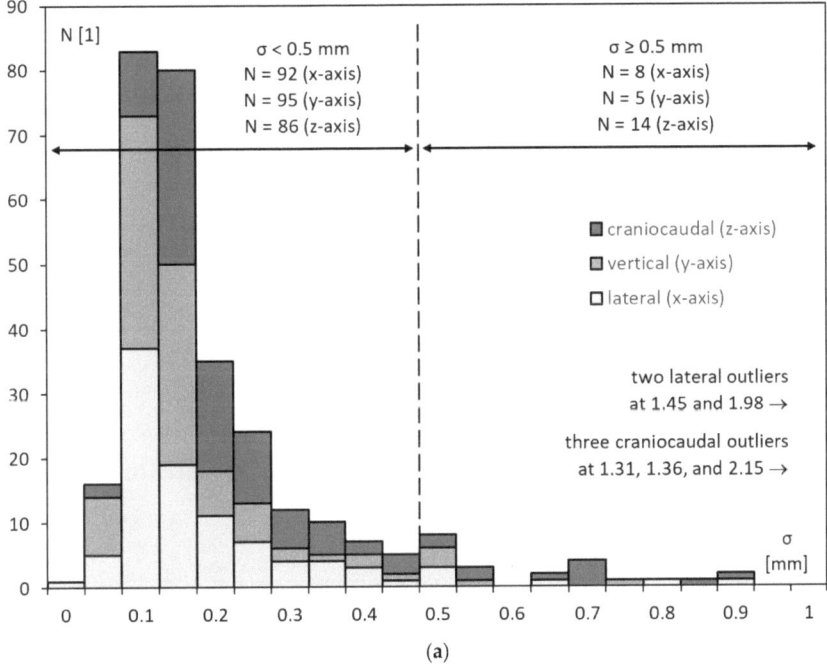

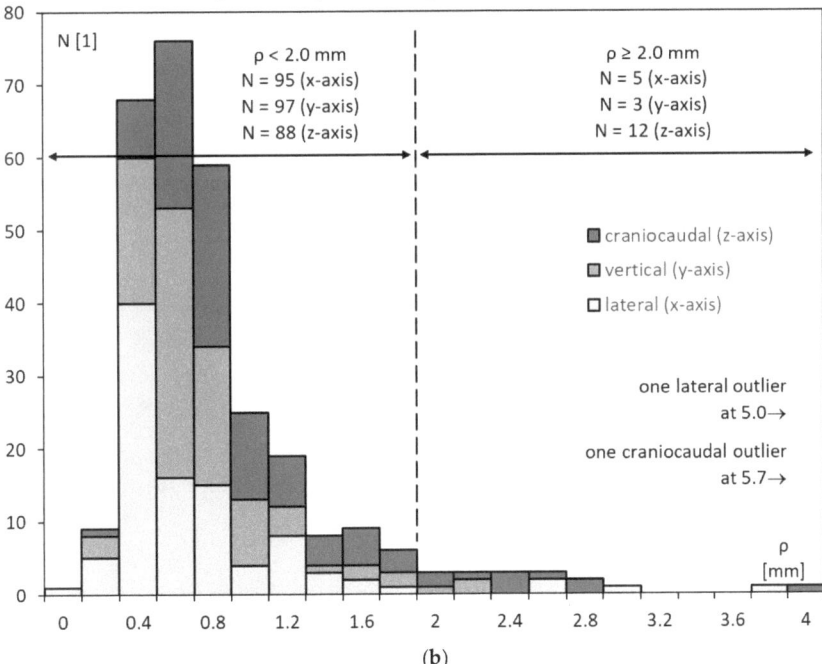

Figure 4. *Cont.*

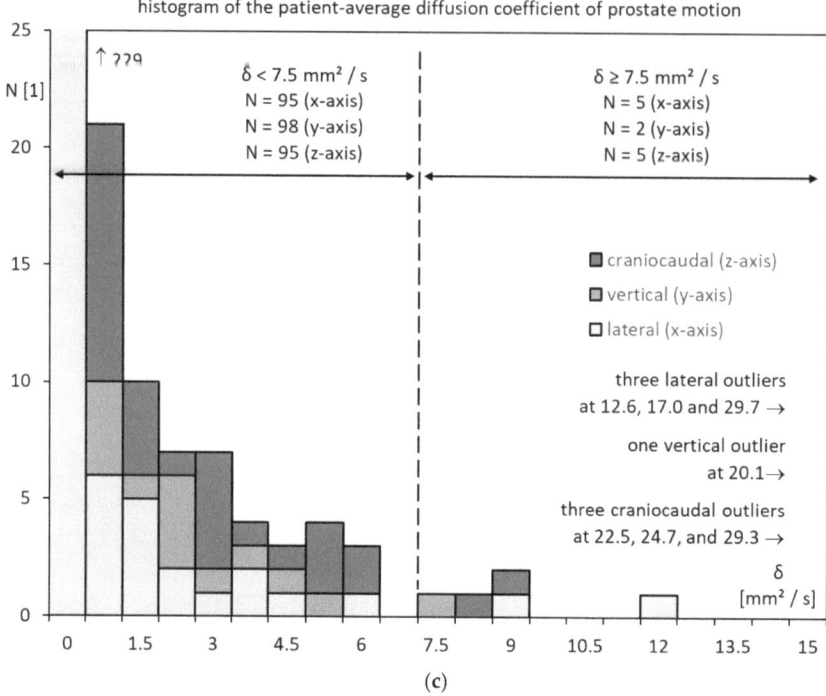

Figure 4. Histogram of patient-average (**a**) standard deviation σ; (**b**) range of motion ρ; (**c**) diffusion coefficient δ.

The lower two quadrants correspond to "low" prostate motility and contain most of the data points. There are a significant number of points both in the lower left and lower right quadrants. This means that there are a significant number of patients with low prostate motility, irrespective of the inner diameter of the lesser pelvis.

The upper two quadrants, however, contain significantly different points. These correspond to patients with "high" prostate motility. And most of them are found in the upper right quadrant, corresponding to high prostate motility and a high inner diameter of the lesser pelvis.

The picture is qualitatively similar for σ, ρ, and δ.

3.5. Receiver Operator Characteristics

Figure 6a (standard deviation), Figure 6b (range of motion), and Figure 6c (diffusion coefficient) show receiver operator curves (ROC) for the suggested test. The tradeoff between sensitivity and specificity is a function of the choice of the cutoff diameter, D. The plots are shown for the patient-average standard deviation σ, patient-average range of motion ρ, and patient-average diffusion coefficient δ, respectively.

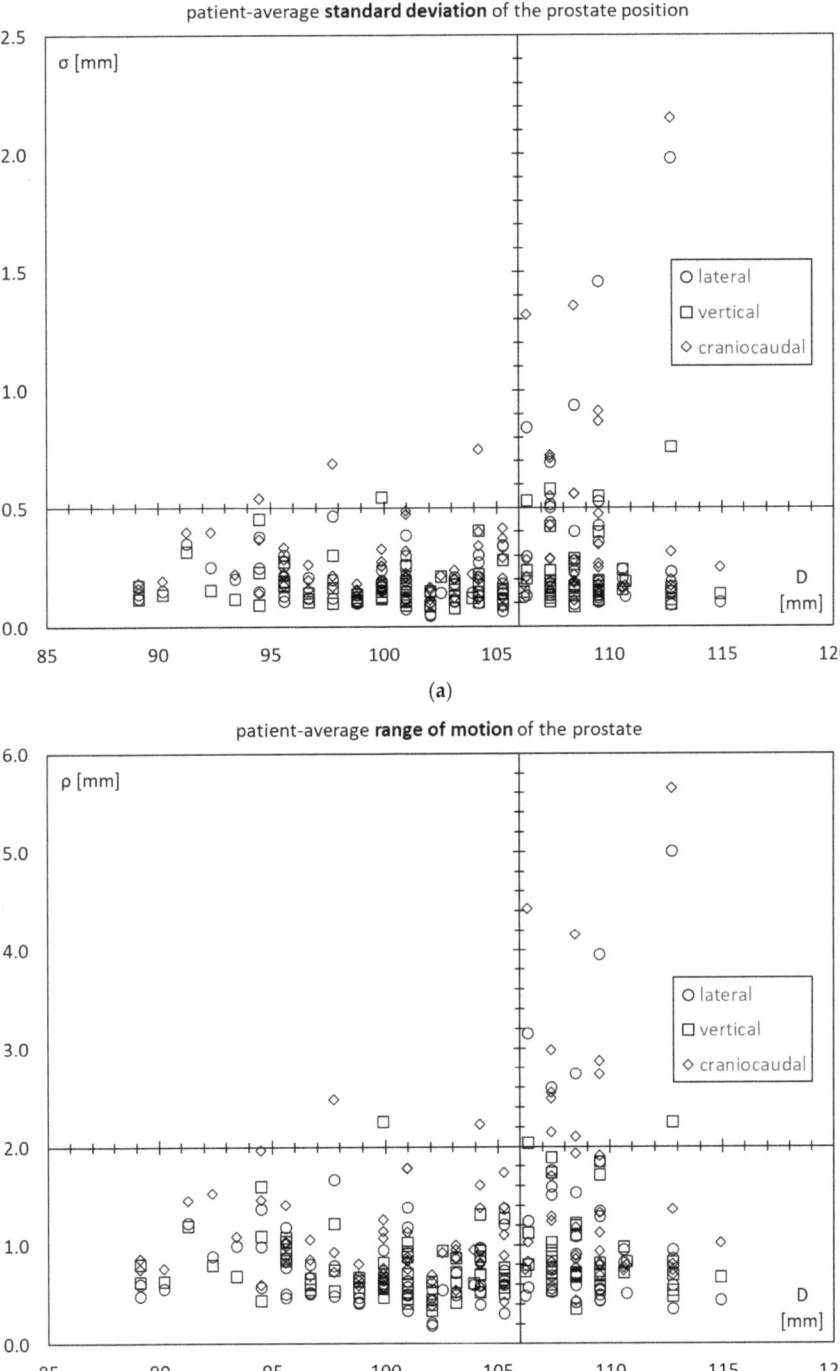

Figure 5. *Cont.*

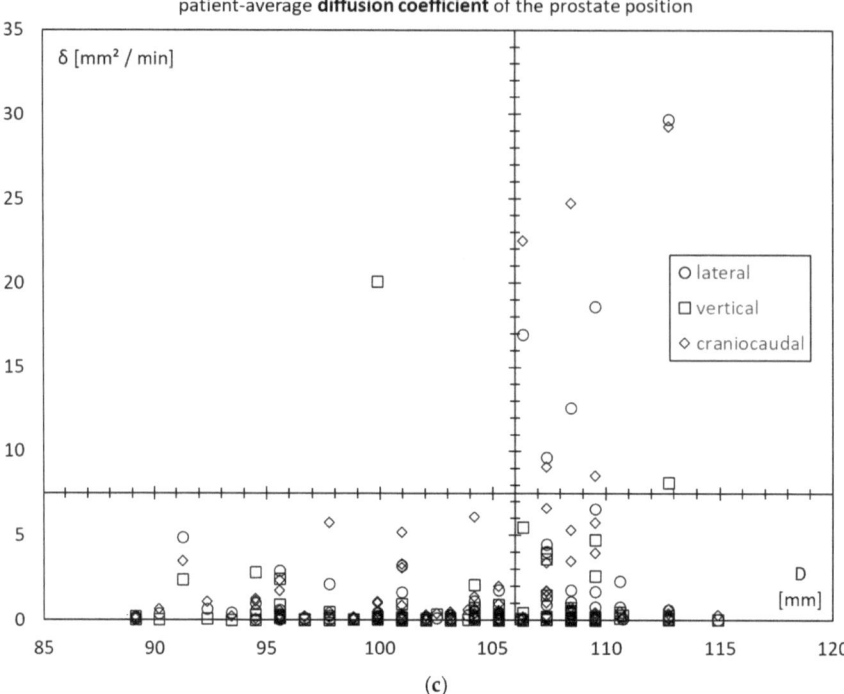

Figure 5. Scatter plots as a function of the inner diameter of the lesser pelvis (D) of the patient-average (**a**) standard deviation σ; (**b**) range of motion ρ; (**c**) diffusion coefficient δ.

The area under the receiver operator curve (AUROC) is 80% in the lateral direction for all three motion characteristics. It is between 68% and 80% in the craniocaudal direction. In the vertical direction, it is only 62% to 70%.

Sensitivity is optimal for a choice of at most D = 106 mm and steeply falls off for higher choices of D, as most patients with high motility are in the range between 106 mm and 110 mm. Specificity, on the other hand, does not benefit from a lower choice of D, as even at high D, there are many patients that do not exhibit high motility.

At values of D lower than 106 mm, sensitivity does not increase anymore, but specificity only decreases further.

This is why D = 106 mm is chosen as the preferred cutoff for the following: As above, the regime D < 106 mm is called "low D" while anything at or above D ≥ 106 mm is considered "high D".

3.6. Prostate Motility for Low D and High D

Figure 7a–c show box plots for the patient-average standard deviation σ, patient-average range of motion ρ, and patient-average diffusion coefficient δ, respectively.

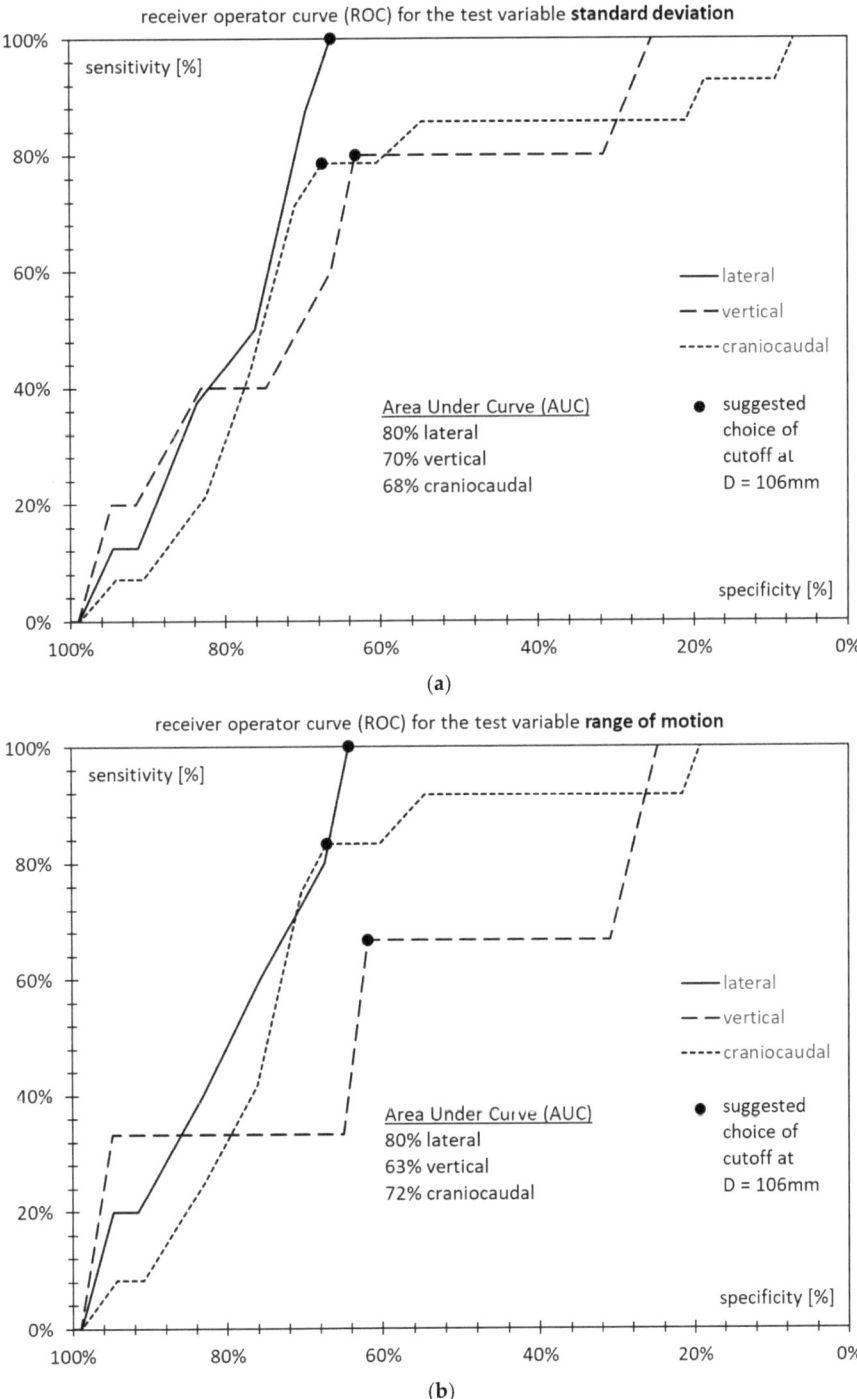

Figure 6. Cont.

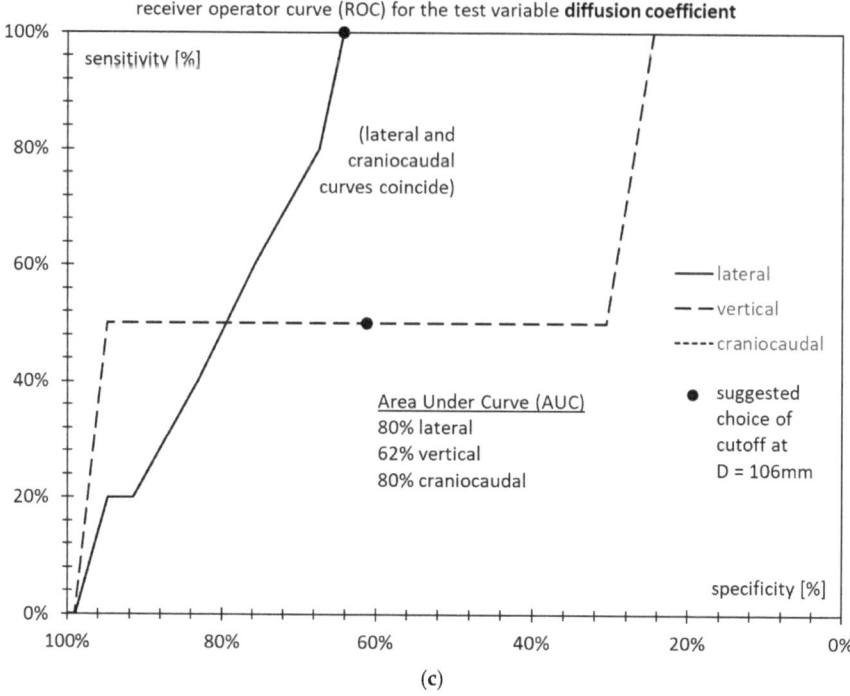

Figure 6. Receiver Operator Curves for the proposed test as a function of diameter D cutoff for (**a**) standard deviation σ; (**b**) range of motion ρ; (**c**) diffusion coefficient δ.

All prostate motility characteristics are visibly higher in cases of high D. The difference (by the unpaired *t*-test) is significant for all situations except for the diffusion coefficient on the vertical axis.

3.7. Test Statistics

Table 3a (standard deviation), Table 3b (range of motion), and Table 3c (diffusion coefficient) show two-by-two contingency tables for low/high D vs. low/high regimes of the prostate motility characteristics.

Fisher's two-sided test fails for the vertical axis but is successful for both the lateral x-axis and the craniocaudal z-axis.

On the lateral x-axis, the proposed test is 100% sensitive and has a 100% negative predictive value for all three characteristics.

On the craniocaudal z-axis, the proposed test is 79% (standard deviation) resp. 83% (range of motion) resp. 100% (diffusion coefficient) sensitive and reaches 95% (standard deviation) resp. 97% (range of motion) resp. 100% (diffusion coefficient) negative predictive value.

On the vertical axis, the proposed test still delivers 98% negative predictive value but is not particularly sensitive.

In general, the proposed test shows little specificity, at only 61% to 67%. Generally, it only has little positive predictive value when <30%.

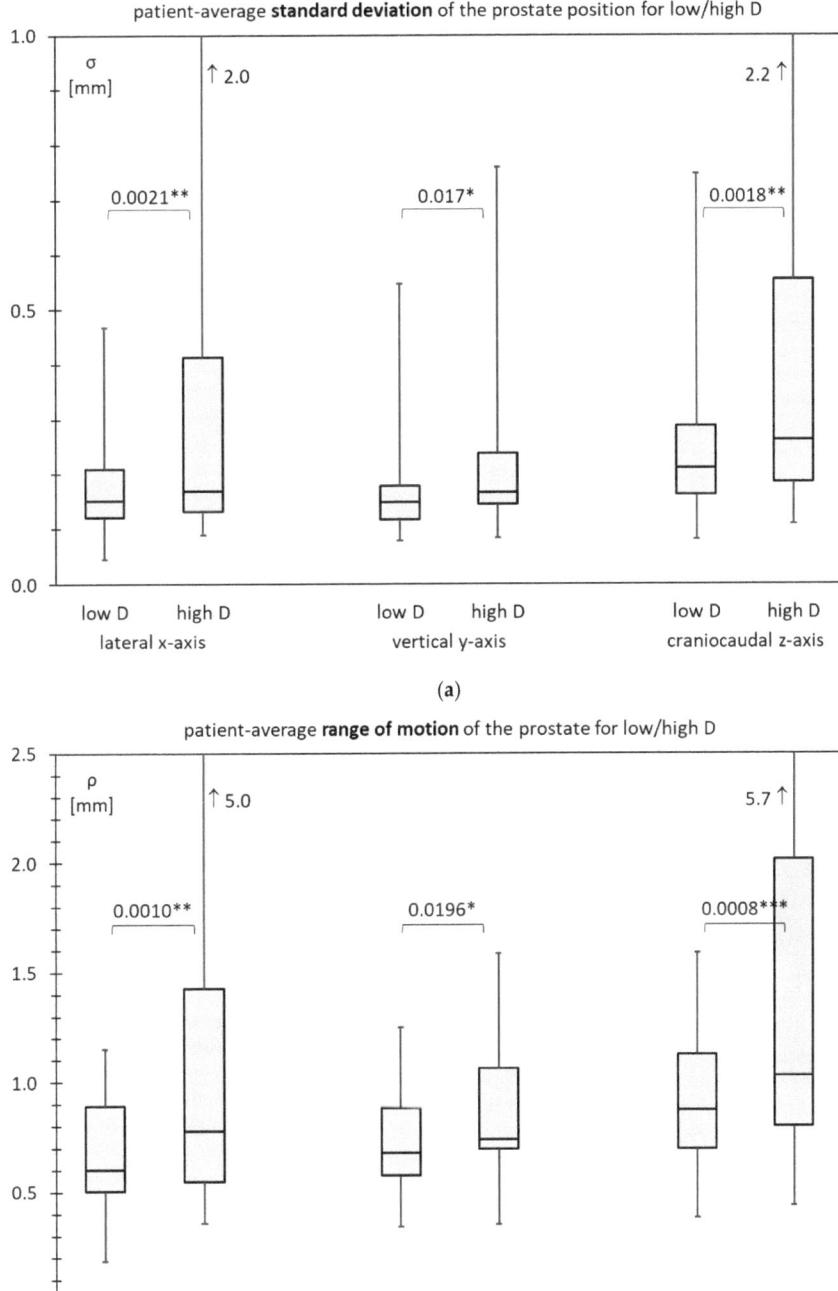

Figure 7. Cont.

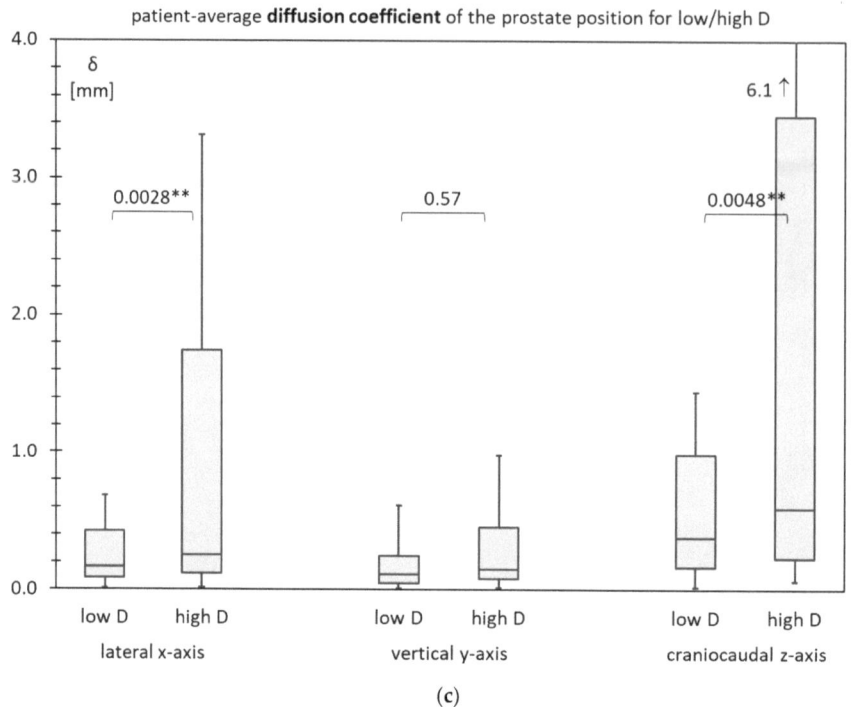

Figure 7. Box plots comparing low and high values of the inner diameter of the lesser pelvis (D) of the patient-average (a) standard deviation σ; (b) range of motion ρ; (c) diffusion coefficient δ. * $p < 0.05$, ** $p < 0.01$, *** $p < 0.001$.

Table 3. (a) Contingency tables, significance, sensitivity, specificity, and negative/positive predictive value for the standard deviation. (b) Contingency tables, significance, sensitivity, specificity, and negative/positive predictive value for the range of motion. (c) Contingency tables, significance, sensitivity, specificity, and negative/positive predictive value for the diffusion coefficient.

Patient-Average Standard Deviation σ [mm]		Inner Diameter of the Lesser Pelvis D [mm]		Significance p-Value	Sensitivity Specificity	NPV PPV
		"Low D" < 106 mm	"High D" ≥ 106 mm			
(a)						
lateral (x-axis)	<0.5	0	8	0.0003	100%	100%
	≥0.5	61	31		66%	21%
vertical (y-axis)	<0.5	1	4	0.0743	80%	98%
	≥0.5	60	35		63%	10%
craniocaudal (z-axis)	<0.5	3	11	0.0020	79%	95%
	≥0.5	58	28		67%	28%

Table 3. Cont.

Patient-Average Range of Motion ρ [mm]		Inner Diameter of the Lesser Pelvis D [mm]		Significance p-Value	Sensitivity Specificity	NPV PPV
		"Low D" < 106 mm	"High D" ≥106 mm			
		(b)				
lateral (x-axis)	<2.0	0	5	0.0076	100%	100%
	≥2.0	61	34		64%	13%
vertical (y-axis)	<2.0	1	2	0.5586	67%	98%
	≥2.0	60	37		62%	5%
craniocaudal (z-axis)	<2.0	2	10	0.0012	83%	97%
	≥2.0	59	29		67%	26%
Patient-Average Diffusion Coefficient δ [mm²/s]		Inner Diameter of the Lesser Pelvis D [mm]		Significance p-Value	Sensitivity Specificity	NPV PPV
		"Low D" < 106 mm	"High D" ≥ 106 mm			
		(c)				
lateral (x-axis)	<7.5	0	5	0.0076	100%	100%
	≥7.5	61	34		64%	13%
vertical (y-axis)	<7.5	1	1	1.0000	50%	98%
	≥7.5	60	38		61%	3%
craniocaudal (z-axis)	<7.5	0	5	0.0076	100%	100%
	≥7.5	61	34		64%	13%

4. Discussion

Anatomical predictors of high prostate interfraction and intrafraction motion have been known before. Several studies have identified factors that are associated with increased prostate motion during radiation therapy, including the size and shape of the prostate gland and the presence of rectal and bladder filling.

For example, [26] found that "large bladder intrafractional filling and a large bladder volume difference from planning CT were more likely to experience bigger longitudinal prostate motion". The study also derived an anatomical predictor where a smaller anterior–posterior size of the bladder and a smaller anterior–posterior to cranio–caudal ratio were favourable.

Perhaps closest in notion to our analysis, [27] uses the maximum rectal diameter (MRD) as a predictor for intrafraction prostate motion. They find that an MRD ≤ 3 cm predicts a prostate displacement ≤ 5 mm with 90% confidence.

Another calculational study derives a population model to estimate the probability of bladder presence during treatment using only the planning computed tomography [28] as in our study. Even earlier studies had already confirmed correlations between planning CT and intrafraction motion [29].

Our results are in line with the naive expectation that a larger prostate lodge and more leeway between the bony anatomy of the pelvis allow for higher prostate intrafraction motion.

In this study, only the center of gravity of the prostate (i.e., its location along the three spatial axes) was recorded by the instrument software. In follow-up work, we would also like to consider the size of the prostate (i.e., its volume) and other anatomical metrics to identify potential further confounding factors [30].

Independent analysis is needed to validate the criterion proposed in this paper in separate patients and unrelated datasets. Further research will be conducted into additional multivariate predictors in our dataset and into their validation by online MR Linac data.

5. Conclusions

An anatomical univariate predictor based on a single planning CT may help identify patients at risk of high prostate motion. While a diameter of the lesser pelvis of less than 106 mm has a high negative predictive value, patients with a larger diameter of the lesser pelvis may still exhibit low prostate motility. On the other hand, patients that are truly at risk are identified by $D \geq 106$ mm with high sensitivity.

Author Contributions: Conceptualization, H.B.; methodology, H.B.; software, H.B. and E.L.; validation, G.L.; formal analysis, H.B.; investigation, M.L. and E.L.; resources, M.L. and E.L.; data curation, H.B. and E.L.; writing—original draft preparation, H.B.; writing—review and editing, H.B., E.L. and G.L.; visualization, H.B.; supervision, C.B.; project administration, C.B.; funding acquisition, C.B. All authors have read and agreed to the published version of the manuscript.

Funding: This research received no external funding.

Institutional Review Board Statement: This study was conducted in accordance with the Declaration of Helsinki and approved by the Institutional Review Board (or Ethics Committee) of the Medical Faculty of LMU Munich (protocol codes 19-351 and 19-361, both on 1 August 2019).

Informed Consent Statement: Informed consent was obtained from all subjects involved in the prospective study starting August 2019. Patient consent was waived due to the provisions of Article 16 Section 3 Number 2 of the law governing the university hospitals in the state of Bavaria ("Gesetz über die Universitätsklinika des Freistaates Bayern") for the retrospective analysis of data older than August 2019.

Data Availability Statement: Anonymous prostate motion datasets generated by 4D ultrasound are available in the Open Data LMU repository at https://data.ub.uni-muenchen.de/265 (accessed on 16 May 2022). A corresponding descriptor has been published at ref. [23]. Planning CT images are not publicly available due to data protection considerations. The lesser pelvis diameter, however, but no images, will be shared upon request with the corresponding author.

Conflicts of Interest: C.B. declares general support for the clinical department and receipt of equipment by manufacturer Elekta. The funders had no role in the design of this study; in the collection, analyses, or interpretation of data; in the writing of the manuscript; or in the decision to publish the results. C.B. also serves in a leadership or fiduciary role as chair of the ESTRO-ACROP committee. The other authors declare no conflict of interest.

References

1. Bagshaw, M.A.; Ray, G.R.; Pistenma, D.A.; Castellino, R.A.; Meares, E.M. External beam radiation therapy of primary carcinoma of the prostate. *Cancer* **1975**, *36*, 723–728. [CrossRef]
2. Terlizzi, M.; Limkin, E.J.; Moukasse, Y.; Blanchard, P. Adjuvant or Salvage Radiation Therapy for Prostate Cancer after Prostatectomy: Current Status, Controversies and Perspectives. *Cancers* **2022**, *14*, 1688. [CrossRef] [PubMed]
3. Kissel, M.; Créhange, G.; Graff, P. Stereotactic Radiation Therapy versus Brachytherapy: Relative Strengths of Two Highly Efficient Options for the Treatment of Localized Prostate Cancer. *Cancers* **2022**, *14*, 2226. [CrossRef] [PubMed]
4. Haisen, S.L.; Chetty, I.J.; Enke, C.A.; Foster, R.D.; Willoughby, T.R.; Kupellian, P.A.; Solberg, T.D. Consequences of Intrafraction Prostate Motion. *Int. J. Radiat. Oncol. Biol. Phys.* **2008**, *71*, 801–812.
5. Faccenda, V.; Panizza, D.; Daniotti, M.C.; Pellegrini, R.; Trivellato, S.; Caricato, P.; Lucchini, R.; De Ponti, E.; Arcangeli, S. Dosimetric Impact of Intrafraction Prostate Motion and Interfraction Anatomical Changes in Dose-Escalated Linac-Based SBRT. *Cancers* **2023**, *15*, 1153. [CrossRef] [PubMed]
6. Litzenberg, D.W.; Balter, J.M.; Hadley, S.W.; Sandler, H.M.; Willoughby, T.R.; Kupelian, P.A.; Levine, L. Influence of intrafraction motion on margins for prostate radiotherapy. *Int. J. Radiat. Oncol. Biol. Phys.* **2006**, *65*, 548–553. [CrossRef]
7. Higuchi, D.; Ono, T.; Kakino, R.; Aizawa, R.; Nakayasu, N.; Ito, H.; Sakamoto, T. Evaluation of internal margins for prostate for step and shoot intensity-modulated radiation therapy and volumetric modulated arc therapy using different margin formulas. *J. Appl. Clin. Med. Phys.* **2022**, *23*, e13707. [CrossRef]
8. Huang, E.; Dong, L.; Chandra, A.; Kuban, D.A.; Rosen, I.I.; Evans, A.; Pollack, A. Intrafraction prostate motion during IMRT for prostate cancer. *Int. J. Radiat. Oncol. Biol. Phys.* **2002**, *53*, 261–268. [CrossRef]
9. Kron, T.; Thomas, J.; Fox, C.; Thompson, A.; Owen, R.; Herschtal, A.; Haworth, A.; Tai, K.-H.; Foroudi, F. Intra-fraction prostate displacement in radiotherapy estimated from pre- and post-treatment imaging of patients with implanted fiducial markers. *Radiother. Oncol.* **2010**, *95*, 191–197. [CrossRef]

10. Huang, K.; Palma, D.A.; Scott, D.; McGregor, D.; Gaede, S.; Yartsev, S.; Bauman, G.; Louie, A.V.; Rodrigues, G. Inter- and intrafraction uncertainty in prostate bed image-guided radiotherapy. *Int. J. Radiat. Oncol. Biol. Phys.* **2012**, *84*, 402–407. [CrossRef]
11. Dang, A.; Kupelian, P.A.; Cao, M.; Agazaryan, N.; Kishan, A.U. Image-guided radiotherapy for prostate cancer. *Transl. Androl. Urol.* **2018**, *7*, 308–320. [CrossRef] [PubMed]
12. Lohr, F.; Boda-Heggemann, J.; Wenz, F.; Wiegel, T. Image-guided radiotherapy for prostate cancer. *Aktuelle Urol.* **2007**, *38*, 386–391. [CrossRef] [PubMed]
13. Pang, E.P.P.; Knight, K.; Hussain, A.; Fan, Q.; Baird, M.; Tan, S.X.F.; Mui, W.H.; Leung, R.W.; Seah, I.K.L.; Master, Z.; et al. Reduction of intra-fraction prostate motion—Determining optimal bladder volume and filling for prostate radiotherapy using daily 4D TPUS and CBCT. *Tech. Innov. Patient Support Radiat. Oncol.* **2018**, *5*, 9–15. [CrossRef]
14. Both, S.; Wang, K.K.; Plastaras, J.P.; Deville, C.; Bar Ad, V.; Tochner, Z.; Vapiwala, N. Real-time study of prostate intrafraction motion during external beam radiotherapy with daily endorectal balloon. *Int. J. Radiat. Oncol. Biol. Phys.* **2011**, *81*, 1302–1309. [CrossRef]
15. Smeenk, R.J.; Louwe, R.J.; Langen, K.M.; Shah, A.P.; Kupelian, P.A.; van Lin, E.N.; Kaanders, J.H. An endorectal balloon reduces intrafraction prostate motion during radiotherapy. *Int. J. Radiat. Oncol. Biol. Phys.* **2012**, *83*, 661–669. [CrossRef]
16. Hedrick, S.G.; Fagundes, M.; Robison, B.; Blakey, M.; Renegar, J.; Artz, M.; Schreuder, N. A comparison between hydrogel spacer and endorectal balloon: An analysis of intrafraction prostate motion during proton therapy. *J. Appl. Clin. Med. Phys.* **2017**, *18*, 106–112. [CrossRef] [PubMed]
17. Ballhausen, H.; Li, M.; Ganswindt, U.; Belka, C. Shorter treatment times reduce the impact of intra-fractional motion: A real-time 4DUS study comparing VMAT vs. step-and-shoot IMRT for prostate cancer. *Strahlenther. Onkol.* **2018**, *194*, 664–674. [CrossRef]
18. Kupelian, P.; Willoughby, T.; Mahadevan, A.; Djemil, T.; Weinstein, G.; Jani, S.; Enke, C.; Solberg, T.; Flores, N.; Liu, D.; et al. Multi-institutional clinical experience with the Calypso system in localization and continuous, real-time monitoring of the prostate gland during external radiotherapy. *Int. J. Radiat. Oncol. Biol. Phys.* **2007**, *67*, 1088–1098. [CrossRef]
19. Richardson, A.K.; Jacobs, P. Intrafraction monitoring of prostate motion during radiotherapy using the Clarity® Autoscan Transperineal Ultrasound (TPUS) system. *Radiography* **2017**, *23*, 310–313. [CrossRef]
20. Sihono, D.S.K.; Ehmann, M.; Heitmann, S.; von Swietochowski, S.; Grimm, M.; Boda-Heggemann, J.; Lohr, F.; Wenz, F.; Wertz, H. Determination of Intrafraction Prostate Motion During External Beam Radiation Therapy with a Transperineal 4-Dimensional Ultrasound Real-Time Tracking System. *Int. J. Radiat. Oncol. Biol. Phys.* **2018**, *101*, 136–143. [CrossRef]
21. Richter, A.; Exner, F.; Weick, S.; Lawrenz, I.; Polat, B.; Flentje, M.; Mantel, F. Evaluation of intrafraction prostate motion tracking using the Clarity Autoscan system for safety margin validation. *Z. Med. Phys.* **2020**, *30*, 135–141. [CrossRef]
22. Ballhausen, H.; Li, M.; Belka, C. The ProMotion LMU dataset, prostate intra-fraction motion recorded by transperineal ultrasound. *Sci. Data* **2019**, *6*, 269. [CrossRef] [PubMed]
23. Ballhausen, H.; Kortmann, E.; Li, M.; Belka, C. The ProMotion LMU dataset (2022 edition), prostate intra-fraction motion recorded by transperineal ultrasound. *Sci. Data* **2022**, *9*, 455. [CrossRef]
24. Ballhausen, H.; Reiner, M.; Kantz, S.; Belka, C.; Söhn, M. The random walk model of intrafraction movement. *Phys. Med. Biol.* **2013**, *58*, 2413–2427. [CrossRef]
25. Ballhausen, H.; Li, M.; Hegemann, N.-S.; Ganswindt, U.; Belka, C. Intra-fraction motion of the prostate is a random walk. *Phys. Med. Biol.* **2015**, *60*, 549–563. [CrossRef]
26. Roch, M.; Zapatero, A.; Castro, P.; Büchser, D.; Pérez, L.; Hernández, D.; Ansón, C.; Chevalier, M.; García-Vicente, F. Impact of rectum and bladder anatomy in intrafractional prostate motion during hypofractionated radiation therapy. *Clin. Transl. Oncol.* **2019**, *21*, 607–614. [CrossRef] [PubMed]
27. Oates, R.; Brown, A.; Tan, A.; Foroudi, F.; Lim Joon, M.; Schneider, M.; Herschtal, A.; Kron, T. Real-time image-guided adaptive-predictive prostate radiotherapy using rectal diameter as a predictor of motion. *Clin. Oncol.* **2017**, *29*, 180–187. [CrossRef] [PubMed]
28. Rios, R.; De Crevoisier, R.; Ospina, J.D.; Commandeur, F.; Lafond, C.; Simon, A.; Haigron, P.; Espinosa, R.; Acosta, O. Population model of bladder motion and deformation based on dominant eigenmodes and mixed-effects models in prostate cancer radiotherapy. *Med. Image Anal.* **2017**, *38*, 133–149. [CrossRef] [PubMed]
29. Shiraishi, K.; Futaguchi, M.; Haga, A.; Sakumi, A.; Sasaki, K.; Yamamoto, K.; Igaki, H.; Ohtomo, K.; Yoda, K.; Nakagawa, K. Validation of planning target volume margins by analyzing intrafractional localization errors for 14 prostate cancer patients based on three-dimensional cross-correlation between the prostate images of planning CT and intrafraction cone-beam CT during volumetric modulated arc therapy. *BioMed Res. Int.* **2014**, *2014*, 960928.
30. Rose, C.; Ebert, M.A.; Mukwada, G.; Skorska, M.; Gill, S. Intrafraction motion during CyberKnife® prostate SBRT: Impact of imaging frequency and patient factors. *Phys. Eng. Sci. Med.* **2023**, *46*, 669–685. [CrossRef]

Disclaimer/Publisher's Note: The statements, opinions and data contained in all publications are solely those of the individual author(s) and contributor(s) and not of MDPI and/or the editor(s). MDPI and/or the editor(s) disclaim responsibility for any injury to people or property resulting from any ideas, methods, instructions or products referred to in the content.

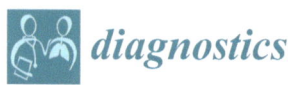

Review

Klotho in Cancer: Potential Diagnostic and Prognostic Applications

Jucileide Mota [1], Alice Marques Moreira Lima [2], Jhessica I. S. Gomes [1], Marcelo Souza de Andrade [1], Haissa O. Brito [1,3], Melaine M. A. Lawall Silva [3], Ana I. Faustino-Rocha [4,5,*], Paula A. Oliveira [4,5], Fernanda F. Lopes [1] and Rui M. Gil da Costa [1,4,5,6,7,8,9]

1. Post-Graduate Programme in Adult Health (PPGSAD), Federal University of Maranhão, São Luís 65085-580, Brazil
2. Health Sciences Center, State University of the Tocantins Region of Maranhão (UEMASUL), Imperatriz 6591-480, Brazil
3. Morphology Department, Federal University of Maranhão, São Luís 65085-580, Brazil
4. Centre for the Research and Technology of Agro-Environmental and Biological Sciences (CITAB), University of Trás-os-Montes and Alto Douro, 5000-801 Vila Real, Portugal
5. Inov4Agro—Institute for Innovation, Capacity Building and Sustainability of Agri-Food Production, University of Trás-os-Montes and Alto Douro, 5000-801 Vila Real, Portugal
6. Laboratory for Process Engineering, Environment, Biotechnology and Energy (LEPABE), Faculty of Engineering, University of Porto, 4200-465 Porto, Portugal
7. Associate Laboratory in Chemical Engineering, Faculty of Engineering (ALiCE), University of Porto, 4200-465 Porto, Portugal
8. Molecular Oncology and Viral Pathology Group, Portuguese Oncology Institute of Porto (IPO Porto), 4200-072 Porto, Portugal
9. Health Research Network, Research Center of Portuguese Oncology Institute of Porto (CIIPOP/RISE@CIIPOP), 4200-072 Porto, Portugal
* Correspondence: anafaustino.faustino@sapo.pt

Abstract: Klotho proteins, αKlotho, βKlotho, and γKlotho, exert tumor-suppressive activities via the fibroblast growth factor receptors and multiple cell-signaling pathways. There is a growing interest in Klotho proteins as potential diagnostic and prognostic biomarkers for multiple diseases. However, recent advances regarding their roles and potential applications in cancer remain disperse and require an integrated analysis. The present review analyzed research articles published between 2012 and 2022 in the Cochrane and Scopus scientific databases to study the role of Klotho in cancer and their potential as tools for diagnosing specific cancer types, predicting tumor aggressiveness and prognosis. Twenty-six articles were selected, dealing with acute myeloid leukemia and with bladder, breast, colorectal, esophageal, gastric, hepatocellular, ovarian, pancreatic, prostatic, pulmonary, renal, and thyroid cancers. αKlotho was consistently associated with improved prognosis and may be useful in estimating patient survival. A single study reported the use of soluble αKlotho levels in blood serum as a tool to aid the diagnosis of esophageal cancer. γKlotho was associated with increased aggressiveness of bladder, breast, and prostate cancer, and βKlotho showed mixed results. Further clinical development of Klotho-based assays will require careful identification of specific tumor subtypes where Klotho proteins may be most valuable as diagnostic or prognostic tools.

Keywords: liquid biopsy; cancer; klotho; prognosis; diagnosis

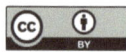

1. Introduction

The Klotho proteins, alpha(α)Klotho [1,2] and beta(β)Klotho [3], are encoded by the *KLA* and *KLB* genes located in chromosomes 4 and 13, respectively. αKlotho was originally identified in mice and elicited great interest due to its anti-aging properties [1]. It is expressed in a variety of tissues and is in the cell membrane as a type I single-pass 135 kDa protein containing an N-terminal sequence, two extracellular domains (designated KL1 and KL2) with glycosidase activity, a transmembrane helix, and an intracellular domain consisting of only 10 amino acids [2].

The αKlotho protein is also present in blood as a secreted protein generated by alternative mRNA splicing containing the KL1 domain only [1] and as a soluble protein that may contain KL1 alone or both the KL1 and Kl2 extracellular domains [4]. Cleavage of the αKlotho extracellular domains is mediated by disintegrin and metalloproteinase domain-containing (ADAM) proteins ADAM10 and ADAM17 [4]. The βKlotho protein shares structural similarities with αKlotho and is also located in the cell's plasma membrane [3,5], and soluble βKlotho has also been reported [6]. Another membrane-bound glycosidase-like protein, designated Klotho-lactase phlorizin hydrolase, was first identified in mice and is encoded by the *LCTL* gene on chromosome 15 in humans [7]. The functions of this protein, also referred to as γKlotho, are less clear than those of αKlotho and βKlotho.

αKlotho binds to FGR receptors, acting as a co-receptor for FGF23 and playing a key role in the renal regulation of phosphate levels [8,9]. βKlotho acts as a co-receptor for fibroblast growth factors 19 and 21 (FGF19 and FGF21) by forming binary complexes with FGFR4 and FGFR1c, respectively [10–12]. The binding of βKlotho with FGFR1c in adipose tissue or FGFR4 in the liver and with endocrine ligands FGF21 and FGF19 triggers multiple intracellular responses, as previously reviewed [5]. Canonically, the binding of FGF21 to the βKlotho-FGFR1c complex activates ERK1/2 downstream signaling and regulates the synthesis of biliary acids in hepatocytes, while FGF19 binds to βKlotho-FGFR4 complexes to downregulate Cyp17a1, also regulating hepatic bile production [11–14].

Loss of αKlotho has been consistently linked with chronic kidney disease and phosphate metabolism dysfunction [15,16]. αKlotho downregulation was also associated with pleiotropic effects involved in aging [1,5] and is proposed to act as a tumor suppressor, as recently reviewed [17]. Interestingly, βKlotho has been associated with both tumorigenic and tumor-suppressive effects in different types of cancer, suggesting a more complex scenario with multiple context-specific activities [18–20]. γKlotho expression has also been studied in multiple types of cancer [21,22]. In cancer, Klotho proteins have been shown to interact with multiple cellular signaling pathways, enhancing or blocking carcinogenesis, as previously reviewed [17,23]. As well as interacting with FGF to activate FGFR, αKlotho (Figure 1) was initially found to downregulate signaling via insulin-like growth factor 1 receptor (IGF-1R), and this may contribute to its effects against some types of cancer [24,25]. βKlotho enhances pro-tumorigenic functions of FGFR in multiple types of cancer [26,27]. The phosphatidylinositol-3-kinase (PI3K) pathway is triggered by multiple membrane-bound receptors and mediates cell proliferation, growth, and survival and is also inhibited by αKlotho [28]. The WNT-β-catenin pathway is activated in multiple cancers where it modulates cell differentiation, survival, and mobility [29]. αKlotho's ability to block this pathway contributes to its anti-tumor properties [30]. Transforming growth factor beta (TGFβ) is also able to modulate cell differentiation and mobility, namely inducing epithelial-to-mesenchymal transition [31], and αKlotho can block those effects [32]. The signaling pathways modulated by γKlotho are less studied, but Hori et al. (2016) implicated this protein in epithelial-to-mesenchymal transition in bladder cancer.

Accumulating data suggests that the tissue expression of Klotho proteins and, especially, the detection and quantitation of their soluble forms in body fluids like blood serum may be useful for establishing the diagnosis and prognosis of some types of cancer [6,33,34]. The present review aims to analyze scientific data regarding the role of Klotho proteins in cancer and to retrieve information regarding their potential use as diagnostic and prognostic biomarkers.

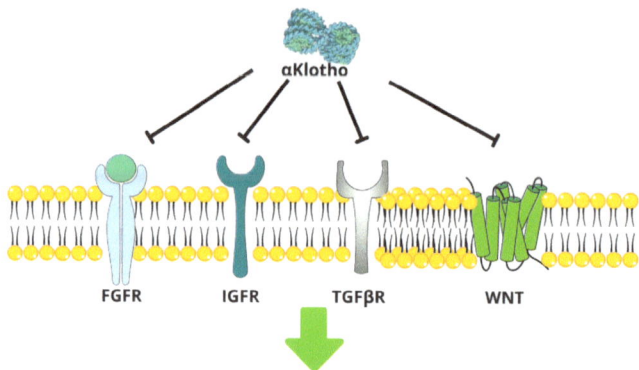

Figure 1. αKlotho downregulates signaling mediated by multiple cell membrane receptors, contributing to its anti-cancer effects.

2. Materials and Methods

The review was performed on three standard databases on biomedicine: PubMed, Scielo, and ScienceDirect, accessed in April 2023, including scientific papers published between 2012 and December 2022. The keywords "cancer AND Klotho" were applied. The following inclusion criteria were established concerning the type of study (case series and case–control studies in humans; experimental in vitro and in vivo studies) and outcomes (effects of Klotho gene products in cancer). Exclusion criteria were lack of clear definition of cancer type or controls, lack of Klotho gene product quantification, case reports, review articles, commentaries, hypothesis and meta-analyses, and languages other than English. The abstracts and, when necessary, the materials and methods were analyzed to apply inclusion and exclusion criteria (Figure 2).

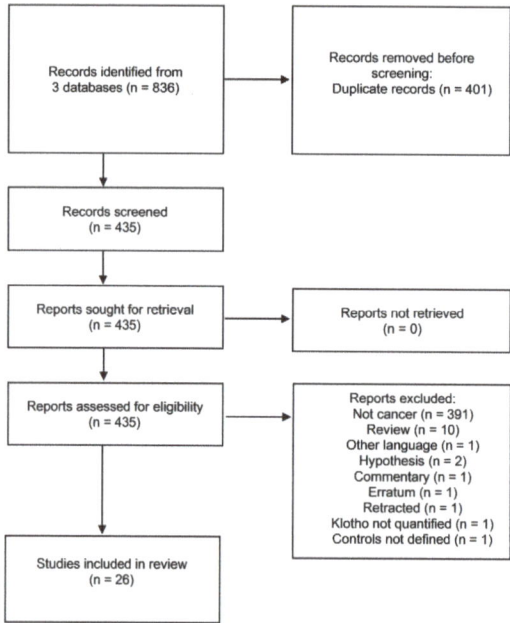

Figure 2. Selection of articles from the PubMed, Scielo, and ScienceDirect databases and resulting publications for analysis.

3. Results

Most publications were excluded due to duplication between databases or by applying exclusion criteria. Many articles have dealt with other pathologies where Klotho proteins are thought to play significant roles, most prominently in renal diseases. Overall, after applying inclusion and exclusion criteria, 26 articles were selected for further analysis (Table 1). Most studies used in vitro and/or clinical observational approaches, with only 7 articles using in vivo studies with animal models. Clinical observational studies often described the expression of Klotho genes at the RNA and/or protein levels and provided correlations between these markers' expression levels and relevant clinical parameters. Caseloads varied between 36 and 313 patients. Remarkably, none of the clinical studies adopted an interventional approach, and most consisted of retrospective cohort studies, while one article included a case–control study. In vitro studies provided insights into the regulation of Klotho protein's expression and its effects on cancer cells. Among the 26 selected articles, 21 dealt with αKlotho, 5 with βKlotho and only 3 with γKlotho, with one article studying α and βKlotho and another studying all the three proteins.

Table 1. Characteristics of the 26 articles included in the review.

Reference	Year	Type of Cancer	In Vitro	In Vivo	Number of Patients	Clinical (Observational)
[26]	2012	Hepatocellular carcinoma	x		56	Retrospective cohort
[27]	2013	Prostate cancer	x		136	Retrospective cohort
[35]	2013	Lung cancer	x	x		-
[36]	2013	Hepatocellular carcinoma	x		64	Retrospective cohort
[28]	2013	Renal cell carcinoma	x		125	Retrospective cohort
[37]	2015	Renal cell carcinoma			160	Retrospective cohort
[38]	2015	Ovarian cancer	x		265	Retrospective cohort
[39]	2015	Acute myeloid leukemia	x		109	Retrospective cohort
[30]	2015	Hepatocellular carcinoma	x			-
[21]	2015	Breast cancer	x		68	Retrospective cohort
[40]	2016	Thyroid cancer	x			-
[41]	2016	Esophageal cancer	x		160	Retrospective case–control
[42]	2017	Pulmonary squamous cell carcinoma	x		40	Retrospective cohort
[43]	2017	Ovarian cancer	x	x	198	Retrospective cohort
[44]	2018	Pancreatic adenocarcinoma	x		313	Retrospective cohort
[22]	2018	Bladder cancer	x	x	205	Retrospective cohort
[45]	2019	Large cell neuroendocrine lung cancer				Retrospective cohort

Table 1. Cont.

Reference	Year	Type of Cancer	In Vitro	In Vivo	Number of Patients	Clinical (Observational)
[46]	2019	Colorectal cancer	x	x	143	Retrospective cohort
[47]	2020	Prostate cancer		x	36	Retrospective cohort
[48]	2020	Colorectal cancer	x			-
[49]	2020	Gastric adenocarcinoma	x			-
[50]	2021	Colorectal cancer	x			-
[51]	2021	Pancreatic cancer		x	178	Retrospective cohort
[52]	2021	Gastric cancer	x		94	Retrospective cohort
[53]	2022	Colorectal cancer	x			-
[54]	2022	Hepatocellular carcinoma	x	x		-

x denotes that in vivo and/or in vitro experiments were performed for each article.

3.1. αKlotho

The main findings of the 21 articles addressing αKlotho in cancer are summarized in Table 2. Four studies were focused on colorectal cancer [46,48,50,53], another three on lung cancer [35,42,45], two on hepatocellular carcinoma [30,36], two on ovarian cancer [38,43], two on renal cell carcinoma [28,37], and two on gastric cancer [49,52]. Prostate cancer [27], acute myeloid leukemia [39], thyroid cancer [40], esophageal cancer [41], breast cancer [21], and pancreatic cancer [51] were each studied by a single article.

Table 2. Studies dealing with αKlotho.

Cancer Type	Reference	Type of Sample	Main Findings	Potential Applications
Prostate cancer	[27]	Frozen and FFPE cancer tissues. PC3, DU145, VCaP, LNCaP cancer cell lines, PNT1a normal prostate cells	KLA gene expression detected in all cell lines by qRT-PCR and FGF19 stimulates PCa cells in vitro. αKlotho detected by IHC in 50% primary and 90% metastatic PCa samples	Screening of patients who may benefit from anti-FGFR therapies and may be using IHC on tumor tissues
Lung cancer	[35]	A549 and H460 tumor cells and xenografts	αKlotho downregulation promotes cisplatin resistance in vitro and in vivo	
	[42]	FFPE cancer tissues (centrally located early lung cancer and SCC), A549, and SQ5 tumor cell lines	αKlotho expressed in 100% centrally located early lung cancer samples but only in 13% SCC using IHC. Inhibited N-cadherin expression in vitro	
	[45]	FFPE cancer tissues (large cell neuroendocrine lung cancer)	αKlotho expressed in 3/4 patients and associated with survival	Tissue expression may predict prognosis (survival)

Table 2. Cont.

Cancer Type	Reference	Type of Sample	Main Findings	Potential Applications
Hepatocellular carcinoma	[36]	Frozen and FFPE tumor and adjacent tissues. HRPG2, BEL-7402, SMMC-7721, HL7702, HUH-7, MHCC-97-H cancer cell lines and L-02 hepatocytes	αKlotho is downregulated at mRNA and protein levels in HCC versus adjacent tissue; promoter methylation and reduced protein expression correlate with reduced survival	αKlotho promoter methylation and protein expression may predict prognosis (survival)
	[30]	HepG2 and SMMC-7721 cancer cell lines, L-02 hepatocytes	Recombinant αKlotho downregulates Wnt/β-catenin signaling, suppressing proliferation and inducing apoptosis	
Renal cell carcinoma	[28]	786-O, OS-RC-2, ACHN, Caki-1 and Renca cancer cell lines. Tumor tissue	αKlotho tissue expression (IHC) is inversely correlated with tumor size, TNM stage, and nuclear grade. In vitro blocked EMT via PI3K/Akt/GSK3 β/Snail	Potential IHC marker of tumor aggressiveness
	[37]	Frozen tumor and adjacent tissue (clear cell RCC). Preoperative blood serum	αKlotho is downregulated in tumor tissue at RNA (qRT-PCR) and protein (IHC) levels. Reduced serum levels (ELISA) associated with higher tumor volume, Fuhrman grade, clinical stage, reduced cancer-specific survival, and progression-free survival	Serum αKlotho levels using ELISA may predict prognosis, including survival.
Ovarian cancer	[38]	Tumor (high-grade papillary-serous adenocarcinoma) and adjacent ovarian tissues. 19 cancer cell lines	αKlotho was reduced in tumor versus adjacent tissues (IHC) and in 16/19 cell lines (qRT-PCR)	
	[43]	FFPE and frozen tumor and adjacent tissues. 7 cancer cell lines	αKlotho was reduced in tumor versus adjacent tissues (IHC). Reduction correlates with low survival. Tumor xenografts expressing αKlotho had a smaller size. $KLA^{-/-}$ mice showed higher IL-6 levels in response to xenografts	Tissue expression using IHC may predict survival
Acute myeloid leukemia	[39]	KG-1 cells	Exposure to miR-126-5p decreased αKlotho levels and induced Akt phosphorylation and cytarabine resistance	αKlotho may predict cytarabine resistance
Breast cancer	[21]	Frozen tumor and adjacent tissues. MDA-MB-231 and H357T cancer cell lines	αKlotho was downregulated in cancer versus adjacent tissue. Undetectable in both cell lines	
Follicular thyroid carcinoma	[40]	FTC133 and FTC238 cancer cell lines	αKlotho reduced cell proliferation and induced apoptosis in vitro	

Table 2. Cont.

Cancer Type	Reference	Type of Sample	Main Findings	Potential Applications
Esophageal cancer	[41]	FFPE cancer and adjacent tissues. Blood serum from patients/controls	αKlotho was downregulated in cancer versus adjacent tissue (IHC). Correlates with improved survival inversely correlated with staging, grade, lymph node metastasis, and β-catenin. Serum levels are higher in patients versus controls	Tissue levels (IHC) may predict prognosis, including survival. Serum 327 pg/mL cut-off (ELISA) is diagnostic with a sensitivity of 81% and specificity of 81%
Colorectal cancer	[46]	FFPE tumor tissue. RKO and LoVo cancer cell lines, Wi-38, and HUVEC cells	Lower αKlotho (IHC) is associated with lower patient survival. αKlotho prevents pro-tumorigenic effects of senescent cells in vitro and in vivo via NFκB/CCL2 blockade	Tissue levels (IHC) may predict survival
	[48]	Six cancer cell lines and normal cells	FL-1 regulates αKlotho expression in cancer cells	
	[50]	CaCo-2 cells	αKlotho induces apoptosis via the TRAIL death receptor	
	[53]	HT29 cancer cell line, CCD841 cells	αKlotho induces apoptosis specifically in cancer cells	
Gastric cancer	[49]	6 cancer cell lines and normal cells	SOX17 regulates αKlotho expression in cancer cells in vitro	
	[52]	HGC-27, AGS, MKN-45, MGC-803, HE-293-T cancer cell lines, GES-1 cells	Circular RNA ITCH upregulates αKlotho by sponging out miR-199-5p, inhibiting cell proliferation, migration, invasion, and EMT	
Pancreatic cancer	[51]	TCGA pancreatic ductal adenocarcinoma datasets, 3 mouse models	Promoter methylation and mRNA downregulation are associated with reduced survival. αKlotho knockdown synergized with Kras mutation to promote carcinogenesis. Soluble αKlotho inhibited xenograft growth and promoted the survival of KPC mice	Methylation and expression levels may predict survival

3.1.1. Clinicopathological Characteristics

αKlotho was generally found to act as a tumor suppressor, and its downregulation was consistently associated with aggressive tumor phenotypes and worse prognosis. In prostate cancer, αKlotho protein expression was detected in 50% of primary and 90% of metastatic samples [27]. In lung cancer, αKlotho was detected in most samples, but its expression pattern seems to be subtype-specific and requires further studies [40,45]. In hepatocellular carcinoma, αKlotho tissue expression is downregulated in tumor versus adjacent tissues and inversely correlates with tumor size, TNM stage, and nuclear grade [36]. Similar findings were obtained when studying renal cell carcinoma [30,39]. In breast [21], esophageal [41] and ovarian [38,43] cancer, αKlotho expression is downregulated compared with normal tissues.

3.1.2. Diagnosis

Soluble αKlotho can be quantified in blood serum using ELISA, and αKlotho levels were also suggested to have diagnostic value for esophageal cancer [41].

3.1.3. Survival and Treatment Response

The quantitation of αKlotho expression levels on tumor tissues using immunohistochemistry (IHC) was of prognostic significance in colorectal, esophageal, hepatocellular, lung, and ovarian cancer [36,41,43,45,46]. *KLA* promoter methylation and mRNA expression levels by quantitative real-time PCR (qRT-PCR) were also reported to have prognostic value in hepatocellular carcinoma and pancreatic cancer [36,51]. Reduced αKlotho serum levels were associated with reduced cancer-specific survival and progression-free survival among renal cell carcinoma patients [37]. Interestingly, reduced αKlotho levels were also suggested to promote cytarabine resistance in acute myeloid leukemia cells [39].

3.2. βKlotho

The 5 articles focused on βKlotho are addressed in Table 3, which summarizes their main findings. Two articles dealt with hepatocellular carcinoma [26,54], while prostate cancer [27], breast cancer [21], and pancreatic adenocarcinoma [44] were studied in one article each.

Table 3. Studies dealing with βKlotho.

Cancer Type	Reference	Type of Sample	Main Findings	Potential Applications
Hepatocellular carcinoma	[26]	Tumor and adjacent tissue in Trizol	*KLB* gene expression is upregulated in cancer tissues. A >2-fold increase correlates with the development of multiple lesions.	Screening of patients who could benefit from anti-FGFR therapies. Prediction of lesion multiplicity.
	[54]	Cell lines and xenograft mouse model	βKlotho mediates FGF9 pro-survival functions via FGFR3 and FGFR4. Inhibiting βKlotho was more effective than inhibiting FGFR4.	Screening of patients who could benefit from anti-FGFR therapies.
Prostate cancer	[27]	Frozen primary tumor tissue, FFPE metastases. PC3, DU145, VCaP, LnCaP cancer cell lines, PNT1a cells	KLB gene expression observed with qRT-PCR in DU145 and VCaP only, and FGF19 showed stimulatory effects. βKlotho was detected in a majority of primary and metastatic lesions using IHC.	βKlotho IHC may be useful for screening patients who could benefit from anti-FGFR therapy.
Breast cancer	[21]	Frozen tumor and adjacent tissue. MDA-MB-231 and HS578T cancer cell lines	βKlotho was downregulated in cancer versus normal tissues and was undetectable in both cell lines, suggesting a tumor-suppressor role.	
Pancreatic adenocarcinoma	[44]	Gene expression data from the Gene Expression Omnibus database	High *KLB* mRNA expression is associated with increased overall survival.	*KLB* gene expression may be useful in predicting patient survival.

3.2.1. Clinicopathological Characteristics

In hepatocellular carcinoma, βKlotho was proposed to mediate tumor aggressiveness via FGFR signaling [26,54]. Conversely, in breast and pancreatic cancers, βKlotho was proposed to act as a tumor suppressor [21,44]. In prostate cancer, βKlotho protein expression was detected in a majority of primary and metastatic lesions [27].

3.2.2. Survival and Treatment Response

Interestingly, one study on hepatocellular carcinoma [26] showed that a >2-fold increase in *KLB* gene expression correlates with the development of multiple versus single lesions. A pre-clinical study [55] suggested that βKlotho mediates FGF9 pro-survival functions in hepatocellular carcinoma via FGFR3 and FGFR4 and may be useful in selecting patients who could benefit from anti-FGFR therapies. A similar scenario was suggested by a single study focused on prostate cancer [27].

3.3. γKlotho

γKlotho was studied in three articles, summarized in Table 4. Breast [21], prostate [47], and bladder cancers [22] were studied in one article each. All three articles found that higher γKlotho expression is associated with cancer aggressiveness and poor prognosis, suggesting that γKlotho levels assessed at the mRNA or the protein level may be useful to predict patient survival and response to therapy.

Table 4. Studies Dealing with γKlotho.

Cancer Type	Reference	Type of Sample	Main Findings	Potential Applications
Breast cancer	[21]	Frozen tumor and adjacent tissue. MDA-MB-231 and HS578T cancer cell lines.	*LCTL* gene expression is upregulated in cancer versus normal tissues, especially in triple-negative lesions, using qRT-PCR, correlating with increased cell proliferation, histological grade, TNM stage, and reduced progression-free survival.	*LCTL* gene expression using qRT-PCR may be useful in predicting patient survival.
Prostate	[47]	FFPE tumor tissue from castration-resistant prostate cancer and cell lines.	Higher γKlotho expression observed by IHC in tumor tissue correlates with reduced overall survival and poor response to docetaxel in patients and in a mouse xenograft model.	γKlotho IHC may predict overall survival and response to docetaxel in castration-resistant prostate cancer.
Bladder cancer	[22]	FFPE pre-treatment tumor tissue. UMUC3, MGH-U3 and J82 cells.	Higher γKlotho expression observed by IHC in muscle-invasive versus non-muscle-invasive lesions. In non-muscle-invasive lesions, γKlotho levels correlated with poor progression-free survival.	γKlotho IHC may predict overall survival in patients with non-muscle-invasive bladder cancer.

3.3.1. Clinicopathological Characteristics

Triple-negative breast cancer is an aggressive breast cancer subtype that poses a significant therapeutic challenge [56]. *LCTL* gene expression was found to be upregulated in triple-negative breast cancer samples, and expression levels correlated with increased cell proliferation, histological grade, and TNM stage [21]. Bladder cancer includes muscle-invasive and non-muscle-invasive forms [57] with distinct biological behavior. Higher γKlotho protein expression was observed in muscle-invasive versus non-muscle-invasive lesions [22].

3.3.2. Survival and Treatment Response

In triple-negative breast cancer, *LCTL* gene expression levels correlated with reduced progression-free survival [21]. Castration-resistant prostate cancer is another challenging malignancy with heterogeneous morphological and molecular phenotypes [55,58]. High γKlotho expression levels, as demonstrated by IHC, were shown to correlate with reduced overall survival and poor response to docetaxel in patients and in a mouse xenograft model [40]. In non-muscle-invasive bladder cancer, γKlotho protein levels were shown to correlate with reduced progression-free survival [22].

4. Discussion

The three Klotho proteins have complex roles in different types of cancer. The role of γKlotho is less well defined than that of its related Klotho proteins, partially because of its unusual molecular structure and because it was discovered more recently. The present review organized data from scientific articles published between 2012 and 2022 regarding the roles of Klotho proteins in cancer and their potential use as diagnostic and prognostic tools.

The role of all three proteins was studied in prostate cancer. This is a highly prevalent disease in middle-aged to older men that usually develops as an androgen-dependent adenocarcinoma but may progress to an androgen-independent castration-resistant phenotype and small-cell neoplasia, often displaying neuroendocrine markers, which are associated with poor patient prognosis [55]. αKlotho and βKlotho expression was detected in prostate cancer cell lines representing prostate adenocarcinoma and small-cell carcinoma, as well as in tumor tissues from primary tumors and metastasis, where they seem to mediate FGFR signaling [27]. It was further suggested that IHC tests for detecting αKlotho and βKlotho in tumor tissue may be of use to predict response to anti-FGFR therapies [27]. γKlotho expression in castration-resistant prostate cancer was associated with reduced survival and resistance to docetaxel [47], which is used as chemotherapy for such advanced cases [59]. Taken together, these results suggest that the immuno-expression patterns of Klotho proteins on prostate cancer tissues may be a valuable tool for tailoring treatment regimens for specific patients.

Lung cancer is also a common and aggressive malignancy, which includes multiple subtypes with distinct biological behavior [60]. Loss of αKlotho expression was consistently associated with increased tumor aggressiveness in three studies using in vitro and in vivo models [35] and clinical observational studies of neuroendocrine tumors [45], early centrally located cancers, and squamous cell carcinomas [42]. The observation that αKlotho may predict survival in patients with large cell neuroendocrine lung cancer is of particular interest, as it suggests that this marker has prognostic value in this specific lung cancer subtype [45]. Additionally, limited in vivo and in vitro data suggest that αKlotho downregulation may predict resistance to cisplatin-based chemotherapy [35], but additional studies are required to confirm this hypothesis.

Hepatocellular carcinoma is the most common type of liver cancer [61]. Although αKlotho was reported to act as a tumor suppressor [30,36], βKlotho showed oncogenic activity via enhanced FGFR signaling [26,54]. Importantly, αKlotho gene promoter methylation and protein expression may be of use as prognostic markers to estimate patient survival [36], while βKlotho may be a useful marker to predict response to anti-FGFR therapies [26].

In renal cell carcinoma, αKlotho downregulation was also reported to act as a tumor suppressor, and its loss was associated with tumor aggressiveness [28,42]. Of particular interest is the use of ELISA tests to detect soluble αKlotho in blood serum samples, as reduced levels of this protein were significantly associated with patients with the clear cell subtype of RCC [37]. These findings suggest that such tests may be used in liquid biopsies to help establish the prognosis of specific RCC patient subgroups.

Ovarian cancer is a frequent malignancy in women [62], and αKlotho was reported to act as a tumor suppressor in this type of cancer using experimental and clinical approaches [38,44]. Importantly, one study suggested that reduced αKlotho immuno-expression in cancer tissues may be useful as a prognostic marker to predict poor patient survival [44]. The same study reported that αKlotho was associated with higher interleukin-6 (IL-6) circulating levels. IL-6 is a pro-inflammatory cytokine that mediates some paraneoplastic syndromes like cancer cachexia [63], so it is interesting to speculate that αKlotho expression levels may also be used to predict the development of such syndromes.

In acute myeloid leukemia, loss of αKlotho was reported to be associated with cytarabine resistance in vitro, suggesting its possible use as a tool to design tailored therapies for leukemia patients [39]. Additional studies are needed to test this hypothesis, as cytarabine remains an important drug for treating this type of leukemia [64].

Breast cancer is highly prevalent in women and is often life-threatening [56]. In one study, αKlotho and βKlotho were downregulated in tumor tissue versus adjacent tissue, suggesting they act as tumor suppressors [21]. Conversely, higher γKlotho (*LCTL*) gene expression levels using qRT-PCR were found in cancer versus adjacent tissue, specifically in the aggressive triple-negative cancer subtype [21,65], suggesting it is associated with tumor aggressiveness. Interestingly, it was suggested that qRT-PCR for *LCTL* may be useful as a prognostic marker to estimate patient survival in patients with triple-negative breast cancer [21].

In papillary thyroid cancer, a single study [40] reported that αKlotho was able to reduce cell proliferation and induce apoptosis in vitro. The potential use of this protein for diagnostic and prognostic purposes in thyroid cancer remains to be determined.

In esophageal cancer, an interesting study [41] reported that the levels of soluble αKlotho in blood serum as detected by ELISA were higher in patients versus healthy controls. A cut-off value was estimated that allowed researchers to distinguish between patients and controls with approximately 81% sensitivity and specificity. Interestingly, in tissue samples, αKlotho was expressed at higher levels in adjacent versus tumor samples, and αKlotho downregulation correlated with increased tumor aggressiveness and reduced patient survival. These data highlight the potential of αKlotho as a marker in liquid biopsies for the diagnosis of esophageal cancer, while tissue levels may have prognostic significance.

Colorectal cancer is highly prevalent in multiple world regions, and large bowel carcinogenesis is associated with chronic inflammation [66]. In this type of cancer, 4 studies consistently reported that αKlotho acts as a tumor suppressor [46,48,50,53]. In vitro tests revealed new regulatory pathways that control αKlotho expression via FL-1 [48] and support the pro-apoptotic role of αKlotho via TRAIL [50]. Interestingly, one study described how αKlotho downregulation promotes a senescence-associated secretory phenotype in mesenchymal cells that may contribute to tumorigenesis via the nuclear factor kappa-light-chain-enhancer of activated B cells (NFκB) signaling pathway [46]. This is a pivotal mediator of inflammation and tissue repair, but also of carcinogenesis in specific settings. Chronic inflammation is a key player in colon cancer, and the secretion of NFκB-controlled C-C motif chemokine ligand 2 (CCL2) by senescent stromal cells was proposed to promote carcinogenesis of the colon. αKlotho abrogated CCL2 signaling and was associated with improved patient survival, suggesting it may be of use as a prognostic marker.

Two in vitro studies addressed the role of αKlotho in gastric cancer, further associating αKlotho downregulation with aggressive cancer phenotypes [49,52]. SOX17 and an epigenetic pathway involving circular RNA ITCH and miR-199-5p were shown to regulate αKlotho expression in gastric cancer cells. Although these findings support the role of αKlotho as a tumor suppressor, further developments are needed to explore its potential role as a diagnostic or prognostic marker in gastric cancer.

A single study addressed the role of αKlotho in pancreatic adenocarcinoma and concluded that *KLA* gene expression levels and promoter methylation may have prognostic value, as increased *KLA* promoter methylation and decreased mRNA expression levels were associated with lower patient survival [51]. This was further supported by tests in three complementary mouse models, where αKlotho decreased cancer growth and improved survival. Another study using expression data from the GEO database also suggested that *KLB* upregulation is associated with improved survival in pancreatic cancer patients [46]. Taken together, these data provide evidence to support the further development of Klotho as a prognostic marker in pancreatic adenocarcinoma.

Urothelial carcinoma of the urinary bladder is a common malignancy that includes highly aggressive forms that invade the bladder's muscular layer and non-muscle-invasive forms associated with local recurrence [67]. One study reported that γKlotho expression was observed in both muscle-invasive and non-muscle-invasive bladder cancer using IHC and that expression levels were associated with poor overall survival among patients with non-muscle-invasive cancer [22].

5. Conclusions

Overall, the datasets published between 2012 and 2022 provide evidence supporting the development of Klotho genes and their mRNA and protein products as potential prognostic markers in multiple types of cancer, especially in the prediction of patient survival. Although αKlotho was consistently associated with improved patient prognosis, γKlotho was associated with increased cancer aggressiveness, and βKlotho showed mixed results. It is critical to accurately identify specific tumor subtypes where Klotho is of interest (muscle-invasive versus non-muscle-invasive urothelial carcinoma) to take the most advantage of its potential. The use of Klotho levels as diagnostic markers was less frequently observed in the literature, although one study provided detailed data regarding soluble αKlotho levels in blood serum and the diagnosis of esophageal cancer. However, most studies still did not present such detailed results, and the clinical use of Klotho will require additional development.

Author Contributions: Conceptualization, R.M.G.d.C. and H.O.B.; methodology, M.S.d.A. and A.M.M.L.; validation, F.F.L. and J.I.S.G., investigation, J.M., M.M.A.L.S. and J.I.S.G.; resources, A.I.F.-R., P.A.O. and R.M.G.d.C.; data curation, M.S.d.A., M.M.A.L.S. and F.F.L.; writing—original draft preparation, R.M.G.d.C. and A.I.F.-R.; writing—review and editing, H.O.B., M.S.d.A., F.F.L., M.M.A.L.S. and P.A.O.; supervision, F.F.L. and R.M.G.d.C.; funding acquisition, M.S.d.A., P.A.O. and H.O.B. All authors have read and agreed to the published version of the manuscript.

Funding: This research was funded by CAPES (grant numbers 001, 0810/2020/88881.510244/2020-01), FAPEMA (IECT-FAPEMA-05796/18, FAPEMA IECT 30/2018—IECT Saúde, PPSUS-02160/20, BPD-01343/23), CI-IPOP (PI86-CI-IPOP-66-2017), FCT (UID/AGR/04033/2020, UIDB/CVT/00772/2020, LA/P/0045/2020, UIDB/00511/2020, UIDP/00511/2020, NORTE-01-0145-FEDER-000054).

Institutional Review Board Statement: Not applicable.

Informed Consent Statement: Not applicable.

Data Availability Statement: The data produced in this study are available in this article.

Conflicts of Interest: The authors declare no conflict of interest. The funders had no role in the design of the study, in the collection, analyses, or interpretation of data, in the writing of the manuscript, or in the decision to publish the results.

References

1. Kuro, O.M.; Matsumura, Y.; Aizawa, H.; Kawaguchi, H.; Suga, T.; Utsugi, T.; Ohyama, Y.; Kurabayashi, M.; Kaname, T.; Kume, E.; et al. Mutation of the mouse klotho gene leads to a syndrome resembling ageing. *Nature* **1997**, *390*, 45–51. [CrossRef] [PubMed]
2. Matsumuraab, Y.; Aizawaab, H.; Shiraki-Iida, T.; Nagaibd, R.; Kuro-M.; Nabeshima, Y.-I. Identification of the HumanKlotho-Gene and Its Two Transcripts Encoding Membrane and SecretedKlothoProtein. *Biochem. Biophys. Res. Commun.* **1998**, *242*, 626–630. [CrossRef] [PubMed]
3. Ito, S.; Kinoshita, S.; Shiraishi, N.; Nakagawa, S.; Sekine, S.; Fujimori, T.; Nabeshima, Y.-I. Molecular cloning and expression analyses of mouse betaβklotho, which encodes a novel Klotho family protein. *Mech. Dev.* **2000**, *98*, 115–119. [CrossRef] [PubMed]
4. Chen, C.-D.; Podvin, S.; Gillespie, E.; Leeman, S.E.; Abraham, C.R. Insulin stimulates the cleavage and release of the extracellular domain of Klotho by ADAM10 and ADAM17. *Proc. Natl. Acad. Sci. USA* **2007**, *104*, 19796–19801. [CrossRef]
5. Kuro-O, M. The Klotho proteins in health and disease. *Nat. Rev. Nephrol.* **2019**, *15*, 27–44. [CrossRef]
6. Bednarska, S.; Fryczak, J.; Siejka, A. Serum β-Klotho concentrations are increased in women with polycystic ovary syndrome. *Cytokine* **2020**, *134*, 155188. [CrossRef]
7. Ito, S.; Fujimori, T.; Hayashizaki, Y.; Nabeshima, Y.-I. Identification of a novel mouse membrane-bound family 1 glycosidase-like protein, which carries an atypical active site structure. *Biochim. Biophys. Acta (BBA)-Gene Struct. Expr.* **2002**, *1576*, 341–345. [CrossRef]
8. Kurosu, H.; Ogawa, Y.; Miyoshi, M.; Yamamoto, M.; Nandi, A.; Rosenblatt, K.P.; Baum, M.G.; Schiavi, S.; Hu, M.-C.; Moe, O.W.; et al. Regulation of Fibroblast Growth Factor-23 Signaling by Klotho. *J. Biol. Chem.* **2006**, *281*, 6120–6123. [CrossRef]
9. Urakawa, I.; Yamazaki, Y.; Shimada, T.; Iijima, K.; Hasegawa, H.; Okawa, K.; Fujita, T.; Fukumoto, S.; Yamashita, T. Klotho converts canonical FGF receptor into a specific receptor for FGF23. *Nature* **2006**, *444*, 770–774. [CrossRef]

10. Lee, S.; Choi, J.; Mohanty, J.; Sousa, L.P.; Tome, F.; Pardon, E.; Steyaert, J.; Lemmon, M.A.; Lax, I.; Schlessinger, J. Structures of β-klotho reveal a 'zip code'-like mechanism for endocrine FGF signalling. *Nature* **2018**, *553*, 501–505. [CrossRef]
11. Lin, B.C.; Wang, M.; Blackmore, C.; Desnoyers, L.R. Liver-specific Activities of FGF19 Require Klotho beta. *J. Biol. Chem.* **2007**, *282*, 27277–27284. [CrossRef] [PubMed]
12. Ogawa, Y.; Kurosu, H.; Yamamoto, M.; Nandi, A.; Rosenblatt, K.P.; Goetz, R.; Eliseenkova, A.V.; Mohammadi, M.; Kuro-O, M. βKlotho is required for metabolic activity of fibroblast growth factor 21. *Proc. Natl. Acad. Sci. USA* **2007**, *104*, 7432–7437. [CrossRef] [PubMed]
13. Kurosu, H.; Choi, M.; Ogawa, Y.; Dickson, A.S.; Goetz, R.; Eliseenkova, A.V.; Mohammadi, M.; Rosenblatt, K.P.; Kliewer, S.A.; Kuro-O, M. Tissue-specific Expression of βKlotho and Fibroblast Growth Factor (FGF) Receptor Isoforms Determines Metabolic Activity of FGF19 and FGF21. *J. Biol. Chem.* **2007**, *282*, 26687–26695. [CrossRef] [PubMed]
14. Kharitonenkov, A.; Dunbar, J.D.; Bina, H.A.; Bright, S.; Moyers, J.S.; Zhang, C.; Ding, L.; Micanovic, R.; Mehrbod, S.F.; Knierman, M.D.; et al. FGF-21/FGF-21 receptor interaction and activation is determined by βKlotho. *J. Cell. Physiol.* **2007**, *215*, 1–7. [CrossRef]
15. Brownstein, C.A.; Adler, F.; Nelson-Williams, C.; Iijima, J.; Li, P.; Imura, A.; Nabeshima, Y.-I.; Reyes-Mugica, M.; Carpenter, T.O.; Lifton, R.P. A translocation causing increased α-Klotho level results in hypophosphatemic rickets and hyperparathyroidism. *Proc. Natl. Acad. Sci. USA* **2008**, *105*, 3455–3460. [CrossRef]
16. Stenvinkel, P.; Painer, J.; Kuro-O, M.; Lanaspa, M.; Arnold, W.; Ruf, T.; Shiels, P.G.; Johnson, R.J. Novel treatment strategies for chronic kidney disease: Insights from the animal kingdom. *Nat. Rev. Nephrol.* **2018**, *14*, 265–284. [CrossRef]
17. Ligumsky, H.; Merenbakh-Lamin, K.; Keren-Khadmy, N.; Wolf, I.; Rubinek, T. The role of α-klotho in human cancer: Molecular and clinical aspects. *Oncogene* **2022**, *41*, 4487–4497. [CrossRef]
18. Ye, X.; Guo, Y.; Zhang, Q.; Chen, W.; Hua, X.; Liu, W.; Yang, Y.; Chen, G. βKlotho Suppresses Tumor Growth in Hepatocellular Carcinoma by Regulating Akt/GSK-3β/Cyclin D1 Signaling Pathway. *PLoS ONE* **2013**, *8*, e55615. [CrossRef]
19. Liu, Z.; Qi, S.; Zhao, X.; Li, M.; Ding, S.; Lu, J.; Zhang, H. Metformin inhibits 17β-estradiol-induced epithelial-to-mesenchymal transition via βKlotho-related ERK1/2 signaling and AMPKα signaling in endometrial adenocarcinoma cells. *Oncotarget* **2016**, *7*, 21315–21331. [CrossRef]
20. Cui, G.; Martin, R.C.; Jin, H.; Liu, X.; Pandit, H.; Zhao, H.; Cai, L.; Zhang, P.; Li, W.; Li, Y. Up-regulation of FGF15/19 signaling promotes hepatocellular carcinoma in the background of fatty liver. *J. Exp. Clin. Cancer Res.* **2018**, *37*, 136. [CrossRef]
21. Trošt, N.; Peña-Llopis, S.; Koirala, S.; Stojan, J.; Potts, P.R.; Tacer, K.F.; Martinez, E.D. γKlotho is a novel marker and cell survival factor in a subset of triple negative breast cancers. *Oncotarget* **2016**, *7*, 2611–2628. [CrossRef] [PubMed]
22. Hori, S.; Miyake, M.; Tatsumi, Y.; Morizawa, Y.; Nakai, Y.; Onishi, S.; Onishi, K.; Iida, K.; Gotoh, D.; Tanaka, N.; et al. Gamma-Klotho exhibits multiple roles in tumor growth of human bladder cancer. *Oncotarget* **2018**, *9*, 19508–19524. [CrossRef] [PubMed]
23. Rubinek, T.; Wolf, I. The Role of Alpha-Klotho as a Universal Tumor Suppressor. *Vitam. Horm.* **2016**, *101*, 197–214. [CrossRef]
24. Kurosu, H.; Yamamoto, M.; Clark, J.D.; Pastor, J.V.; Nandi, A.; Gurnani, P.; McGuinness, O.P.; Chikuda, H.; Yamaguchi, M.; Kawaguchi, H.; et al. Suppression of Aging in Mice by the Hormone Klotho. *Science* **2005**, *309*, 1829–1833. [CrossRef] [PubMed]
25. Sachdeva, A.; Gouge, J.; Kontovounisios, C.; Nikolaou, S.; Ashworth, A.; Lim, K.; Chong, I. Klotho and the Treatment of Human Malignancies. *Cancers* **2020**, *12*, 1665. [CrossRef]
26. Poh, W.; Wong, W.; Ong, H.; Aung, M.O.; Lim, S.G.; Chua, B.T.; Ho, H.K. Klotho-beta overexpression as a novel target for suppressing proliferation and fibroblast growth factor receptor-4 signaling in hepatocellular carcinoma. *Mol. Cancer* **2012**, *11*, 14. [CrossRef]
27. Feng, S.; Dakhova, O.; Creighton, C.J.; Ittmann, M. Endocrine Fibroblast Growth Factor FGF19 Promotes Prostate Cancer Progression. *Cancer Res.* **2013**, *73*, 2551–2562. [CrossRef] [PubMed]
28. Zhu, Y.; Xu, L.; Zhang, J.; Xu, W.; Liu, Y.; Yin, H.; Lv, T.; An, H.; Liu, L.; He, H.; et al. Klotho suppresses tumor progression via inhibiting PI3K/Akt/GSK3β/Snail signaling in renal cell carcinoma. *Cancer Sci.* **2013**, *104*, 663–671. [CrossRef]
29. Suzuki, H.; Watkins, D.N.; Jair, K.-W.; Schuebel, K.E.; Markowitz, S.D.; Chen, W.D.; Pretlow, T.P.; Yang, B.; Akiyama, Y.; van Engeland, M.; et al. Epigenetic inactivation of SFRP genes allows constitutive WNT signaling in colorectal cancer. *Nat. Genet.* **2004**, *36*, 417–422. [CrossRef] [PubMed]
30. Sun, H.; Gao, Y.; Lu, K.; Zhao, G.; Li, X.; Li, Z.; Chang, H. Overexpression of Klotho suppresses liver cancer progression and induces cell apoptosis by negatively regulating wnt/β-catenin signaling pathway. *World J. Surg. Oncol.* **2015**, *13*, 307. [CrossRef] [PubMed]
31. Pickup, M.; Novitskiy, S.; Moses, H.L. The roles of TGFβ in the tumour microenvironment. *Nat. Rev. Cancer* **2013**, *13*, 788–799. [CrossRef]
32. Doi, S.; Zou, Y.; Togao, O.; Pastor, J.V.; John, G.B.; Wang, L.; Shiizaki, K.; Gotschall, R.; Schiavi, S.; Yorioka, N.; et al. Klotho Inhibits Transforming Growth Factor-β1 (TGF-β1) Signaling and Suppresses Renal Fibrosis and Cancer Metastasis in Mice. *J. Biol. Chem.* **2011**, *286*, 8655–8665. [CrossRef] [PubMed]
33. Hori, S.; Miyake, M.; Onishi, S.; Tatsumi, Y.; Morizawa, Y.; Nakai, Y.; Anai, S.; Tanaka, N.; Fujimoto, K. Clinical significance of α- and β-Klotho in urothelial carcinoma of the bladder. *Oncol. Rep.* **2016**, *36*, 2117–2125. [CrossRef] [PubMed]
34. Zhou, J.; Ben, S.; Xu, T.; Xu, L.; Yao, X. Serum β-klotho is a potential biomarker in the prediction of clinical outcomes among patients with NSCLC. *J. Thorac. Dis.* **2021**, *13*, 3137–3150. [CrossRef] [PubMed]

35. Wang, Y.; Chen, L.; Huang, G.; He, D.; He, J.; Xu, W.; Zou, C.; Zong, F.; Li, Y.; Chen, B.; et al. Klotho Sensitizes Human Lung Cancer Cell Line to Cisplatin via PI3k/Akt Pathway. *PLoS ONE* **2013**, *8*, e57391. [CrossRef] [PubMed]
36. Xie, B.; Zhou, J.; Yuan, L.; Ren, F.; Liu, D.-C.; Li, Q.; Shu, G. Epigenetic silencing of Klotho expression correlates with poor prognosis of human hepatocellular carcinoma. *Hum. Pathol.* **2013**, *44*, 795–801. [CrossRef]
37. Gigante, M.; Lucarelli, G.; Divella, C.; Netti, G.S.; Pontrelli, P.; Cafiero, C.; Grandaliano, G.; Castellano, G.; Rutigliano, M.; Stallone, G.; et al. Soluble Serum αKlotho Is a Potential Predictive Marker of Disease Progression in Clear Cell Renal Cell Carcinoma. *Medicine* **2015**, *94*, e1917. [CrossRef]
38. Lojkin, I.; Rubinek, T.; Orsulic, S.; Schwarzmann, O.; Karlan, B.Y.; Bose, S.; Wolf, I. Reduced expression and growth inhibitory activity of the aging suppressor klotho in epithelial ovarian cancer. *Cancer Lett.* **2015**, *362*, 149–157. [CrossRef]
39. Shibayama, Y.; Kondo, T.; Ohya, H.; Fujisawa, S.-I.; Teshima, T.; Iseki, K. Upregulation of microRNA-126-5p is associated with drug resistance to cytarabine and poor prognosis in AML patients. *Oncol. Rep.* **2015**, *33*, 2176–2182. [CrossRef]
40. Dai, D.; Wang, Q.; Li, X.; Liu, J.; Ma, X.; Xu, W. Klotho inhibits human follicular thyroid cancer cell growth and promotes apoptosis through regulation of the expression of stanniocalcin-1. *Oncol. Rep.* **2015**, *35*, 552–558. [CrossRef]
41. Tang, X.; Fan, Z.; Wang, Y.; Ji, G.; Wang, M.; Lin, J.; Huang, S. Expression of klotho and β-catenin in esophageal squamous cell carcinoma, and their clinicopathological and prognostic significance. *Dis. Esophagus* **2016**, *29*, 207–214. [CrossRef] [PubMed]
42. Ibi, T.; Usuda, J.; Inoue, T.; Sato, A.; Takegahara, K. Klotho expression is correlated to molecules associated with epithelial-mesenchymal transition in lung squamous cell carcinoma. *Oncol. Lett.* **2017**, *14*, 5526–5532. [CrossRef] [PubMed]
43. Yan, Y.; Wang, Y.; Xiong, Y.; Lin, X.; Zhou, P.; Chen, Z. Reduced Klotho expression contributes to poor survival rates in human patients with ovarian cancer, and overexpression of Klotho inhibits the progression of ovarian cancer partly via the inhibition of systemic inflammation in nude mice. *Mol. Med. Rep.* **2017**, *15*, 1777–1785. [CrossRef] [PubMed]
44. Haq, F.; Sung, Y.-N.; Park, I.; Kayani, M.A.; Yousuf, F.; Hong, S.-M.; Ahn, S.-M. FGFR1 expression defines clinically distinct subtypes in pancreatic cancer. *J. Transl. Med.* **2018**, *16*, 374. [CrossRef] [PubMed]
45. Brominska, B.; Gabryel, P.; Jarmołowska-Jurczyszyn, D.; Janicka-Jedyńska, M.; Kluk, A.; Trojanowski, M.; Brajer-Luftmann, B.; Woliński, K.; Czepczyński, R.; Gut, P.; et al. Klotho expression and nodal involvement as predictive factors for large cell lung carcinoma. *Arch. Med. Sci.* **2019**, *15*, 1010–1016. [CrossRef] [PubMed]
46. Liu, Y.; Pan, J.; Pan, X.; Wu, L.; Bian, J.; Lin, Z.; Xue, M.; Su, T.; Lai, S.; Chen, F.; et al. Klotho-mediated targeting of CCL 2 suppresses the induction of colorectal cancer progression by stromal cell senescent microenvironments. *Mol. Oncol.* **2019**, *13*, 2460–2475. [CrossRef]
47. Onishi, K.; Miyake, M.; Hori, S.; Onishi, S.; Iida, K.; Morizawa, Y.; Tatsumi, Y.; Nakai, Y.; Tanaka, N.; Fujimoto, K. γ-Klotho is correlated with resistance to docetaxel in castration-resistant prostate cancer. *Oncol. Lett.* **2020**, *19*, 2306–2316. [CrossRef]
48. Xie, B.; Hu, F.; Li, M.; Mo, L.; Xu, C.; Xiao, Y.; Wang, X.; Nie, J.; Yang, L.; He, Y. FLI-1 mediates tumor suppressor function via Klotho signaling in regulating CRC. *Cell Biol. Int.* **2020**, *44*, 1514–1522. [CrossRef]
49. Yang, L.; Wu, Y.; He, H.; Hu, F.; Li, M.; Mo, L.; Xiao, Y.; Wang, X.; Xie, B. Delivery of BR2-SOX17 fusion protein can inhibit cell survival, proliferation, and invasion in gastric cancer cells through regulating Klotho gene expression. *Cell Biol. Int.* **2020**, *44*, 2011–2020. [CrossRef]
50. GGunes, S.; Soykan, M.N.; Sariboyaci, A.E.; Uysal, O.; Sevimli, T.S. Enhancement of Apo2L/TRAIL signaling pathway receptors by the activation of Klotho gene with CRISPR/Cas9 in Caco-2 colon cancer cells. *Med. Oncol.* **2021**, *38*, 146. [CrossRef]
51. Rubinstein, T.A.; Reuveni, I.; Hesin, A.; Klein-Goldberg, A.; Olauson, H.; Larsson, T.E.; Abraham, C.R.; Zeldich, E.; Bosch, A.; Chillón, M.; et al. A Transgenic Model Reveals the Role of Klotho in Pancreatic Cancer Development and Paves the Way for New Klotho-Based Therapy. *Cancers* **2021**, *13*, 6297. [CrossRef] [PubMed]
52. Wang, Y.; Wang, H.; Zheng, R.; Wu, P.; Sun, Z.; Chen, J.; Zhang, L.; Zhang, C.; Qian, H.; Jiang, J.; et al. Circular RNA ITCH suppresses metastasis of gastric cancer via regulating miR-199a-5p/Klotho axis. *Cell Cycle* **2021**, *20*, 522–536. [CrossRef] [PubMed]
53. Sariboyaci, A.E.; Uysal, O.; Soykan, M.N.; Gunes, S. The potential therapeutic effect of klotho on cell viability in human colorectal adenocarcinoma HT-29 cells. *Med. Oncol.* **2022**, *39*, 191. [CrossRef] [PubMed]
54. Tao, Z.; Cui, Y.; Xu, X.; Han, T. FGFR redundancy limits the efficacy of FGFR4-selective inhibitors in hepatocellular carcinoma. *Proc. Natl. Acad. Sci. USA* **2022**, *119*, e2208844119. [CrossRef]
55. Labrecque, M.P.; Coleman, I.M.; Brown, L.G.; True, L.D.; Kollath, L.; Lakely, B.; Nguyen, H.M.; Yang, Y.C.; Gil da Costa, R.M.; Kaipainen, A.; et al. Molecular profiling stratifies diverse phenotypes of treatment-refractory metastatic castration-resistant prostate cancer. *J. Clin. Investig.* **2019**, *129*, 4492–4505. [CrossRef]
56. Harbeck, N.; Gnant, M. Breast cancer. *Lancet* **2017**, *389*, 1134–1150. [CrossRef]
57. Gil da Costa, R.M.; Levesque, C.; Bianchi-Frias, D.; Chatterjee, P.; Lam, H.; Santos, C.; Coleman, I.M.; Ferreirinha, P.; Vilanova, M.; da Cunha, N.P.; et al. Pharmacological NF-κB inhibition decreases cisplatin chemoresistance in muscle-invasive bladder cancer and reduces cisplatin-induced toxicities. *Mol. Oncol.* **2023**. [CrossRef]
58. DeLucia, D.C.; Cardillo, T.M.; Ang, L.S.; Labrecque, M.P.; Zhang, A.; Hopkins, J.E.; De Sarkar, N.; Coleman, I.; Gil da Costa, R.M.; Corey, E.; et al. Regulation of CEACAM5 and Therapeutic Efficacy of an Anti-CEACAM5-SN38 Antibody–drug Conjugate in Neuroendocrine Prostate Cancer. *Clin. Cancer Res.* **2021**, *27*, 759–774. [CrossRef]
59. Tannock, I.F.; De Wit, R.; Berry, W.R.; Horti, J.; Pluzanska, A.; Chi, K.N.; Oudard, S.; Théodore, C.; James, N.D.; Turesson, I.; et al. Docetaxel plus Prednisone or Mitoxantrone plus Prednisone for Advanced Prostate Cancer. *N. Engl. J. Med.* **2004**, *351*, 1502–1512. [CrossRef]

60. Rodriguez-Canales, J.; Parra-Cuentas, E.; Wistuba, I.I. Diagnosis and Molecular Classification of Lung Cancer. *Cancer Treat. Res.* **2016**, *170*, 25–46. [CrossRef]
61. Forner, A.; Reig, M.; Bruix, J. Hepatocellular carcinoma. *Lancet* **2018**, *391*, 1301–1314. [CrossRef] [PubMed]
62. Lheureux, S.; Braunstein, M.; Oza, A.M. Epithelial ovarian cancer: Evolution of management in the era of precision medicine. *CA A Cancer J. Clin.* **2019**, *69*, 280–304. [CrossRef] [PubMed]
63. Santos, J.M.O.; Costa, A.C.; Dias, T.R.; Satari, S.; e Silva, M.P.C.; Gil da Costa, R.M.; Medeiros, R. Towards Drug Repurposing in Cancer Cachexia: Potential Targets and Candidates. *Pharmaceuticals* **2021**, *14*, 1084. [CrossRef] [PubMed]
64. Liu, H. Emerging agents and regimens for AML. *J. Hematol. Oncol.* **2021**, *14*, 49. [CrossRef]
65. Bianchini, G.; De Angelis, C.; Licata, L.; Gianni, L. Treatment landscape of triple-negative breast cancer—Expanded options, evolving needs. *Nat. Rev. Clin. Oncol.* **2022**, *19*, 91–113. [CrossRef]
66. Patel, S.G.; Karlitz, J.J.; Yen, T.; Lieu, C.H.; Boland, C.R. The rising tide of early-onset colorectal cancer: A comprehensive review of epidemiology, clinical features, biology, risk factors, prevention, and early detection. *Lancet Gastroenterol. Hepatol.* **2022**, *7*, 262–274. [CrossRef]
67. Compérat, E.; Amin, M.B.; Cathomas, R.; Choudhury, A.; De Santis, M.; Kamat, A.; Stenzl, A.; Thoeny, H.C.; Witjes, J.A. Current best practice for bladder cancer: A narrative review of diagnostics and treatments. *Lancet* **2022**, *400*, 1712–1721. [CrossRef]

Disclaimer/Publisher's Note: The statements, opinions and data contained in all publications are solely those of the individual author(s) and contributor(s) and not of MDPI and/or the editor(s). MDPI and/or the editor(s) disclaim responsibility for any injury to people or property resulting from any ideas, methods, instructions or products referred to in the content.

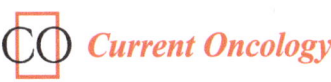

Review

A Literature Review of Racial Disparities in Prostate Cancer Research

Matthieu Vermeille [1], Kira-Lee Koster [2], David Benzaquen [3], Ambroise Champion [3], Daniel Taussky [3,4,*], Kevin Kaulanjan [5] and Martin Früh [2,6]

1. Genolier Swiss Radio-Oncology Network, Clinique de Genolier, 1272 Genolier, Switzerland; vermeille@hin.ch
2. Department of Medical Oncology and Hematology, Cantonal Hospital St. Gallen, 9007 St. Gallen, Switzerland; kira-lee.koster@kssg.ch (K.-L.K.); martin.frueh@kssg.ch (M.F.)
3. Radiation Oncology, Hôpital de La Tour, 1217 Meyrin, Switzerland; david.benzaquen@latour.ch (D.B.); ambroise.champion@latour.ch (A.C.)
4. Department of Radiation Oncology, Centre Hospitalier de l'Université de Montréal, Montreal, QC H3Y2V4, Canada
5. Department of Urology, Université des Antilles, CHU de Guadeloupe, 97110 Pointe-à-Pitre, France; kevin.kaulanjan@gmail.com
6. Department of Medical Oncology, Inselspital, University Hospital Bern, 3010 Bern, Switzerland
* Correspondence: daniel.taussky.chum@ssss.gouv.qc.ca; Tel.: +514-890-8254; Fax: +514-412-7537

Abstract: Background: Despite recent awareness of institutional racism, there are still important racial disparities in prostate cancer medical research. We investigated the historical development of research on racial disparities and bias. Methods: PubMed was searched for the term 'prostate cancer race' and added key terms associated with racial disparity. As an indicator of scientific interest in the topic, we analyzed whether the number of publications increased linearly as an indicator of growing interest. The linearity is expressed as R^2. Results: The general search term "prostate cancer race" yielded 4507 publications. More specific search terms with ≥ 12 publications showing a higher scientific interest were found after 2005. The terms with the most publications when added to the general term were "genetic" (n = 1011), "PSA" (n = 995), and "detection" (n = 861). There was a linear increase in publications for "prostate cancer race" ($R^2 = 0.75$) since 1980. Specific terms added to the general terms with a high linear increase ($R^2 \geq 0.7$) were "screening" ($R^2 = 0.82$), "detection" ($R^2 = 0.72$), "treatment access" ($R^2 = 0.71$), and "trial underrepresentation" ($R^2 = 0.71$). However, only a few studies have investigated its association with sexual activity. A combination with "sexual" showed 157 publications but only two years with ≥ 12 publications/year. Conclusion: The terms "genetic", "PSA", and "detection" have been the focus of recent research on racial differences in prostate cancer. We found that old stereotypes are still being mentioned but seem to find little interest in the current literature. Further research interest was found in "treatment access". Recently, interest in socioeconomic factors has decreased.

Keywords: prostate cancer; racial disparity; detection; treatment access; socioeconomic factors

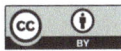

1. Introduction

There are large disparities in the incidence and mortality rates of prostate cancer among Black men [1,2]. It has been well-researched and the literature is vast. Black men are an average of two years younger than White men at diagnosis. Many studies have investigated the factors which might explain this racial difference. More recent publications concentrate not only on biological factors, such as genetics or environmental factors, but also on the structural and social determinants of health and equity, cultural mistrust, knowledge and communication, and other socioeconomic factors, such as insurance status and the interactions amongst different factors [2,3].

Scientific literature as far back as the 1930s has investigated the difference in the incidence of prostatic blockage between Black and White men. When reviewing the literature, it seems that in the 1980s and the 1990s there were few studies investigating racial disparities, and the few articles investigating the subject were probably written mainly by White authors, focusing on biological differences in testosterone levels and sexual activity or sexually transmitted infections (STIs). This focus was based on the understanding that Black men have higher serum and intraprostatic tissue androgen concentrations [4–6].

Race and ethnicity are social constructs with limited utility in understanding medical research, but these terms may be useful for studying and viewing racism and disparities [7]. Historically, racial disparities have been attributed to biological differences. With time, there has been acknowledgment that racial differences in prostate cancer are rooted in many factors that are not only biological [8], but also starting with more subtle forms of racism and even going as far as institutional racism and systematic discrimination by the government, enterprises, schools, or other organizations.

First, we provide an overview of how the medical literature has evolved in recent years. Then, we investigate the factors over time that were of interest in explaining racial disparities in the medical community. Research on etiological factors for prostate cancer was analyzed and how it has changed over the years by analyzing differences in culture and sexual behavior in more scientific subjects, such as genetic and socioeconomic disparities.

In the second section, research papers on racial differences were cited, which in our opinion, are particularly biased. Racially biased research was frequent in the past but has continued to play a role until today.

2. Material and Methods

First, we reviewed the literature to find common key words associated with "prostate cancer" and "race". We then identified several historical articles in key publications that were among the first to report racial inequality in cancer detection and survival.

We accessed PubMed (https://pubmed.ncbi.nlm.nih.gov/) on 19 and 22 May 2023 and entered different search terms that have been in the past or are still attributed to racial disparities in prostate cancer.

We first searched the term "prostate cancer race", which yielded 4507 publications and then added additional more specific terms such as "genetic", "PSA", and "detection". Compared with the term "prostate cancer race", the search term "prostate cancer African descent" yielded 175 publications, and "prostate cancer ethnicity" yielded 3976 publications (Figure 1).

No limit was applied to the years analyzed. PubMed covers articles dating back to 1966 and selectively to 1865. Search terms were based on analyzing all 129 review articles on the terms "prostate cancer race" as accessed on 19 May 2023. While the number of citations an article generates would be a much better indicator of the interest that an article generates, we chose to use the number of publications on a certain topic as an indicator of scientific interest in a scientific subject. In our opinion, the number of publications equally represents interest in a subject. We chose to utilize PubMed and not other services such as for example the Web of Science, because a publication listed in PubMed means that the National Library of Medicine (NLM) deemed the scientific and editorial character and quality of a journal as meriting inclusion. We searched for each term, and recorded the number of publications. The year in which the term was first listed on PubMed was recorded, and then was analyzed at ≥ 6 and ≥ 12 publications. These numbers represent a certain interest in the scientific community in a subject indicated by there being at least one publication per month or per every other month in a year. We calculated the number of years between publication of ≥ 6 and ≥ 12 publications. A shorter time represents a rapid increase in interest in the subject's knowledge.

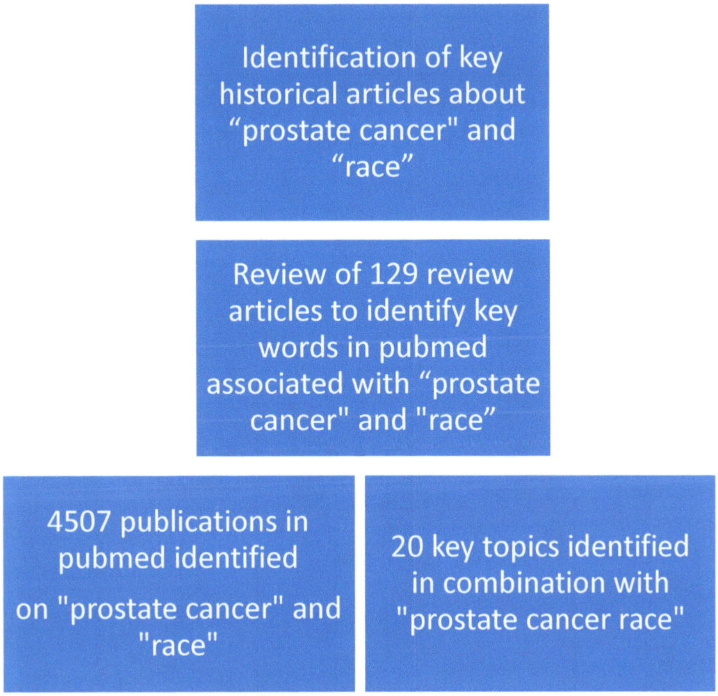

Figure 1. Flowchart of methods and materials.

Then, a graph based on the number of publications per year was created. The number of publications per year can easily be exported from PubMed to an Excel spreadsheet. Finally, Excel was used to calculate whether the increase in publications was linear. A linear increase represented an increase in interest and knowledge of the subject. Linearity is expressed as R^2, a measure of how well a linear regression model "fits" a dataset. The strong linearity was $R^2 > 0.7$, moderate 0.5–0.7, and weak was $R^2 = 0.3–<0.5$.

3. Results

First, we researched when awareness of racial differences must have begun. While reviewing the literature, we found that in general, the fact that there was an increasing incidence of prostate cancer in Black patients had been well-documented in large studies since at least 1980. Increasing incidence of prostate cancer in Black patients has been reported in several epidemiologic studies. An analysis of voluntary data supplied by hospitals in 1979 showed that Black patients presented with more advanced clinical stage and poorer survival rates. The first listed publication on "prostate cancer black mortality increase" appeared in PubMed in 1977. And the first time that there were >1 publications on the subject was in 1985. But only from 2008 on were there consistently >12 publications per year.

In our analysis of the literature in PubMed, we found among the 4507 publications on "prostate cancer race", most of the analyzed terms reached ≥6 publications/year beginning in 1994 (Table 1). Most search terms with ≥12 publications were identified after 2005. In recent years, publications with the terms "genetic" and "socioeconomic," for example, have more than 40 publications per year, showing that these subjects have been extensively researched.

Table 1. Factors researched on PubMed in combination with search terms added to "prostate cancer race" ordered according to number of publications.

Term/Term Added	Publications May, 2023	First Year Listed in Pubmed	Year First Time 6 Publicat.	Year First Time 12 Publicat.	Diff. in Years	R^2
prostate cancer race	4507	1964	1979	1990	11	0.75
screening	2246	1968	1983	1994	11	0.82
genetic	1011	1972	1995	1997	2	0.65
PSA	995	1991	1995	1995	0	0.48
detection rate	861	1980	1994	1997	3	0.72
socioeconomic	690	1971	2008	2013	5	0.80
treatment outcome	457	1993	1998	2000	2	0.43
clinical trial	355	1983	1996	2006	10	0.52
treatment access	311	1983	1996	2007	11	0.71
active surveillance	233	1996	2012	2012	0	0.57
marital	204	1972	1999	2013	14	0.58
obesity	191	1993	2005	2005	0	0.20
diet	185	1979	2003	2007	4	0.35
belief	177	1964	1998	2006	8	0.26
testosterone	112	1977	2004	--	--	0.09
inflammation	86	1996	2009	--	--	0.56
immune	77	2001	2014	2021	7	0.39
microenvironnement	26	2004	2021	--	--	0.25
underrepresentation	11	2001	--	--	--	0.71
microbiome	9	2016	--	--	--	--
stigma	7	2015	--	--	--	--

Table 1 shows the number of publications per search term in descending order of the number of publications. The following terms: "PSA" (1995), "obesity" (2005), and "active surveillance" (2012), combined with "prostate cancer race" were picked up quickly by the scientific community, meaning that their number of publications immediately went from <6 to ≥12 per year.

In general, terms investigating an association with sexual activity, a term that could indicate a bias towards Black men, had few publications. Only two terms associated with sexual activity had >50 publications: the combination with "sexual" had 157 publications but only in two years (2011 and 2022) with exactly 12 publications, and "sexual factors" had 93 publications, but always <12 publications/year and a maximum of eight publications per year in 2013. The term "genetics testosterone" has been used in only 36 publications. This term is sometimes used to investigate genetic differences between the testosterone receptors. First publications about "testosterone", "sexual", and "marital" could be found in the 1970s (Table 2), while subjects that are still much discussed such as "treatment access", "clinical trial", and "treatment outcome" began only in the 1980s (Table 1).

Several search terms showed a strong linear increase ($R^2 > 0.7$) in publications, representing a continuous interest, such as the general search term "prostate cancer race" ($R^2 = 0.75$), "socioeconomic" (a factor that has recently been identified as a key factor for racial disparities in 690 publications), and a strong linear increase ($R^2 = 0.80$). Other specific terms added to the general term with a strong linear increase were "screening" ($R^2 = 0.82$), "detection" ($R^2 = 0.72$), "treatment access" ($R^2 = 0.71$), and "trial underrepresentation"

($R^2 = 0.71$). Interest in "genetics" has plateaued ($R^2 = 0.65$), but with more than 50 publications every year since 2015, after reaching ≥12 publications in 1997. Figure 2 lists some graphs illustrating the increase in publications of the four selected terms added to the general search term "prostate cancer race".

Table 2. Search terms added to "prostate cancer race" with sexual subjects that had <100 publications.

Term Added	Publications May, 2023	First Year Listed in Pubmed	Year First Time 6 Publicat.	Year First Time 12 Publicat.	Diff in Years	R^2
sexual	157	1971	2005	2011	6	0.36
sexual factors	93	1971	2005	--	--	0.33
sexual activity	45	1973	2011	--	--	0.14
intercourse	16	1974	--	--	--	0.007
STD	4	1992	--	--		

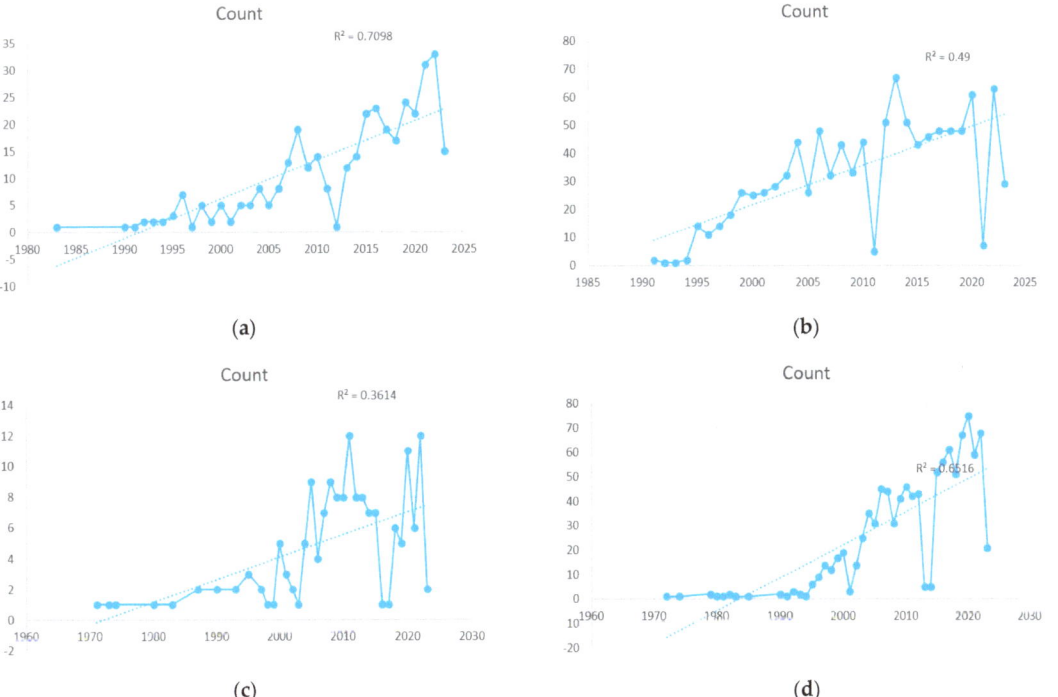

Figure 2. Selected terms added to the general search term "prostate cancer race". (**a**) "Treatment access"; (**b**) "PSA"; (**c**) "Sexual"; (**d**) "genetic".

4. Discussion

We found that Black men had more advanced disease and worse survival since at least 1980 when larger studies were published. But the subject of increased mortality only really gained interest in the scientific community from 2008 on, when there were consistently >12 publications per year on the topic.

Today, we found that there is a strong awareness of racial disparities in prostate cancer with >4500 publications in PubMed on the subject of "prostate cancer race". Interest in racial disparities seems to have begun around 1954, and most of the search terms with

≥12 publications were found after 2005. In the last years, publications with the terms "genetic" and "socioeconomic", for example, have had more than 40 publications/year, thereby implying that these subjects are thoroughly researched. Most articles deal with genetics, as well as terms associated with prostate cancer detection such as "PSA" and "detection" of prostate cancer. Recently, there has been a large and linear increase in the subject of "socioeconomic" factors and prostate cancer detection as well as "treatment access" and "trial underrepresentation". Factors traditionally associated with bias against Black men, such as sexual activity and testosterone levels, were of little but persistent interest.

4.1. Race in Prostate Cancer Research

Race has been recognized as a social construct defined by how one group perceives another [9]. However, a more recent publication argued that race has both genetic and social components. The authors embraced genetic studies in African populations to better understand these diseases [8,10]. In their 1992 review, Burks and Littleton, from the Henry Ford Hospital in Detroit [11], who focused on the epidemiology of prostate cancer in Black men, had already shown that significant racial differences are related to factors such as access to medical care, genetic and environmental factors, and cultural differences, including diet and social habits. They stated that most reports presented conflicting data with no clear positive correlations, and their conclusions are often speculative. Better controlled prospective studies of epidemiologic variables and a comprehensive genetic evaluation of Black families with prostate cancer are needed, to more thoroughly understand the racial disparity affecting American Black men and the biology of this disease in all men.

4.2. Comparison to Cervical Cancer

Compared to prostate cancer, cervical cancer is clearly associated with STIs such as **Human papillomavirus (HPV)** [12]. Interestingly, the search term "cervical cancer race" yielded 1990 publications compared with the 4500 terms for prostate cancer. Adding the search term "sexual" to cervical cancer resulted in 225 publications, compared with 157 publications for prostate cancer.

4.3. A Short History of the Importance of Race in Prostate Cancer Research

We examined the historical development of research on racial disparity. The opinion that hormonal and sexual factors play a role in the differences between Black and White men probably originated in the fact that since the early 1940s it has been known that prostate cancer is hormonally dependent [13]. Additionally, STIs had been investigated as an etiological factor for prostate cancer. One study found that circumcision appeared to be protective only among Black men [14] and another study found that HSV-2 might be implicated in prostate cancer development [15,16]. The theory that the presence of sexually transmitted infectious agents cause prostate cancer and thereby a history of venereal disease posing as a risk factor for prostate cancer, suggesting that racial disparity might be due to differences in sexual activity between Black and White men [6] has been abandoned [17].

Another factor contributing to the bias in the medical establishment regarding Black men is that Black patients are sometimes seen as more tolerant to pain in general [18] and urinary symptoms in particular, and therefore are significantly less likely than White patients to receive prescriptions for opioids [19]. A telling publication from South Africa published in 1966 reported that nearly two-thirds of African and half of Asiatic patients delayed coming to the hospital until forced to do so by the retention of urine. The reason given by the authors was the greater tolerance to dysuria [13].

Even back then, the much more obvious cause of delayed doctor visits would have likely been restricted access to the medical system or the perception of unequal treatment by Black patients, resulting in distrust in the system.

4.4. Bias against Black Patients in Prostate Cancer Research

A factor that has gained little interest today is that Black men seem, despite similar care settings, to be generally less satisfied with their treatment [20]. In their 2008 publication, one of >700 publications, Sanda et al. studied the quality of life of patients with prostate cancer. One of their findings was that "Black patients reported lower satisfaction with the degree of overall treatment outcomes". We were unable to identify the reasons for this discrepancy between Black and non-Black patients. However, this finding has received little research attention. The authors were unable to determine whether these differences were biological, a reflection of disparities in the quality of care, or differences in patient expectations. One could hypothesize that within the trial setting, patients may have felt uncomfortable, and their expectations and interaction with the research staff were not optimal, or there were other cultural or socioeconomic differences. This is one of the reasons why the Black population in clinical trials in general is underrepresented [21].

One could argue that the fact that they were treated in a trial could have created mistrust in patients, that their interaction with the research staff was not optimal, or that there were other cultural or socioeconomic differences in Black patients [22].

Some of the biased literature may stem from previous research on benign prostatic hyperplasia (BPH) in Black men. Derbes et al. in their findings published in 1937 in the *Journal of Urology* [23] showed that some of the biased literature may stem from previous research on BPH in Black men, which examined 1405 cases of BPH treated at the State of Louisiana Charity Hospital. They found that Black men possibly have a higher frequency of BPH and are, on average, five years younger than White men. They attributed these findings to the fact that it is generally supposed that the Black man "accepts physical discomfort, especially that associated with the genito-urinary tract, as a natural event in the course of life and would be slower in seeking medical aid than the White man". They cited other reasons that are not reproduced here.

There were studies without any racial prejudice such as the publication by Burns, read before the Southeastern Section, American Urological Association, in Biloxi, Miss, in 1939 [24].

Ross et al. published a rather strongly biased example in May 1987 in the *Journal of the National Cancer Institute* [6]. They stated that they investigated the reason for the higher risk of prostate cancer in Black men and stated that a history of venereal disease, as well as the frequency of sexual intercourse, was higher in Black men. Later on, they explained that these differences were because the two groups were dissimilar in "social class characteristics".

In 2022, Basourakos et al. [25] found that the age-specific frequencies of definitive treatment were similar for men of all races. Additionally, they found that "Black men have a higher incidence of and mortality from prostate cancer compared to men of other races, and that the Black race does not appear to be associated with inferior long-term outcomes as long as there is equal access to care and standardized treatment". There is increasing awareness of the necessity to include Black men in prostate cancer trials in general and specifically in cancer prevention trials [26].

4.5. Limitations of Our Study

The limitation of our study is that we did not separate publications about Black men only but included the term "race" without specifying further. It would have been a herculean task to analyze 4500 abstracts and classify each publication according to one main topic. Therefore, some publications have appeared in several searches although they have no direct importance to the subject of the publication. Furthermore, we did not include the search term "ethnicity" with nearly 4000 publications. We have, therefore, included some patients of origins other than African, although most studies on race and prostate cancer deal with disparities between Black men and other races. In general, little research has been conducted on other racial disparities outside North America. Therefore, our data are mostly US-specific and cannot necessarily be applied to other countries. There is a growing number of journals, and therefore, publications and research, over the years. Therefore, more recent topics have more publications and a faster uptake per definition than older topics. Healthcare professionals have been shown to exhibit the same level of implicit bias as that of the wider population. It has been observed that patients who experience racism lack trust and experience a delay in seeking healthcare [27].

5. Conclusions

In conclusion, interest in the influence of race on prostate cancer began in the mid-1990s and has become a more researched subject since 2005. Biased terms dealing with racial sex differences have gained little but persistent interest. Recently, terms such as "genetic", "PSA", and "detection" have become the focus of research.

Author Contributions: Conceptualization: M.V., D.T., K.-L.K., and M.F.; Methodology: M.V., D.T., K.-L.K., and M.F.; Software: D.T.; Validation: D.T.; Formal Analysis: D.T.; Investigation: M.V., D.T., K.-L.K., and M.F.; Resources: D.T., A.C., and D.B.; Data Curation: D.T.; Writing—Original Draft Preparation: M.V., D.T., K.-L.K., M.F., A.C., D.B., and K.K.; Writing—Review and Editing: M.V., D.T., K.-L.K., M.F., A.C., D.B., and K.K.; Visualization: M.V., D.T., K.-L.K., M.F., A.C., D.B., and K.K.; Supervision: D.T.; Project Administration: D.T.; All authors have read and agreed to the published version of the manuscript.

Funding: This research received no external funding.

Conflicts of Interest: The authors declare no conflict of interest.

Abbreviations

STIs: sexually transmitted infections; HPV: Human papillomavirus; BPH: benign prostatic hyperplasia.

References

1. Lillard, J.W., Jr.; Moses, K.A.; Mahal, B.A.; George, D.J. Racial disparities in B lack men with prostate cancer: A literature review. *Cancer* **2022**, *128*, 3787–3795. [CrossRef] [PubMed]
2. Mahal, B.A.; Gerke, T.; Awasthi, S.; Soule, H.R.; Simons, J.W.; Miyahira, A.; Halabi, S.; George, D.; Platz, E.A.; Mucci, L. Prostate cancer racial disparities: A systematic review by the prostate cancer foundation panel. *Eur. Urol. Oncol.* **2022**, *5*, 18–29. [CrossRef] [PubMed]
3. Nyame, Y.A.; Cooperberg, M.R.; Cumberbatch, M.G.; Eggener, S.E.; Etzioni, R.; Gomez, S.L.; Haiman, C.; Huang, F.; Lee, C.T.; Litwin, M.S. Deconstructing, addressing, and eliminating racial and ethnic inequities in prostate cancer care. *Eur. Urol.* **2022**, *82*, 341–351. [CrossRef] [PubMed]
4. Marks, L.S.; Hess, D.L.; Dorey, F.J.; Macairan, M.L. Prostatic tissue testosterone and dihydrotestosterone in African-American and white men. *Urology* **2006**, *68*, 337–341. [CrossRef]
5. Ross, R.; Bernstein, L.; Judd, H.; Hanisch, R.; Pike, M.; Henderson, B. Serum testosterone levels in healthy young black and white men. *J. Natl. Cancer Inst.* **1986**, *76*, 45–48.
6. Ross, R.; Shimizu, H.; Paganini-Hill, A.; Honda, G.; Henderson, B. Case-control studies of prostate cancer in blacks and whites in southern California. *J. Natl. Cancer Inst.* **1987**, *78*, 869–874.
7. Flanagin, A.; Frey, T.; Christiansen, S.L.; Committee AMoS. Updated guidance on the reporting of race and ethnicity in medical and science journals. *JAMA* **2021**, *326*, 621–627. [CrossRef]
8. Bhardwaj, A.; Srivastava, S.K.; Khan, M.A.; Prajapati, V.K.; Singh, S.; Carter, J.E.; Singh, A.P. Racial disparities in prostate cancer: A molecular perspective. *Front. Biosci.* **2017**, *22*, 772. [CrossRef]
9. Freeman, H.; Payne, R. Editorial: Racial injustice in health care. *N. Engl. J. Med.* **2000**, *342*, 1045–1047. [CrossRef]
10. Oni-Orisan, A.; Mavura, Y.; Banda, Y.; Thornton, T.A.; Sebro, R. Embracing genetic diversity to improve black health. *Mass. Med. Soc.* **2021**, *384*, 1163–1167. [CrossRef]
11. Burks, D.A.; Littleton, R.H. The epidemiology of prostate cancer in black men. *Henry Ford Hosp. Med. J.* **1992**, *40*, 89–92.
12. Dunne, E.F.; Park, I.U. HPV and HPV-associated diseases. *Infect. Dis. Clin.* **2013**, *27*, 765–778. [CrossRef] [PubMed]
13. Movsas, S. Prostatic obstruction in the African and Asiatic. *Br. J. Surg.* **1966**, *53*, 538–543. [CrossRef] [PubMed]
14. Spence, A.R.; Rousseau, M.C.; Karakiewicz, P.I.; Parent, M.É. Circumcision and prostate cancer: A population-based case-control study in M ontréal, C anada. *BJU Int.* **2014**, *114*, E90–E98. [CrossRef] [PubMed]

15. Dennis, L.K.; Coughlin, J.A.; McKinnon, B.C.; Wells, T.S.; Gaydos, C.A.; Hamsikova, E.; Gray, G.C. Sexually transmitted infections and prostate cancer among men in the US military. *Cancer Epidemiol. Biomark. Prev.* **2009**, *18*, 2665–2671. [CrossRef]
16. Ge, X.; Wang, X.; Shen, P. Herpes simplex virus type 2 or human herpesvirus 8 infection and prostate cancer risk: A meta-analysis. *Biomed. Rep.* **2013**, *1*, 433–439. [CrossRef]
17. Mordukhovich, I.; Reiter, P.L.; Backes, D.M.; Family, L.; McCullough, L.E.; O'Brien, K.M.; Razzaghi, H.; Olshan, A.F. A review of African American-white differences in risk factors for cancer: Prostate cancer. *Cancer Causes Control.* **2011**, *22*, 341–357. [CrossRef]
18. Jagsi, R.; Griffith, K.A.; Vicini, F.; Boike, T.; Dominello, M.; Gustafson, G.; Hayman, J.A.; Moran, J.M.; Radawski, J.D.; Walker, E. Identifying patients whose symptoms are underrecognized during treatment with breast radiotherapy. *JAMA Oncol.* **2022**, *8*, 887–894. [CrossRef]
19. Morrison, R.S.; Wallenstein, S.; Natale, D.K.; Senzel, R.S.; Huang, L.-L. "We don't carry that"—Failure of pharmacies in predominantly nonwhite neighborhoods to stock opioid analgesics. *N. Engl. J. Med.* **2000**, *342*, 1023–1026. [CrossRef]
20. Sanda, M.; Dunn, R.; Michalski, J. Quality of Quality of Life in Men Treated for Early Prostate Cancer: A Prospective Patient Preference Cohort Study 457 Life and Satisfaction with Outcome among Prostate-Cancer Survivors. *N. Engl. J. Med.* **2008**, *358*, 1250–1261. [CrossRef]
21. Xiao, H.; Vaidya, R.; Liu, F.; Chang, X.; Xia, X.; Unger, J.M. Sex, racial, and ethnic representation in COVID-19 clinical trials: A systematic review and meta-analysis. *JAMA Intern. Med.* **2023**, *183*, 50–60. [CrossRef] [PubMed]
22. Roy, E.; Chino, F.; King, B.; Madu, C.; Mattes, M.; Morrell, R.; Pollard-Larkin, J.; Siker, M.; Takita, C.; Ludwig, M. Increasing diversity of patients in radiation oncology clinical trials. *Int. J. Radiat. Oncol. Biol. Phys.* **2023**, *116*, 103–114. [CrossRef] [PubMed]
23. Derbes, V.d.P.; Leche, S.M.; Hooker, C.W. The Incidence of Benign Prostatic Hypertrophy among the Whites and Negroes in New Orleans. Available online: https://doi.org/10.1016/S0022-5347(17)71966-0 (accessed on 5 November 2023).
24. Burns, E. Prostatic Obstruction In Negroes. Available online: https://www.auajournals.org/doi/abs/10.1016/S0022-5347%2817%2971256-6 (accessed on 5 November 2023).
25. Basourakos, S.P.; Gulati, R.; Vince, R.A.; Spratt, D.E.; Lewicki, P.J.; Hill, A.; Nyame, Y.A.; Cullen, J.; Markt, S.C.; Barbieri, C.E. Harm-to-benefit of three decades of prostate cancer screening in Black men. *NEJM Evid.* **2022**, *1*, EVIDoa2200031. [CrossRef] [PubMed]
26. Moinpour, C.M.; Atkinson, J.O.; Thomas, S.M.; Underwood, S.M.; Harvey, C.; Parzuchowski, J.; Lovato, L.C.; Ryan, A.M.; Hill, M.S.; Deantoni, E. Minority recruitment in the prostate cancer prevention trial. *Ann. Epidemiol.* **2000**, *10*, S85–S91. [CrossRef]
27. FitzGerald, C.; Hurst, S. Implicit bias in healthcare professionals: A systematic review. *BMC Med. Ethics* **2017**, *18*, 19. [CrossRef]

Disclaimer/Publisher's Note: The statements, opinions and data contained in all publications are solely those of the individual author(s) and contributor(s) and not of MDPI and/or the editor(s). MDPI and/or the editor(s) disclaim responsibility for any injury to people or property resulting from any ideas, methods, instructions or products referred to in the content.

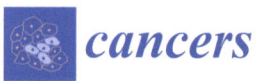

Article

Robot-Assisted Radical Prostatectomy by Lateral Approach: Technique, Reproducibility and Outcomes

Moisés Rodríguez Socarrás *, Juan Gómez Rivas, Javier Reinoso Elbers, Fabio Espósito, Luis Llanes Gonzalez, Diego M. Carrion Monsalve, Julio Fernandez Del Alamo, Sonia Ruiz Graña, Jorge Juarez Varela, Daniel Coria, Vanesa Cuadros Rivera, Richard Gastón and Fernando Gómez Sancha

Instituto de Cirugía Urológica Avanzada (ICUA), Clínica CEMTRO, 28035 Madrid, Spain; juangomezr@gmail.com (J.G.R.); jre@icua.es (J.R.E.); fabioesposito025@gmail.com (F.E.); lll@icua.es (L.L.G.); dcm@icua.es (D.M.C.M.); jfa@icua.es (J.F.D.A.); srg@icua.es (S.R.G.); daniel.coria@live.cl (D.C.); vcr@icua.es (V.C.R.); fgs@icua.es (F.G.S.)
* Correspondence: mrs@icua.es

Simple Summary: Robotic radical prostatectomy is a treatment for prostate cancer. The lateral approach radical prostatectomy technique allows total preservation of the anterior pubovesical complex, as well as vascular and nervous structures in close contact with the prostate, involved in continence and male potency. We analyzed more than 500 patients undergoing robotic radical prostatectomy using the lateral approach technique, operated by two surgeons at our institution, from January 2015 to March 2021. The technique is reproduced by both surgeons, the oncological and functional results are outstanding with this technique, which means that it is a successful treatment to cure prostate cancer, preserving excellent urinary continence and sexual function.

Abstract: Background: Radical prostatectomy by lateral approach allows performing a prostatectomy through a buttonhole, with direct access to the seminal vesicle and fully sparing the anterior pubovesical complex. Our aim is to show the results of reproducing the technique of robotic radical prostatectomy by lateral approach, in terms of intraoperative, postoperative, oncological and functional parameters. Methods: We analyzed 513 patients submitted to robotic radical prostatectomy by lateral approach from January 2015 to March 2021, operated on by two surgeons in our institution. The oncological and functional results of both surgeons were compared. Results: When comparing both surgeons, the rate of positive surgical margins (PSM) was 32.87% and 37.9% and significant surgical margins (PSM > 2 mm) were 5.88% and 7.58% ($p = 0.672$) for surgeon 1 and surgeon 2, respectively. Immediate continence was 86% and 85% and sexual potency at one year 73% and 72%, with a similar rate of complications for surgeon 1 and 2. Conclusions: Radical prostatectomy by the lateral approach technique with preservation of the anterior pubovesical complex is reproducible and offers good oncological and functional results.

Keywords: robot-assisted radical prostatectomy; radical prostatectomy technique; lateral approach; prostate cancer

Citation: Rodríguez Socarrás, M.; Gómez Rivas, J.; Reinoso Elbers, J.; Espósito, F.; Llanes Gonzalez, L.; Monsalve, D.M.C.; Fernandez Del Alamo, J.; Ruiz Graña, S.; Juarez Varela, J.; Coria, D.; et al. Robot-Assisted Radical Prostatectomy by Lateral Approach: Technique, Reproducibility and Outcomes. *Cancers* 2023, *15*, 5442. https://doi.org/10.3390/cancers15225442

Academic Editor: Emmanuel S. Antonarakis

Received: 8 September 2023
Revised: 8 November 2023
Accepted: 10 November 2023
Published: 16 November 2023

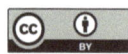

Copyright: © 2023 by the authors. Licensee MDPI, Basel, Switzerland. This article is an open access article distributed under the terms and conditions of the Creative Commons Attribution (CC BY) license (https://creativecommons.org/licenses/by/4.0/).

1. Introduction

There are different surgical techniques for performing robotic radical prostatectomy for the treatment of localized prostate cancer [1–3]. The lateral approach is a technique, developed by Dr. Richard Gaston, is based on the dissection of the prostate through a lateral buttonhole, offering maximum preservation of the anterior pubovesical complex and neurovascular bundles, and keeping the use of thermal energy to a minimum [4–7].

The evolution in imaging techniques such as mpMRI, Positron emission tomography (PET), and microultrasound (MUS), among others, allows better identification of tumours and their localization, increasing the diagnostic yield of biopsy systems and influencing the planning of the surgical strategy [8]. However, surgical technique and surgeon experience impact on positive surgical margins (PSM) and functional and oncologic outcomes [9–14]. Some surgeons say that the lateral approach technique is difficult to reproduce, but like any technique [15], reproducing it requires knowledge of the appropriate anatomical landmarks.

The aim of our study is to show the results, in terms of intraoperative, postoperative, oncological and functional parameters, of reproducing the technique of robotic radical prostatectomy by lateral approach.

2. Materials and Methods

We analysed 513 patients submitted to robotic radical prostatectomy by lateral approach from January 2015 to March 2021, operated on by two surgeons in our institution. Surgeon 1, RG (the inventor of the technique and with extensive experience in robotic surgery, 289 patients), and surgeon 2, FGS (224 patients). The primary endpoint is reproducibility of the surgical technique. Intraoperative and postoperative results were assessed as surgical time, bleeding, days of hospitalization, days of catheterization, and complications according to Clavien–Dindo classification. Oncological outcomes include surgical margins, biochemical recurrence (BR) and functional parameters in terms of urinary continence and potency rates. Significant positive surgical margins (significant PSM) were defined as >2 mm [16,17].

Patients with clinically localized or locally advanced prostate cancer undergoing RARP with more than one year of follow-up were included, staging was based on bone scan and preoperative CT, if necessary, based on the current European Association of Urology guidelines at the time of surgery. Multiparametric prostate resonance imaging (mpMRI) was requested for all patients unless contraindicated (pacemaker, phobia, contrast allergy). Preoperatively, all patients were assessed using the Briganti's and Memorial Sloan–Kettering PCa nomograms to measure the risk of lymph node involvement.

Patients without follow-up, no definitive pathology data or missing records were excluded. Patients in whom it was not possible to perform the lateral approach technique due to tumour, prostate, patient characteristics, and surgeon's choice (Sugeon 1: n = 16 and surgeon 2: n = 23) were excluded from the final analysis. Patients who required adjuvant or salvage radiotherapy were excluded from urine continence analysis, and patients with erectile dysfunction present before surgery that limited intercourse without response to medication were also excluded from potency analysis.

A comparison of the results of surgeon 1 and surgeon 2 was performed using the Student's t-test for quantitative variables, chi-square for qualitative variables, the Kaplan–Meier and log-rank test for power analysis, continence and biochemical recurrence; SPSS software version 25.0 (IBM Corp., Armonk, NY, USA) was used for statistical analysis.

2.1. Surgical Technique

All patients were operated on under general anaesthesia in a modified Trendelemburg position at 30° tilt. Following this technique, the first trocar is placed by direct supraumbilical approach pulling the abdominal wall, unless there is a history of previous abdominal surgery and scars with suspected adhesion. In these cases, the left paramedial trocar must be placed first and the other trocars are placed under direct vision. Once all the trocars are placed, the robot could be mounted. We used the Da Vinci Xi robotic system (Intuitive Surgical Inc, Sunnyvale, CA, USA) in all procedures, while the AirSeal® Intelligent Flow System (CONMED Corporation, Largo, FL, USA) was used for the pneumoperitoneum.

In the classic right lateral approach (Figure 1), the Retzius space is partially preserved by the section of the right umbilical ligament and the peritoneum, keeping the left portion of the bladder in place. Exposition of the right pubovesical ligament and endopelvic fascia was performed with dissection close to the bladder and the prostate wall, keeping the fat tissue in place.

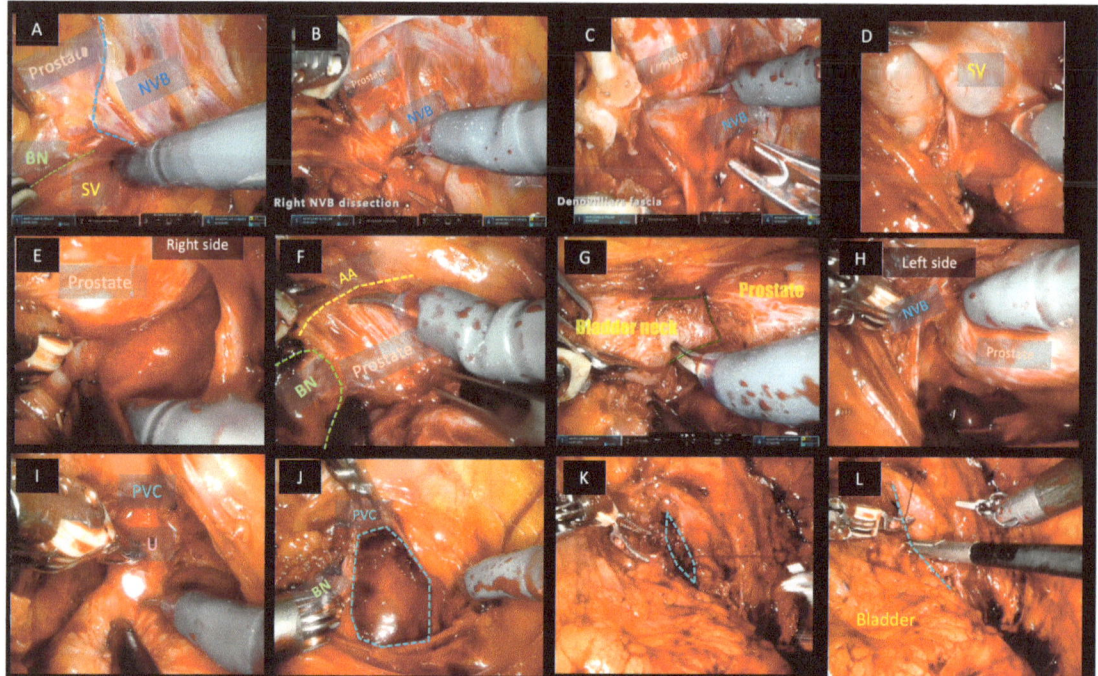

Figure 1. Robotic radical prostatectomy by the lateral approach technique. (**A**) direct access to the seminal vesicle in the triangle formed medially by the bladder neck, anteriorly by the prostate, laterally by the pedicle and nerovascular bundle. (**B**) dissection of neurovascular bundle. (**C**) dissection of right lateral face. (**D**) dissection of seminal vesicles. (**E**) dissection of posterior face from right to left. (**F**) dissection of the plane between the Detrusor's Apron and the anterior aspect of the prostate. (**G**) dissection and preservation of the bladder neck. (**H**) dissection of the left surface of the prostate and left NVB. (**I**) dissection of the apex preserving the anterior pubovesical complex. (**J–L**) closing the buttonhole (BN: bladder neck SV = seminal vesicle NVB = neurovascular bundle AA = anterior apron PVC = anterior pubovesical complex U = urethra).

One of the fundamental characteristics of this technique is the direct access to the seminal vesicle, performing the dissection through the triangular space covered by fat and through which the veins of the vesico-prostatic venous plexus run, in a triangular space delimited on its internal side by the bladder, anteriorly by the base of the prostate and laterally by the neurovascular bundle. The venous vessels found in this space are clipped with 3 mm mini-clips. The neurovascular bundle must be dissected carefully and bluntly, avoiding the use of thermal energy. Then, the dissection of the vesicles and ligation of the vas deferens and posterior plane of the prostate could be performed, reaching the bladder neck and allowing perfect preservation of the bladder neck. The anterior apron, composed of fibrous tissue and muscle fibres of the detrusor muscle that runs along the anterior aspect of the prostate, has to be dissected until it reaches the bladder neck cranially and the apex distally, saving and completely preserving the anterior pubovesical complex and the Santorini plexus. In the next step, the entire posterior plane has to be dissected from right to left in the right approach, until the left bandelette is reached and separated. Then, it is only necessary to clip perforating prostatic nourishing vessels at the base and medial–lateral zone.

The next step is mobilizing the prostate and leaving the pubovesical complex anteriorly. Now, the apex is dissected, with skill and patience, the urethra is sectioned, preserving the sphincter and saving the verumontanum. Urethrovesical end-to-end anastomosis was performed using of V-lock® suture, the first stitch starts at 5 o'clock and continues through the posterior late in a running fashion finishing at 3 o'clock.

After confirmation of hemostasis and bagging of the specimen, the pneumoperitoneum is deflated and the specimen is removed by supraumbilical incision, usually a 20 Ch Foley catheter will be left without leaving drainage in most cases.

2.2. Postoperative Management and Follow-Up

The urinary catheter was removed between 7 and 10 days after surgery and the complications were classified according to the Clavien–Dindo classification.

Surgical margins, biochemical recurrence (BCR), continence and potency were then evaluated. BCR was understood as two consecutive values of PSA >0.2 ng/mL; urinary continence was assessed on the day of catheter removal (immediate), at 3 (early) and 12 months after surgery. Patients are considered fully continent when they used no pads. Patients have been considered potent after surgery if they could achieve sexual intercourse. Patients taking PDE5 inhibitors to achieve intercourse were considered potent with drugs. Patients for whom intercourse depended on a vacuum erection device, penile injection of alprostadil, or a penile prosthesis were not considered as potent. The rate of erectile function recovery was defined considering only patients who were potent before RARP.

3. Results

Table 1 summarizes the baseline characteristics of the 513 patients (Surgeon 1, $n = 289$, Surgeon 2, $n = 224$). Mean age (years) was 62.12 ± 7.49 (IQR = 56–68) and 63.23 ± 6.51 (IQR = 58–64), PSA (ng/mL) = 7.98 ± 5.89 (5.01–8.21) and 7.41 ± 3.47 (5.00–8.21), prostatic volume (mL) 42.30 ± 21.66 (28–50.5) and 47.27 ± 27.7 (28–50), furthermore 199 (69%) and 159 (71%) were clinically significant prostate cancer (csPCa) (GG 2 or higher) for surgeon 1 and surgeon 2, respectively.

Regarding operative and postoperative results: surgical time (min) was 126.28 ± 36.652 and 180.56 ± 57.427 ($p < 0.001$); the lateral approach was possible in 273 (94.5%) and 201 (90.5%) ($p = 0.6$) patients; intraoperative bleeding (mL) 266.08 ± 125.16 and 372.45 ± 135 mL ($p < 0.001$); lymphadenectomy was performed in 117 (42.2%) and 73 (43.2%); the extracapsular extension was found in 62 (21.4%) and 61 (27.3%); positive lymph nodes 13 (4.5%) and 11 (4.9%). The rate of PSM was 95 (32.9%) and 85 (37.9%) for surgeon 1 and surgeon 2, respectively, and significant PSM (>2 mm) was 17 (5.9%) and 17 (7.6%) ($p = 0.6$). BCR rate was 34 (11.7%) and 27 (12%) for surgeon 1 and surgeon 2, respectively, the average follow-up period was 1728 ± 89.31 days, while the Clavien–Dindo complication rate >2, was 11 (3.8%) and 5 (2.2%).

Regarding continence and potency rates, 86% and 85% of patients were fully continent at day 0 of bladder catheter removal (totally dry), 93 and 91% at 1 month and 96 and 98% at 1 year for surgeons 1 and 2, respectively (Figure 2A). Sexual potency rates were 60% and 66% at 3 months, 73% and 72% at 1 year for surgeons 1 and 2, respectively. Kaplan–Meier curves and log-rank test are shown in Figure 2, no difference between the surgeons was found for urinary incontinence $p = 0.080$, erectile dysfunction $p = 0.2$ and biochemical recurrence (BR) $p = 0.7$ (Figure 2C–E). Stage pT3a and pT3b data are shown in Supplementary Table S1.

Table 1. Pre- and postoperative results n = 513 patients submitted to robot-assisted radical prostatectomy by lateral approach.

	Surgeon 1 (n = 289)	Surgeon 2 (n = 224)	p
Baseline characteristics:			
Age, mean ± SD, IQR	62.12 ± 7.498 (56–68)	63.23 ± 6.512 (58–64)	0.84
PSA ng/mL, ± SD, IQR	7.98 ± 5.89 (5.01–8.21)	7.41 ± 3.47 (5.00–8.21)	0.283
Prostate volume gr, ± SD, IQR	42.30 ± 21.66 (28–50.5)	47.27 ± 27.7 (28–50)	0.077
ED, n%	11.10%	25.00%	0.001
csPCa (ISUP ≥ 2), n%	199 (69%)	159 (71%)	0.121
TRUS /Fusion Bx/Mapeo (MRI + MicroUS)	117/80/90	38/82/103	<0.001
Postoperative Outcomes:			
Surgical Time min ± SD, IQR	126.28 ± 36.652	180.56 ± 57.427	<0.001
Lateral approach, n%	273 (94.5%)	201 (90.5%)	0.650
Lymphadenectomy; Yes, n%	117 (42.23%)	73 (43.19%)	0.84
NVB preservation; No/Unilateral/Bilateral, n%	25 (8.66%)/76 (26.35%)/188 (64.98%)	32 (14.2%)/29 (13.01%)/163 (72.78%)	<0.001
Intraoperative Bleeding ml ± SD, IQR	266.08 ± 125.16	372.45 ± 135 mL	<0.001
Conversion to open/laparoscopy, Yes/No, n%	0	1	-
Hospital stay days, mean ± SD(IQR)	2.84 ± 0.744 (2–3)	3.34 ± 1.022 (3–4)	0.90
Blood Transfusion, Yes/No, n%	9 (3.11%)	5 (2.23%)	0.170
csPCa (ISUP ≥ 2), n%	271 (93.1%)	207 (92.4%)	0.681
Extracapsular extension, n%	62 (21.4%)	61 (27.23%)	0.273
Positive lymp nodes, n%	13 (4.49%)	12 (4.9%)	0.533
PSM focal/significant, n%.	95 (32.87%)/17 (5.88%)	85 (37.9%)/17 (7.58%)	0.262
BR: Persistence/BR	9 (3.11%)/34 (11.7%)	8 (3.57%)/27 (12.05%)	0.815
Complications (Clavien III/IV), n%.	11 (3.8%)	5 (2.23%)	0.763

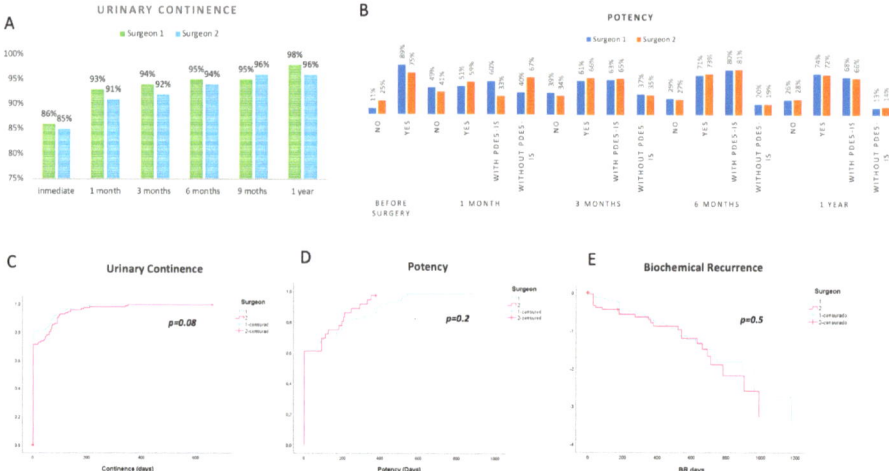

Figure 2. (**A**) Urine continence rates, (**B**) potency. Kaplan–Meier curves and log rank of (**C**) incontinence. (**D**) potency. (**E**) biochemical recurrence, comparing both surgeons.

4. Discussion

Robotic radical prostatectomy by the lateral approach technique can be reproduced with similar results in oncological and functional terms according to our data. When comparing both surgeons, the rate of positive surgical margins was 95 (32.9%) and 85 (37.9%) and significant PSM was 17 (5.9%) and 17 (7.6%) ($p = 0.2$) for surgeon 1 and surgeon 2, respectively; immediate continence was 86% and 85% and sexual potency at one year 73% and 72%, with a similar rate of complications for surgeon 1 and 2, respectively.

Clearly, preservation of the bladder neck and neurovascular bundles plays a direct role in the functional outcomes of continence and sexual potency [18]. However, modern prostatic anatomy studies have shown that most of the nerves involved in penile innervation run anterior to the prostate [19].

The technique of radical prostatectomy by lateral approach developed by Dr R. Gaston is characterized by some distinctive steps including the direct approach to the seminal vesicle (classically right), which allows the dissection of the homolateral neurovascular bundle, excellent preservation of the vesical neck of the contralateral neurovascular bundle and the complete preservation of the anterior pubovesical complex [1,4–6].

Other techniques with preservation of the pubovesical complex and Retzius space have also shown excellent results, indicating that preservation of the pubovesical complex seems to play a crucial role in maintaining sexual potency [14,15,20–24]. However, to our knowledge, this is the first series of patients with reproducible results of the lateral approach technique.

Asimakopoulos et al. previously reported in a small sample of 30 patients undergoing robotic radical prostatectomy with lateral approach technique 10% PSM, 80% of patients were dry at catheter removal, and after 3 months 73% presented an International Index of Erectile Function score > 17 [4].

De Carvalho et al. published a pubovesical complex preservation technique with a median skin-to-skin operative time of 78 min, BCR of 7% and overall PSM rate of 13.3% and 27% in patients with stage pT3. Immediate continence was 85.9% and 98.4% at one year, potency at one month was 53% and 86% at one year [21].

The Bocciardi Retzius-sparing technique claims PSMs of 10.1%, immediate continence was achieved in 92% of the patients, the 1-year continence rate was 96% and potency was 77% [20].

However, according to some authors, these results are extraordinary because, according to data from specialized tertiary care centres, around half of the patients reported altered erectile function before radical prostatectomy, 80% of the patients are totally continent after Foley catheter removal and only 53% recover full sexual function [25]. Furthermore, the same authors state that up to 50% of patients show extracapsular extension at the final pathology specimen, 20–35% seminal vesicle invasion, 35–60% of cT3 patients had PSM at the final pathology regardless of nerve-sparing status and >40% PSM in patients with seminal vesicle invasion [25].

The direct approach to the right seminal vesicle may seem strange to surgeons unfamiliar with the technique. Still, with the experience we have gained in reproducing the technique, we think that apart from the bladder neck, posterior border of the prostate and neurovascular bundle, the vesicoprostatic veins that run in this triangular space are crucial as an anatomical landmark to follow the path to the seminal vesicle behind these veins that often need to be clipped with mini-clips and avoiding the use of thermal energy.

Based on the principle that the anterior pubovesical complex is fundamental for the preservation of sexual potency, this lateral approach technique through a buttonhole represents a longitudinal incision which is less disruptive than a transverse incision on the fibres of the anterior apron and the pubovesical complex. However, as a result, a contraindication to performing the technique due to the risk of increased margins in this location, according to the recommendation of its creator, are anterior prostate tumours with extraprostatic extension [15].

Of course, the evolution in imaging techniques and biopsy systems has improved the characterization and localization of tumours before surgery [26,27]. Therefore, in our practice we request mpMRI for all patients unless contraindicated, and we also perform a prostate-mapping biopsy protocol based on mpMRI fusion biopsy and MUS [9].

With surgical expertise and the best possible knowledge of the location of the tumours, it is possible to perform a personalized surgery tailored to the patient. However, several studies indicate that mpMRI is not an accurate indicator of prostatic extracapsular extension, which influences the surgeon's decision to unnecessarily perform more aggressive surgeries that do not decrease PSM or result in better oncological results with the risk of worse functional outcomes [10,11,28–30]. Some nomograms and algorithms, for example, those recently based on MUS, seem to increase the accuracy of predicting the extracapsular location, but more extensive studies are needed on this matter [31].

Surgical technique and experience do matter and seem to have an impact on oncological results in terms of PSM, but surprisingly the impact of surgical experience in BCR is unclear [10,11]. The number of cases needed to reach a plateau in terms of margins is variable, it might be ~200 cases; however, in highly experienced centres with structured learning and mentoring from a very experienced surgeon, proficiency can be achieved early [10,11]. Thus, we think that, with surgical experience, a seasoned surgeon mastering a technique develops the ability to "run away from the tumour" by sorting out sites of extracapsular extension, reducing surgical margins.

As a single-centre retrospective study, our study has several limitations including inherent selection bias, data collection bias, no use of validated questionnaires to objectively measure functional outcomes, no long-term oncological outcomes. Although the results are similar between the two surgeons, we have not performed a stratified analysis of the patients, nor randomisation or propensity score matching techniques, which will be the subject of subsequent studies.

However, we compare the results of a surgeon who is the creator of the technique, with very extensive experience (more than 5000 cases of robotic surgery), which would be the best possible reference for the procedure, and another surgeon who reproduces the technique learned first-hand directly from surgeon 1.

5. Conclusions

Radical prostatectomy by the lateral approach technique with preservation of the anterior pubovesical complex is reproducible and offers good oncological and functional results.

Supplementary Materials: The following supporting information can be downloaded at: https://www.mdpi.com/article/10.3390/cancers15225442/s1, Table S1: pT3 stage in radical prostatectomy specimens n = 513 patients submitted to robot-assisted radical prostatectomy by lateral approach.

Author Contributions: Conceptualization, M.R.S., J.G.R. and F.G.S.; methodology, M.R.S., J.G.R., V.C.R. and F.G.S.; software, M.R.S. and F.E.; validation, M.R.S. and J.G.R.; formal analysis, M.R.S.; investigation, M.R.S., D.M.C.M., S.R.G. and V.C.R.; data curation, M.R.S., F.E., J.J.V. and D.C.; writing—original draft preparation, M.R.S., J.G.R.; writing—review and editing, M.R.S., J.R.E., L.L.G. and F.G.S.; visualization, J.F.D.A., V.C.R. and F.G.S.; supervision, V.C.R., F.G.S. and R.G. All authors have read and agreed to the published version of the manuscript.

Funding: This research received no external funding.

Institutional Review Board Statement: Ethical review and approval were waived for this study due to "Non-drug observational studies that do not involve interventions or the use of biological samples of human origin using only anonymised or anonymised clinical records or other personal data do not require IRB/IEC authorisation" (https://www.sergas.es/docs/ceic/preguntas%20frecuentes%20cas_20101112.htm (14 September 2023)).

Informed Consent Statement: Not applicable.

Data Availability Statement: The data presented in this study can be shared up on request.

Conflicts of Interest: The authors declare no conflict of interest.

References

1. Martini, A.; Falagario, U.G.; Villers, A.; Dell'oglio, P.; Mazzone, E.; Autorino, R.; Moschovas, M.C.; Buscarini, M.; Bravi, C.A.; Briganti, A.; et al. Contemporary Techniques of Prostate Dissection for Robot-assisted Prostatectomy. *Eur. Urol.* **2020**, *78*, 583–591. [CrossRef] [PubMed]
2. Schuetz, V.; Reimold, P.; Goertz, M.; Hofer, L.; Dieffenbacher, S.; Nyarangi-Dix, J.; Duensing, S.; Hohenfellner, M.; Hatiboglu, G. Evolution of Salvage Radical Prostatectomy from Open to Robotic and Further to Retzius Sparing Surgery. *J. Clin. Med.* **2021**, *11*, 202. [CrossRef] [PubMed]
3. Cochetti, G.; Del Zingaro, M.; Ciarletti, S.; Paladini, A.; Felici, G.; Stivalini, D.; Cellini, V.; Mearini, E. New Evolution of Robotic Radical Prostatectomy: A Single Center Experience with PERUSIA Technique. *Appl. Sci.* **2021**, *11*, 1513. [CrossRef]
4. Asimakopoulos, A.D.; Annino, F.; D'Orazio, A.; Pereira, C.F.T.; Mugnier, C.; Hoepffner, J.-L.; Piechaud, T.; Gaston, R. Complete Periprostatic Anatomy Preservation During Robot-Assisted Laparoscopic Radical Prostatectomy (RALP): The New Pubovesical Complex-Sparing Technique. *Eur. Urol.* **2010**, *58*, 407–417. [CrossRef]
5. Asimakopoulos, A.D.; Montes, V.E.C.; Gaston, R. Robot-Assisted Laparoscopic Radical Prostatectomy with Intrafascial Dissection of the Neurovascular Bundles and Preservation of the Pubovesical Complex: A Step-By-Step Description of the Technique. *J. Endourol.* **2012**, *26*, 1578–1585. [CrossRef]
6. Asimakopoulos, A.D.; Miano, R.; Galfano, A.; Bocciardi, A.M.; Vespasiani, G.; Spera, E.; Gaston, R. Retzius-sparing robot-assisted laparoscopic radical prostatectomy: Critical appraisal of the anatomic landmarks for a complete intrafascial approach: Retzius-Sparing Robot-Assisted Laparoscopic Radical Prostatectomy. *Clin. Anat.* **2015**, *28*, 896–902. [CrossRef]
7. Asimakopoulos, A.D.; Annino, F.; Colalillo, G.; Gaston, R.; Piechaud, T.; Mauriello, A.; Anceschi, U.; Borri, F. "Urethral-Sparing" Robotic Radical Prostatectomy: Critical Appraisal of the Safety of the Technique Based on the Histologic Characteristics of the Prostatic Urethra. *Curr. Oncol.* **2023**, *30*, 1065–1076. [CrossRef]
8. Oderda, M.; Calleris, G.; D'agate, D.; Falcone, M.; Faletti, R.; Gatti, M.; Marra, G.; Marquis, A.; Gontero, P. Intraoperative 3D-US-mpMRI Elastic Fusion Imaging-Guided Robotic Radical Prostatectomy: A Pilot Study. *Curr. Oncol.* **2022**, *30*, 110–117. [CrossRef]
9. Socarrás, M.E.R.; Rivas, J.G.; Rivera, V.C.; Elbers, J.R.; González, L.L.; Mercado, I.M.; del Alamo, J.F.; del Dago, P.J.; Sancha, F.G. Prostate Mapping for Cancer Diagnosis: The Madrid Protocol. Transperineal Prostate Biopsies Using Multiparametric Magnetic Resonance Imaging Fusion and Micro-Ultrasound Guided Biopsies. *J. Urol.* **2020**, *204*, 726–733. [CrossRef]
10. Bravi, C.A.; Tin, A.; Vertosick, E.; Mazzone, E.; Martini, A.; Dell'Oglio, P.; Stabile, A.; Gandaglia, G.; Fossati, N.; Suardi, N.; et al. The Impact of Experience on the Risk of Surgical Margins and Biochemical Recurrence after Robot-Assisted Radical Prostatectomy: A Learning Curve Study. *J. Urol.* **2019**, *202*, 108–113. [CrossRef]
11. Gandi, C.; Totaro, A.; Bientinesi, R.; Marino, F.; Pierconti, F.; Martini, M.; Russo, A.; Racioppi, M.; Bassi, P.; Sacco, E. A multi-surgeon learning curve analysis of overall and site-specific positive surgical margins after RARP and implications for training. *J. Robot. Surg.* **2022**, *16*, 1451–1461. [CrossRef] [PubMed]
12. Esperto, F.; Cacciatore, L.; Tedesco, F.; Testa, A.; Callè, P.; Ragusa, A.; Deanesi, N.; Minore, A.; Prata, F.; Brassetti, A.; et al. Impact of Robotic Technologies on Prostate Cancer Patients' Choice for Radical Treatment. *J. Pers. Med.* **2023**, *13*, 794. [CrossRef] [PubMed]
13. Carbonell, E.; Matheu, R.; Muní, M.; Sureda, J.; García-Sorroche, M.; Ribal, M.J.; Alcaraz, A.; Vilaseca, A. The Effect of Adverse Surgical Margins on the Risk of Biochemical Recurrence after Robotic-Assisted Radical Prostatectomy. *Biomedicines* **2022**, *10*, 1911. [CrossRef] [PubMed]
14. Luan, Y.; Ding, X.-F.; Lu, S.-M.; Huang, T.-B.; Chen, J.; Xiao, Q.; Wang, L.-P.; Chen, H.-P.; Han, Y.-X. The Efficacy of Urinary Continence in Patients Undergoing Robot-Assisted Radical Prostatectomy with Bladder-Prostatic Muscle Reconstruction and Bladder Neck Eversion Anastomosis. *Medicina* **2022**, *58*, 1821. [CrossRef]
15. Checcucci, E.; Veccia, A.; Fiori, C.; Amparore, D.; Manfredi, M.; Di Dio, M.; Morra, I.; Galfano, A.; Autorino, R.; Bocciardi, A.M.; et al. Retzius-sparing robot-assisted radical prostatectomy vs the standard approach: A systematic review and analysis of comparative outcomes. *BJU Int.* **2020**, *125*, 8–16. [CrossRef]
16. Shikanov, S.; Song, J.; Royce, C.; Al-Ahmadie, H.; Zorn, K.; Steinberg, G.; Zagaja, G.; Shalhav, A.; Eggener, S. Length of Positive Surgical Margin After Radical Prostatectomy as a Predictor of Biochemical Recurrence. *J. Urol.* **2009**, *182*, 139–144. [CrossRef]
17. John, A.; Lim, A.; Catterwell, R.; Selth, L.; O'callaghan, M. Length of positive surgical margins after radical prostatectomy: Does size matter?—A systematic review and meta-analysis. *Prostate Cancer Prostatic Dis.* **2023**, 1–8. [CrossRef]
18. Gacci, M.; De Nunzio, C.; Sakalis, V.; Rieken, M.; Cornu, J.-N.; Gravas, S. Latest Evidence on Post-Prostatectomy Urinary Incontinence. *J. Clin. Med.* **2023**, *12*, 1190. [CrossRef]
19. Eichelberg, C.; Erbersdobler, A.; Michl, U.; Schlomm, T.; Salomon, G.; Graefen, M.; Huland, H. Nerve Distribution along the Prostatic Capsule. *Eur. Urol.* **2007**, *51*, 105–111. [CrossRef]
20. Galfano, A.; Di Trapani, D.; Sozzi, F.; Strada, E.; Petralia, G.; Bramerio, M.; Ascione, A.; Gambacorta, M.; Bocciardi, A.M. Beyond the Learning Curve of the Retzius-sparing Approach for Robot-assisted Laparoscopic Radical Prostatectomy: Oncologic and Functional Results of the First 200 Patients with ≥1 Year of Follow-up. *Eur. Urol.* **2013**, *64*, 974–980. [CrossRef]
21. de Carvalho, P.A.; Barbosa, J.A.; Guglielmetti, G.B.; Cordeiro, M.D.; Rocco, B.; Nahas, W.C.; Patel, V.; Coelho, R.F. Retrograde Release of the Neurovascular Bundle with Preservation of Dorsal Venous Complex During Robot-assisted Radical Prostatectomy: Optimizing Functional Outcomes. *Eur. Urol.* **2020**, *77*, 628–635. [CrossRef] [PubMed]

22. Lambert, E.; Allaeys, C.; Berquin, C.; De Visschere, P.; Verbeke, S.; Vanneste, B.; Fonteyne, V.; Van Praet, C.; Lumen, N. Is It Safe to Switch from a Standard Anterior to Retzius-Sparing Approach in Robot-Assisted Radical Prostatectomy? *Curr. Oncol.* **2023**, *30*, 3447–3460. [CrossRef]
23. Flammia, R.S.; Bologna, E.; Anceschi, U.; Tufano, A.; Licari, L.C.; Antonelli, L.; Proietti, F.; Alviani, F.; Gallucci, M.; Simone, G.; et al. "Single Knot–Single Running Suture" Vesicourethral Anastomosis with Posterior Musculofascial Reconstruction during Robot-Assisted Radical Prostatectomy: A Step-by-Step Guide of Surgical Technique. *J. Pers. Med.* **2023**, *13*, 1072. [CrossRef]
24. Olivero, A.; Tappero, S.; Maltzman, O.; Vecchio, E.; Granelli, G.; Secco, S.; Caviglia, A.; Bocciardi, A.M.M.; Galfano, A.; Dell'oglio, P. Urinary Continence Recovery after Retzius-Sparing Robot Assisted Radical Prostatectomy and Adjuvant Radiation Therapy. *Cancers* **2023**, *15*, 4390. [CrossRef]
25. Montorsi, F.; Gandaglia, G.; Würnschimmel, C.; Graefen, M.; Briganti, A.; Huland, H. Re: Paolo Afonso de Carvalho, João ABA Barbosa, Giuliano B. Guglielmetti, et al. Retrograde Release of the Neurovascular Bundle with Preservation of Dorsal Venous Complex During Robot-assisted Radical Prostatectomy: Optimizing Functional Outcomes. Eur Urol 2020;77:628-35: Incredible Results for Robot-assisted Nerve-sparing Radical Prostatectomy in Prostate Cancer Patients. *Eur. Urol.* **2021**, *79*, e44–e46. [CrossRef]
26. Yang, C.-H.; Chen, L.-H.; Lin, Y.-S.; Hsu, C.-Y.; Tung, M.-C.; Huang, S.-W.; Wu, C.-H.; Ou, Y.-C. Incorporating VR-RENDER Fusion Software in Robot-Assisted Partial Prostatectomy: The First Case Report. *Curr. Oncol.* **2023**, *30*, 1699–1707. [CrossRef] [PubMed]
27. Rodler, S.; Kidess, M.A.; Westhofen, T.; Kowalewski, K.-F.; Belenchon, I.R.; Taratkin, M.; Puliatti, S.; Rivas, J.G.; Veccia, A.; Piazza, P.; et al. A Systematic Review of New Imaging Technologies for Robotic Prostatectomy: From Molecular Imaging to Augmented Reality. *J. Clin. Med.* **2023**, *12*, 5425. [CrossRef]
28. Rud, E.; Baco, E.; Klotz, D.; Rennesund, K.; Svindland, A.; Berge, V.; Lundeby, E.; Wessel, N.; Hoff, J.-R.; Berg, R.E.; et al. Does Preoperative Magnetic Resonance Imaging Reduce the Rate of Positive Surgical Margins at Radical Prostatectomy in a Randomised Clinical Trial? *Eur. Urol.* **2015**, *68*, 487–496. [CrossRef]
29. Kozikowski, M.; Malewski, W.; Michalak, W.; Dobruch, J. Clinical utility of MRI in the decision-making process before radical prostatectomy: Systematic review and meta-analysis. *PLoS ONE* **2019**, *14*, e0210194. [CrossRef]
30. Kim, S.H.; Cho, S.H.; Kim, W.H.; Kim, H.J.; Park, J.M.; Kim, G.C.; Ryeom, H.K.; Yoon, Y.S.; Cha, J.G. Predictors of Extraprostatic Extension in Patients with Prostate Cancer. *J. Clin. Med.* **2023**, *12*, 5321. [CrossRef]
31. Pedraza, A.M.; Parekh, S.; Joshi, H.; Grauer, R.; Wagaskar, V.; Zuluaga, L.; Gupta, R.; Barthe, F.; Nasri, J.; Pandav, K.; et al. Side-specific, Microultrasound-based Nomogram for the Prediction of Extracapsular Extension in Prostate Cancer. *Eur. Urol. Open Sci.* **2023**, *48*, 72–81. [CrossRef] [PubMed]

Disclaimer/Publisher's Note: The statements, opinions and data contained in all publications are solely those of the individual author(s) and contributor(s) and not of MDPI and/or the editor(s). MDPI and/or the editor(s) disclaim responsibility for any injury to people or property resulting from any ideas, methods, instructions or products referred to in the content.

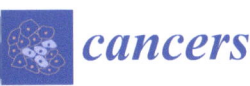 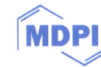

Article

Imaging GRPr Expression in Metastatic Castration-Resistant Prostate Cancer with [^{68}Ga]Ga-RM2—A Head-to-Head Pilot Comparison with [^{68}Ga]Ga-PSMA-11

René Fernández [1,*], Cristian Soza-Ried [1,2], Andrei Iagaru [3], Andrew Stephens [4], Andre Müller [4], Hanno Schieferstein [5,6], Camilo Sandoval [7], Horacio Amaral [1,2] and Vasko Kramer [1,2]

1 Nuclear Medicine and PET/CT Center PositronMed, Providencia, Santiago 7501068, Chile; csoza@positronmed.cl (C.S.-R.); hamaral@positronmed.cl (H.A.); vkramer@positronpharma.cl (V.K.)
2 Positronpharma SA, Providencia, Santiago 7501068, Chile
3 Department of Radiology, Division of Nuclear Medicine and Molecular Imaging, Stanford University, Stanford, CA 94305, USA; aiagaru@stanford.edu
4 Life Molecular Imaging GmbH, 13353 Berlin, Germany; a.stephens@life-mi.com (A.S.); a.mueller@life-mi.com (A.M.)
5 Formerly Piramal Imaging GmbH, 13353 Berlin, Germany; hanno.schieferstein@gmx.de
6 Merck Healthcare KGaA, 64293 Darmstadt, Germany
7 Fundación Arturo López Pérez, Providencia, Santiago 750069, Chile; camilo.sandoval@falp.org
* Correspondence: rfernandez@positronmed.cl

Citation: Fernández, R.; Soza-Ried, C.; Iagaru, A.; Stephens, A.; Müller, A.; Schieferstein, H.; Sandoval, C.; Amaral, H.; Kramer, V. Imaging GRPr Expression in Metastatic Castration-Resistant Prostate Cancer with [^{68}Ga]Ga-RM2—A Head-to-Head Pilot Comparison with [^{68}Ga]Ga-PSMA-11. *Cancers* **2024**, *16*, 173. https://doi.org/10.3390/cancers16010173

Academic Editors: Paula A. Oliveira, Ana Faustino and Lúcio Lara Santos

Received: 8 November 2023
Revised: 18 December 2023
Accepted: 24 December 2023
Published: 29 December 2023

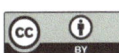

Copyright: © 2023 by the authors. Licensee MDPI, Basel, Switzerland. This article is an open access article distributed under the terms and conditions of the Creative Commons Attribution (CC BY) license (https://creativecommons.org/licenses/by/4.0/).

Simple Summary: Prostate cancer is the most prevalent cancer among men. Patients diagnosed with metastatic, castration-resistant prostate cancer (mCRPC) face a highly aggressive disease and reduced overall survival. For these patients, [^{177}Lu]Lu-PSMA-617 has shown promising results. However, this therapy may not benefit patients with low or heterogeneous PSMA expression. The gastrin-releasing peptide receptor (GRPr) is highly expressed in prostate cancer and other cancer cells, and [^{177}Lu]Lu-labeled GRPr-ligands have demonstrated good tumor uptake and retention, with minimal uptake in healthy tissues. However, the level of GRPr expression in advanced mCRPC patients remains elusive. In this study, we compared [^{68}Ga]Ga-RM2 with [^{68}Ga]Ga-PSMA-11 in a Latin American mCRPC cohort to evaluate the clinical utility of [^{68}Ga]Ga-RM2 in this group of patients. Although GRPr is overexpressed in the early stages of prostate cancer, our results indicate that in more advanced stages, such as mCRPC, the expression is lower than PSMA.

Abstract: Background: The gastrin-releasing peptide receptor (GRPr) is highly overexpressed in several solid tumors, including treatment-naïve and recurrent prostate cancer. [^{68}Ga]Ga-RM2 is a well-established radiotracer for PET imaging of GRPr, and [^{177}Lu]Lu-RM2 has been proposed as a therapeutic alternative for patients with heterogeneous and/or low expression of PSMA. In this study, we aimed to evaluate the expression of GRPr and PSMA in a group of patients diagnosed with castration-resistant prostate cancer (mCRPC) by means of PET imaging. Methods: Seventeen mCRPC patients referred for radio-ligand therapy (RLT) were enrolled and underwent [^{68}Ga]Ga-PSMA-11 and [^{68}Ga]Ga-RM2 PET/CT imaging, 8.8 ± 8.6 days apart, to compare the biodistribution of each tracer. Uptake in healthy organs and tumor lesions was assessed by SUV values, and tumor-to-background ratios were analyzed. Results: [^{68}Ga]Ga-PSMA-11 showed significantly higher uptake in tumor lesions in bone, lymph nodes, prostate, and soft tissues and detected 23% more lesions compared to [^{68}Ga]Ga-RM2. In 4/17 patients (23.5%), the biodistribution of both tracers was comparable. Conclusions: Our results show that in our cohort of mCRPC patients, PSMA expression was higher compared to GRPr. Nevertheless, RLT with [^{177}Lu]Lu-RM2 may be an alternative treatment option for selected patients or patients in earlier disease stages, such as biochemical recurrence.

Keywords: mCRPC; GRPr; PSMA; [^{68}Ga]Ga-RM2; [^{68}Ga]Ga-PSMA-11; PET imaging

1. Introduction

Prostate cancer (PCa) is the most common cancer in men, with an incidence of approximately 30.7 per 100,000 inhabitants (age standardized) [1]. While the five-year survival rate of localized, low-volume prostate cancer is close to 100%, metastatic, castration-resistant prostate cancer (mCRPC) is a highly aggressive disease with a significantly reduced median overall survival, accounting for 3.8% of all cancer deaths in men [1–3]. Although taxane-based chemotherapy and other available treatments can mitigate the effects of the disease, mCRPC can eventually progress, leaving the patients without further treatment options.

Recently, radioligand therapy (RLT) with [^{177}Lu]Lu-PSMA-617, targeting the prostate-specific membrane antigen (PSMA), has emerged as a promising treatment for advanced PCa patients. RLT with [^{177}Lu]Lu-PSMA-617 has demonstrated a remarkable capacity to improve quality of life and overall survival in most patients with mCRPC [4]. Nonetheless, the evidence indicates that approximately 30% of patients already show progression after the first or second treatment cycle [5,6], which might in part be related to a heterogeneous PSMA expression and low, insufficient absorbed doses in individual lesions.

The gastrin-releasing peptide (GRP) can be found in the nervous system and peripheral tissues, such as the gastrointestinal tract. GRP binds to its receptor (gastrin-releasing peptide receptor (GRPr)), a G-coupled protein from the bombesin family. GRPr is overexpressed in different cancers, such as breast cancer, small-cell lung cancer, and gastrointestinal stromal tumors. However, GRPr is also highly expressed in tumoral vessels of urinary tract cancers, particularly treatment-naïve and recurrent prostate cancer [7–9], and during early and advanced stages of PCa [10,11]. Therefore, positron emission tomography (PET) imaging with the synthetic GRPr antagonist [^{68}Ga]Ga-RM2 has emerged as a useful tool for biopsy guidance in patients with suspected PCa [12] and for staging and localization of disease in patients with primary PCa and patients with biochemical recurrence (BCR) and negative findings on conventional imaging and evaluation of treatment response [8,13–16]. Thus both, PSMA and GRPr are relevant diagnostic biomarkers for PET imaging in PCa at different stages of the disease [9,14,17–20]. Nevertheless, the biological mechanisms underlying PCa progression are complex and PET imaging of PSMA and GRPr might provide different insights into the heterogeneity of the disease. For instance, several studies support the notion that not all prostate cancer lesions present high levels of PSMA expression [20–23]. Interestingly, some metastases are exclusively detected by GRPr-targeted compounds and others are positive only for PSMA-targeted radiotracers, suggesting a complementary role between PSMA- and GRPR-targeted compounds [19,24,25]. However, determining the expression behavior of GRPr in the advanced stages of PCa remains a challenge. On the other hand, both tracers have renal elimination; however, PSMA presents increased physiological uptake in the liver parenchyma, a feature not observed with RM2. The low hepatobiliary uptake of ^{68}Ga-RM2 enables the detection of liver metastasis.

Due to the high GRPr expression in PCa, [^{177}Lu]Lu-labeled GRPr-ligands have been proposed as a therapeutic alternative for patients with low PSMA expression. This was exemplified in a proof-of-concept study evaluating the biodistribution and dosimetry of [^{177}Lu]Lu-RM2 in mCRPC patients showing good tumor uptake, retention, and rapid clearance from healthy tissues [26]. The low hepatobiliary, salivary, and lacrimal gland uptake might represent an advantage of [^{177}Lu]Lu-labeled GRPr ligands currently under development considering the high frequency of xerostomia as an adverse effect in patients under RLT with [^{177}Lu]Lu-PSMA-617 [27,28]. Furthermore, given the high expression of GRPr in several cancer types, it is a relevant pan-tumor target for RLT [29–31]. However, a drawback for RLT may emerge due to the high uptake in the pancreas, leading to undesired side effects attributed to the high radiation dose. Thus, the pancreas is considered a dose-limiting organ for GRPr-mediated treatment. Nonetheless, preliminary data indicate that the uptake is not persistent and cleared within 24 h [26–28], and the pancreas is considered radioresistant [32]. However, the extent of GRPr expression in the advanced stages of PCa remains unclear [33,34], and ongoing investigations are evaluating what criteria are appropriate to select patients for GRPr-targeting RLT [35]. In this study, we compared

[^{68}Ga]Ga-RM2 and [^{68}Ga]Ga-PSMA-11 in a cohort of Latin American patients diagnosed with mCRCP to further understand the potential clinical utility of GRPr-targeting RLT in these patients.

2. Materials and Methods

2.1. Patient Population

This prospective study was approved by the regional ethics committee board (Servicio de Salud Metropolitano Oriente, ethics committee, permit 26042016) and was conducted following the Declaration of Helsinki, Good Clinical Practices, and Chilean regulations. Seventeen subjects (median 66, IQR 8 years of age) with biopsy-proven mCRPC, rising PSA > 2 ng/mL, Gleason score of 8 to 10, testosterone < 20 ng/mL, a performance status score ECOG of 0–3, without further conventional treatment options, and who have been referred for RLT with either [^{177}Lu]Lu-PSMA-617 or [^{177}Lu]Lu-RM2, were enrolled in the study and gave written informed consent. Previous treatments included surgery (33%), androgen receptor signaling inhibitors (ARSI) (78%), radiotherapy (RT) (67%), and a combination of systemic therapies (ARSI, RT, and chemotherapy) (33%) (Table 1). Patients had PSA levels of 292 ± 465 ng/mL (range 0.05–1365 ng/mL) measured within 4 ± 3 days (range: 1–7 days) prior to PET imaging. Further blood biomarkers were evaluated as inclusion criteria (alkaline phosphatases > 2.5 upper normal limits in the absence of bone metastases; glutamic-oxaloacetic transaminase (GOT) and glutamic pyruvic transaminase (GPT) < 2.5 upper normal limits and up to 5 times if liver metastases are present; and creatinine clearance $\geq$ 40 mL/min/1.73 m^2) for all patients included in the study and prior to the intervention. Exclusion criteria included the inability to sign the informed consent, not complying with the inclusion criteria, severe claustrophobia, or being diagnosed with a malignancy other than adenocarcinoma of the prostate.

Table 1. Patient characteristics, previous treatments, and PET findings in the prostate (P), lymph nodes (LN), bone (B), and soft tissue (ST).

Patient No.	Age (y)	Gleason Score	PSA (ng/mL)	Previous Treatments	[^{68}Ga]Ga-PSMA-11 *	[^{68}Ga]Ga-RM2	Delay (Days)
1	63	NA	NA	QT + RT + ARSI	B + P	B + P	1
2	65	NA	1206	RT + ARSI	B + LN + P + ST	B + LN + P	2
3	71	NA	7.94	S + QT + RT + ARSI	LN	LN	14
4	53	7	NA	ARSI	LN + B + P	LN + B + P	1
5	76	NA	88.4	S + RT + ARSI	B	B	18
6	54	7 (4 + 3)	470	ARSI	B + LN + P + ST	B + LN + P + ST	1
7	75	NA	NA	QT + RT + ARSI	B + P	B + P	7
8	73	NA	660	QT + RT + ARSI	B + LN + P	B + LN + P	2
9	53	8	1	RT **	P + LN	P	6
10	70	6	7.11	NA	P + LN	P + LN	14
11	68	NA	40.1	S + QT + RT + ARSI	B + LN + P	P	14
12	64	NA	1365	RT + ARSI	B + LN + P + ST	B + LN	3
13	55	8	0.05	S + RT + ARSI	B + LN + ST	B + LN + ST	18
14	71	NA	NA	NA	LN + P	P	6
15	66	NA	79.37	S + ARSI	B	B	4
16	64	4 + 3	3.6	S + RT + ARSI	B	B	33
17	71	NA	18	QT + RT + ARSI	B	NL	6

* All patients had metastatic disease at the moment of the study. ** The patient rejected ARSI therapy due to personal reasons. NA: not available.

2.2. Radiotracer Preparation

Production of [^{68}Ga]Ga-PSMA-11 and [^{68}Ga]Ga-RM2 was performed in accordance with local GMP regulations and using a similar procedure as published previously [14]. Briefly, radiolabeling of [^{68}Ga]Ga-PSMA-11 and [^{68}Ga]Ga-RM2 was performed using a cassette-based module (Gaia, Elysia-Raytest, Straubenhardt, Germany), PSMA-11, cassettes and reagent kits (Advanced biochemical compounds ABX, Dresden, Germany), RM2 (kindly provided from Life Molecular Imaging, Berlin, Germany), and a 2 GBq ^{68}Ge/^{68}Ga-generator (iThemba Labs, Somerset West 7129, Cape Town, South Africa).

The eluted gallium-68, was trapped on a strong cation exchange cartridge, rinsed with ultrapure water, and eluted with 450 µL eluent (5 M NaCl in 5.5 M HCl) into a mixture of 40 µL precursor (1 mg/mL in ultrapure water) in 3.85 mL buffer (0.08 M ammonium acetate, pH 4.5) and 200 µL ethanol. After radiolabeling at 95 °C for 8 min., the reaction mixture was diluted with 5 mL water. The crude product was extracted using a C18 cartridge and rinsed with water. The purified product was eluted with 1.5 mL 60 vol% ethanol followed by 8.5 mL saline and passed through a 0.22 µm sterile filter (Millex-GV, Merck Millipore, Darmstadt, Germany). Quality control was performed, including controls for visual inspection, pH, radiochemical purity by HPLC, radionuclidic identity, residual solvents, endotoxins, filter integrity (prior release), and sterility (post-release).

2.3. PET/CT Imaging and Analysis

All subjects had two PET/CT scans performed on separate days using a Biograph mCT Flow scanner (Siemens Healthineers, Erlangen, Germany) within 8.8 ± 8.6 days (range 1–33 days), without any medical intervention between the scans. The order of [^{68}Ga]Ga-PSMA-11 and [^{68}Ga]Ga-RM2 PET scans was random and according to the availability of the radiotracer. A contrast-enhanced CT scan and low-dose CT scan were performed for anatomical localization and attenuation correction prior to [^{68}Ga]Ga-PSMA-11 and [^{68}Ga]Ga-RM2 PET scans, respectively. PET/CT images were acquired head-to-mid-thigh at 60 ± 5 min post-injection of 191 ± 25 MBq (range 122–229 MBq) [^{68}Ga]Ga-PSMA-11 and 166 ± 39 MBq (range: 63–243 MBq) [^{68}Ga]Ga-RM2, respectively, starting at the pelvis.

Volumes of interest (VOIs) were drawn around tumor lesions, visually distinguished as regions of increased radiotracer uptake relative to adjacent background uptake and outside areas of expected physiological radiotracer uptake. To perform semi-quantitative analysis, mean and maximum standard uptake values (SUVmean and max, respectively) were calculated using Siemens SyngoVia software (SV60). Tumor-to-background ratios (TBRs) were calculated by dividing the SUVmax of different tumor lesions by the SUVmean of the blood pool in the left ventricle of the heart.

2.4. Statistical Analysis

The normal distribution of continuous variables was determined with Q-Q plots and histograms. In the case of non-parametric quantitative data, the Wilcoxon signed-rank test was used to compare SUVmax values and TBRs between scans. The test was two-sided, and a p-value < 0.05 was considered statistically significant. All statistical analyses were performed using R software version 4.2.0 (22 April 2022) [36]. The sample size for the study considered a minimum of 16 patients (17 were finally included). The sample size calculation was based on the difference between means and standard deviations of SUVmean ratios to the normal background (blood pool) for both tracers (9.2 ± 7.2 for [^{68}Ga]Ga-PSMA-11 and 5.2 ± 3.5 for [^{68}Ga]Ga-RM2), reported by Minamimoto et al. (2016). The calculation considered a confidence of 95% and a power of 80%, with a correlation of 60%. The analysis was performed using G*power [37].

3. Results

3.1. Patient Characteristics

Seventeen participants (65.3 ± 7.4 years of age; range: 53–76 years) were enrolled (Table 1) and both PET/CT scans were performed 8.8 ± 8.6 days (range: 1–33 days) apart.

3.2. Uptake Comparison between [^{68}Ga]Ga-PSMA-11 and [^{68}Ga]Ga-RM2

The administration of [^{68}Ga]Ga-PSMA-11, [^{68}Ga]Ga-RM2, and the imaging procedure were well tolerated and no adverse events, discomfort, or change in vital signs was observed. The excretion profile of both tracers was similar with a predominant renal clearance via the kidneys observed for [^{68}Ga]Ga-PSMA-11 and [^{68}Ga]Ga-RM2 (Figures 1 and 2). However, we observed differences in the physiological biodistribution between the two tracers in the submandibular, parotid, and lacrimal glands, liver, and small intestine, where unlike [^{68}Ga]Ga-PSMA-11, [^{68}Ga]Ga-RM2 showed no uptake. In contrast, [^{68}Ga]Ga-RM2 showed high uptake in the pancreas, whereas no uptake of [^{68}Ga]Ga-PSMA-11 was observed.

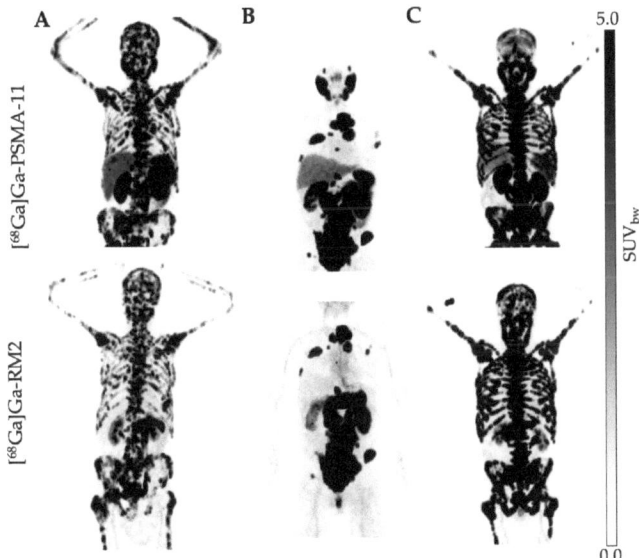

Figure 1. (**A–C**) Maximum-intensity projections (MIP) of [^{68}Ga]Ga-PSMA-11 (**upper row**) and [^{68}Ga]Ga-RM2 (**lower row**) PET images of patients with similar biodistribution and tumor uptake (n = 14).

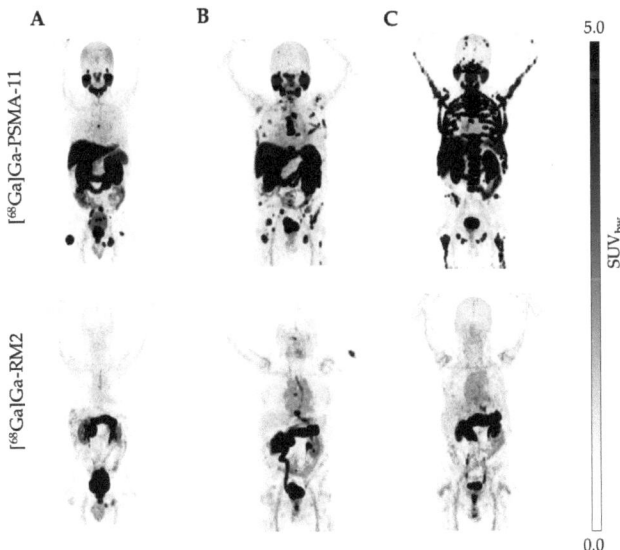

Figure 2. (**A–C**) Maximum-intensity projections (MIP) of [^{68}Ga]Ga-PSMA-11 (**upper row**) and [^{68}Ga]Ga-RM2 (**lower row**) PET images of patients with high PSMA but low GRPr expression (n = 13).

[^{68}Ga]Ga-RM2 presents an absence of physiological uptake in the liver, contrary to what was observed with [^{68}Ga]Ga-PSMA-11, which favors the detection of possible hepatic metastasis lesions. This was validated in one patient, who exhibited a hepatic lesion with [^{68}Ga]Ga-RM2 that was not visible on [^{68}Ga]Ga-PSMA-11 scan (Figure 3).

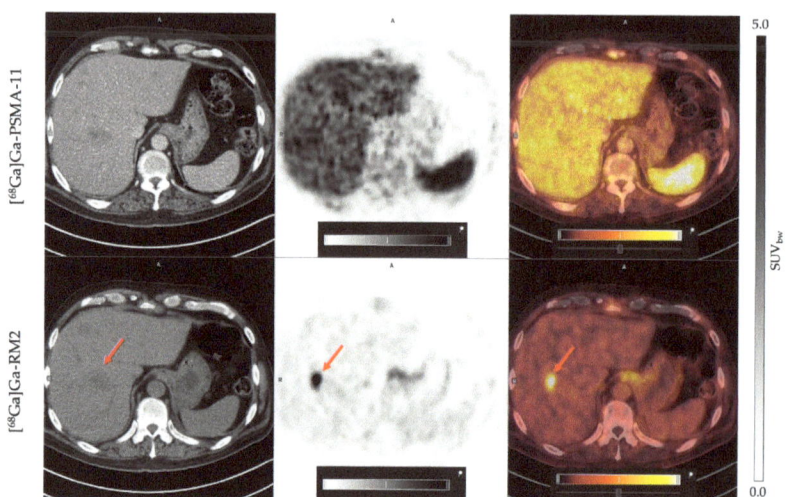

Figure 3. Patient 13: PET/CT [^{68}Ga]Ga-PSMA-11 (**upper row**) and [^{68}Ga]Ga-RM2 (**lower row**). Red arrows indicates a liver metastasis visible with [^{68}Ga]Ga-RM2 and not detected with [^{68}Ga]Ga-PSMA-11.

Specific uptake in tumor lesions in the prostate, lymph nodes, bone, and soft tissue was evident with both radioligands; however, the SUVmax values of [^{68}Ga]Ga-PSMA-11 were statistically higher compared to [^{68}Ga]Ga-RM2 in most lesions. Indeed, only 23.5% of the patients showed a high GRPr expression (Figures 1, 2 and 4).

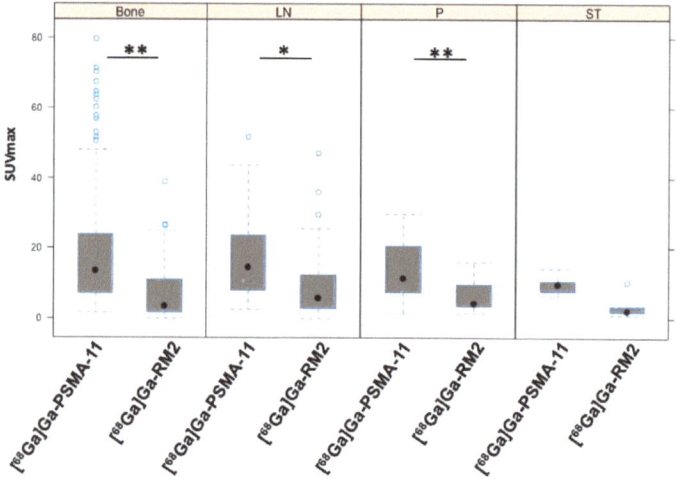

Figure 4. Average SUVmax values of [^{68}Ga]Ga-PSMA-11 and [^{68}Ga]Ga-RM2 in bone, lymph node (LN), prostate (P), and soft tissue (ST) lesions across all patients. * $p < 0.05$, ** $p < 0.01$. Light blue dots represent outlier values. Black dots represent median values.

As for the SUVmax values, the same trend was observed when evaluating TBRs for bone, lymph node, prostate, and soft tissue lesions, which were significantly higher for [^{68}Ga]Ga-PSMA-11 compared to [^{68}Ga]Ga-RM2 (Table 2).

Table 2. SUVmax values and TBRs for [^{68}Ga]Ga-PSMA-11 and [^{68}Ga]Ga-RM2 in bone, lymph node, prostate, and soft tissue lesions.

Region	Parameter	[^{68}Ga]Ga-PSMA-11	[^{68}Ga]Ga-RM2	p-Value
Bone	SUVmax	17.0 ± 5.2	11.0 ± 5.9	0.0029
	TBR	15.9 ± 10.9	4.3 ± 5.4	0.0023
LN	SUVmax	15.7 ± 10.7	3.5 ± 6.0	0.028
	TBR	16.0 ± 12.4	5.7 ± 5.2	0.038
Prostate	SUVmax	16.8 ± 12.2	4.8 ± 4.2	0.002
	TBR	16.5 ± 13.0	5.9 ± 4.6	0.002
Soft tissue	SUVmax	9.8 ± 3.2	1.7 ± 2.1	0.06
	TBR	13.7 ± 11.4	1.5 ± 1.7	0.11

TBR: tumor-to-background ratio. LN: lymph node.

Next, we analyzed whether both tracers were able to detect the same number of lesions considering the total number of lesions found in each patient. In line with our previous results, [^{68}Ga]Ga-PSMA-11 detected 23.2% more tumor lesions compared to [^{68}Ga]Ga-RM2.

4. Discussion

Prostate cancer, and in particular mCRPC, shows high levels of PSMA expression which also correlates with disease stage and severity [38,39]. However, due to the unstable genomic nature of cancerous cells, a tumor may present a great variability of PSMA expression levels resulting in different grades of malignancy and outcomes [40]. For instance, results from the Vision Trial indicate that 50–60% of patients with mCRPC respond with a PSA decline of >50% and an improvement in their overall survival of 15.3 months compared to 11.3 months in standard care. Likewise, imaging-based progression-free survival is also increased in those patients compared to standard care (median, 8.7 vs. 3.4 months) [4,5]. However, approximately 30–40% of mCRPC patients do not respond to [^{177}Lu]Lu-PSMA therapy [5,6], which might be due to a heterogeneous PSMA expression or a decrease in PSMA triggered by an aggressive trans-differentiation process, resulting in cancerous cells resistant to therapies. Typically, these patients display visceral metastasis, and adenocarcinoma features are reduced or lost [41,42]. This variance or decrease in PSMA expressions affects the patient selection process and subsequently results in low absorbed doses in individual tumor lesions, ultimately reducing the therapeutic efficacy of [^{177}Lu]Lu-PSMA therapy [40,43]. Variability in PSMA expression might depend on many different factors. For example, inflammation NF-κB has been involved in resistance to ADT, contributing to mCRPC progression [44]. Signaling pathways such as PI3K/AKT influence the tumor niche inducing different downstream events, including the expression of the H19 gene [45,46] and hypoxia [47]. The interaction between hypoxia and other pathways is, however, complex. The evidence suggests that hypoxia drives transdifferentiation toward an NE-like phenotype promoting tumor resistance [48].

Similar to PSMA, GRPr is a membrane-bound tumor biomarker, which is found to be overexpressed in 84% of prostate cancer cells [49]. While expression of both PSMA and GRPr is increased in prostate cancer cells, the underlying biological mechanisms responsible for this abnormal behavior are distinct. Previous work has shown that in androgen–dependent prostate cancer xenografts, GRPr is highly expressed, but this expression is drastically reduced after castration. These findings suggested that the expression of GRPr may be regulated by the action of androgen [50] and therefore associated with earlier phases of the disease. In contrast, PSMA expression is higher in later and poorly differentiated stages of the disease [51], suggesting inverse expression profiles of GRPr and PSMA. In a pilot study including six biochemically recurrent prostate cancer patients,

Minamimoto et al. (2016) compared [^{68}Ga]Ga-PSMA-11 with [^{68}Ga]Ga-RM2, revealing distinctive biodistribution patterns for both tracers. However, in tumoral tissue, the study concluded that there were no significant differences in uptake between the two tracers [14].

More recently, Minamimoto et al. (2018) demonstrated a detection rate of approximately 72% using [^{68}Ga]Ga-RM2 in a prospective study including 32 patients with biochemical recurrence of prostate cancer and negative findings on conventional imaging [15]. In addition, other reports have shown the expression of GRPr in metastatic lymph nodes, bones, and advanced tumor stages [11,52], suggesting the clinical potential of GRPr as a target for PET imaging and RLT and as an alternative to PSMA.

Consequently, the objective of this study was to compare the uptake and performance of [^{68}Ga]Ga-RM2 and [^{68}Ga]Ga-PSMA-11, with the aim of evaluating their potential as therapeutic targets for RLT in patients with advanced mCRPC.

We and others have shown that PSMA is highly expressed in prostate tumoral lesions and also in kidneys, spleen, lacrimal, parotid, and submandibular glands, small intestine, and bladder [14,40,53]. This is consistent with what we observed in the present study. The physiological expression of GRPr shows a different pattern compared to PSMA and is high in the pancreas, bladder [14], lymph node metastases, and bone lesions of prostate cancer [11]. Interestingly, the low uptake of [^{68}Ga]Ga-RM2 in hepatic tissue allowed the detection of a malignant lesion in the liver, while this lesion was not observed in the [^{68}Ga]Ga-PSMA-11 PET/CT scan (Figure 4). This observation is in line with results reported by Verhoeven et al. (2023) [54].

In our study, [^{68}Ga]Ga-PSMA-11 outperformed [^{68}Ga]Ga-RM2 in terms of lesion detection rate, uptake, and imaging contrast in tumor lesions in bone, lymph nodes, and prostate in patients with advanced mCRPC. The SUVmax values for [^{68}Ga]Ga-PSMA-11 were significantly higher than for [^{68}Ga]Ga-RM2 in most lesions (Table 2). We obtained the same results using tumor-to-background ratios, allowing for the standardization of the image analysis, providing reproducible, consistent and accurate data across different PET scanners and patients [55,56]. Although both tracers detected tumoral lesions in each patient, [^{68}Ga]Ga-PSMA-11 detected 23.2% more lesions than [^{68}Ga]Ga-RM2. Both tracers show a high affinity for their targets and it is unlikely that the lower detection rate and uptake values of are related to differences in affinity (Ki = 9.3 nM for [^{68}Ga]Ga-RM2 and Ki = 7.5 ± 2.2 nM for [^{68}Ga]Ga-RM2, respectively, [57,58]). Furthermore, several reports have shown that GRP derivatives present a high affinity to GRPr, demonstrating its potential in clinical applications [7,57,59].

Interestingly, in some patients with advanced disease, both tracers showed a similar biodistribution in tumor lesions (Figure 1). For those patients, alternating cycles between PSMA- and GRPr-targeted RLT may lead to the same treatment response but with less toxicity from each drug. The expression of PSMA in some healthy tissues, such as salivary and lacrimal glands, the kidney, and bone marrow, produces temporary side effects. Our studies, alongside others, have demonstrated that hematological side effects such as pancytopenia are transient and mainly limited to grade 2. Commonly, patients treated with PSMA-targeted RLT experience xerostomia, fatigue, and nausea [60]. In contrast, GRPr-targeted RLT does not affect salivary or lacrimal glands, and the first-in-human dosimetry study has reported that the treatment was well tolerated and showed no side effects. The most intensive uptake, however, is in the pancreas, which is considered a critical organ. Nonetheless, akin to other RLTs with Lutetium-177, the bone marrow is acknowledged as a critical organ, and no significant differences with PSMA-targeted therapies have been noted [26]. Nevertheless, for mCRPC the clinical benefit of using [^{177}Lu]Lu-RM2 is limited to patients who have high expression of GRPr and experienced xerostomia as a dose-limiting event after PSMA-targeted RLT.

Previous works have suggested that GRPr expression is higher in initial disease stages and that [^{68}Ga]Ga-RM2 may be particularly valuable for detecting well-differentiated, slow-growing prostate cancer lesions [14,34,49,51]. This is further supported by several head-to-head comparison studies with [^{68}Ga]Ga-RM2 and [^{68}Ga]Ga-PSMA-11 in preoperative intermediate and high-risk PCa and biochemical recurrent PCa where both tracers performed equally [8,24]. Furthermore, a recent clinical trial showed that [^{68}Ga]Ga-RM2 is a promising PET tracer to improve the characterization of patients and guide biopsy, particularly in intermediate-risk patients with intraprostatic prostate cancer [61].

While these results support the notion that GRPr expression is reduced in most cases of advanced mCRPC, individual patients with low PSMA but high GRPr expression may still find benefit in GRPr-targeted RLT. In fact, we have recently published a case report series with clinical results of 4 patients included in our study (4 out of 17, 23.5%) who showed high [^{68}Ga]Ga-RM2 uptake and were subsequently treated with a single dose of 5.6 GBq [^{177}Lu]Lu-RM2. The 3D SPECT/CT and planar images revealed high tumor uptake and stable binding for up to seven days. In this report, we showed that [^{177}Lu]Lu-RM2 uptake in pancreatic tissue was high but showed a rapid clearance after 24–48 h. Furthermore, there were no significant differences between baseline levels of red blood cells, leukocytes, platelets, creatinine, or amylase levels pre-therapy and after 1, 4, and 8 weeks of therapy. Two patients showed a partial response during the initial weeks, and no adverse effects were observed, demonstrating the feasibility of [^{177}Lu]Lu-RM2 RLT [62]. These results align with the study conducted by Kurth et al. (2019). In their study, 35 patients with mCRPC without further treatment alternatives were imaged using [^{68}Ga]Ga-RM2. Subsequently, four patients were selected to receive [^{177}Lu]Lu-RM2 treatment. The therapy was well tolerated by all patients, and no side effects were evident. Most of the [^{177}Lu]Lu-RM2 uptake was observed in the pancreas where GRPr expression is high. However, due to the rapid clearance of the radiotracer from this organ, the mean absorbed dose for the pancreas was low [26]. Thus, [^{177}Lu]Lu-RM2 therapy was considered to be safe and tolerable for mCRPC patients without any other treatment options.

A very recent clinical study (LuTectomy Trial) investigated the use of [^{177}Lu]Lu-PSMA-617 as neo-adjuvant therapy prior to radical prostatectomy in patients with localized, high-risk prostate cancer [63]. The study evaluated the dosimetry and safety of [^{177}Lu]Lu-PSMA-617 in this indication and the evaluation of long-term oncological benefits is ongoing and might result in a prolonged time until recurrence. Likewise, considering the high expression of GRPr in early stages of prostate cancer, this could also be a potential, clinical indication for [^{177}Lu]Lu-RM2.

5. Conclusions

In conclusion, our results confirm previous reports [11,14,34,49] that although PSMA and GRPr are both expressed in mCRPC, GRPr expression is reduced in advanced mCRPC patients and [^{68}Ga]Ga-PSMA-11 shows significantly higher uptake compared to [^{68}Ga]Ga-RM2. Nevertheless, the low physiological uptake of [^{68}Ga]Ga-RM2 in the liver allowed the detection of a hepatic lesion in one patient that was not observable with [^{68}Ga]Ga-PSMA-11. GRPr-targeted RLT remains a therapeutic alternative for those patients who have limited treatment options and exhibit high GRPr expression. This might include different oncologic indications such as PCa, mCRPC, and lung and breast cancer.

Author Contributions: Study design and conceptualization, V.K., R.F., A.S., C.S. and H.A.; radiochemistry, V.K., A.M. and H.S.; data collection, image acquisition and reconstruction, R.F.; formal analysis, R.F., C.S. and C.S.-R.; data interpretation and statistical analysis, C.S.-R.; original manuscript preparation, C.S.-R.; review and editing, all; supervision, R.F., A.I. and A.S. All authors have read and agreed to the published version of the manuscript.

Funding: This research received no external funding.

Institutional Review Board Statement: All procedures performed in studies involving human participants were in accordance with the ethical standards of the institutional and national research committee and with the principles of the 1964 Declaration of Helsinki and its later amendments or comparable ethical standards. The study was approved by the regional ethics committee board (CEC SSM Oriente, permit 26042016) and written informed consent has been obtained from all participants.

Informed Consent Statement: Informed consent was obtained from all subjects involved in the study.

Data Availability Statement: The data presented in this study are available on request from the corresponding author. The data are not publicly available due to restrictions regarding the privacy of the patients and ethical reasons.

Acknowledgments: We would like to thank all patients and their families for participating and supporting the study. Further, we would like to thank Johanna Wettlin for coordinating patient and imaging visits.

Conflicts of Interest: A.S. and A.M. are employees of Life Molecular Imaging GmbH and H.S. was employee of Piramal Imaging GmbH during the conduct of this study. The authors declare no further conflict of interest.

References

1. Ferlay, J.; Ervik, M.; Lam, F.; Colombet, M.; Mery, L.; Piñeros, M.; Znaor, A.; Soerjomataram, I.; Bray, F. *Global Cancer Observatory: Cancer Today*; International Agency for Research on Cancer: Lyon, France, 2020. Available online: https://gco.iarc.fr/today (accessed on 2 August 2022).
2. Mateo, J.; McKay, R.; Abida, W.; Aggarwal, R.; Alumkal, J.; Alva, A.; Feng, F.; Gao, X.; Graff, J.; Hussain, M.; et al. Accelerating precision medicine in metastatic prostate cancer. *Nat. Cancer* **2020**, *1*, 1041–1053. [CrossRef] [PubMed]
3. Beer, T.M.; Armstrong, A.J.; Rathkopf, D.; Loriot, Y.; Sternberg, C.N.; Higano, C.S.; Iversen, P.; Evans, C.P.; Kim, C.S.; Kimura, G.; et al. Enzalutamide in Men with Chemotherapy-naive Metastatic Castration-resistant Prostate Cancer: Extended Analysis of the Phase 3 PREVAIL Study. *Eur. Urol.* **2017**, *71*, 151–154. [CrossRef] [PubMed]
4. Sartor, O.; de Bono, J.; Chi, K.N.; Fizazi, K.; Herrmann, K.; Rahbar, K.; Tagawa, S.T.; Nordquist, L.T.; Vaishampayan, N.; El-Haddad, G.; et al. Lutetium-177-PSMA-617 for Metastatic Castration-Resistant Prostate Cancer. *N. Engl. J. Med.* **2021**, *385*, 1091–1103. [CrossRef] [PubMed]
5. Rahbar, K.; Schmidt, M.; Heinzel, A.; Eppard, E.; Bode, A.; Yordanova, A.; Claesener, M.; Ahmadzadehfar, H. Response and Tolerability of a Single Dose of 177Lu-PSMA-617 in Patients with Metastatic Castration-Resistant Prostate Cancer: A Multicenter Retrospective Analysis. *J. Nucl. Med.* **2016**, *57*, 1334–1338. [CrossRef] [PubMed]
6. Ahmadzadehfar, H.; Wegen, S.; Yordanova, A.; Fimmers, R.; Kurpig, S.; Eppard, E.; Wei, X.; Schlenkhoff, C.; Hauser, S.; Essler, M. Overall survival and response pattern of castration-resistant metastatic prostate cancer to multiple cycles of radioligand therapy using [(177)Lu]Lu-PSMA-617. *Eur. J. Nucl. Med. Mol. Imaging* **2017**, *44*, 1448–1454. [CrossRef] [PubMed]
7. Jensen, R.T.; Battey, J.F.; Spindel, E.R.; Benya, R.V. International Union of Pharmacology. LXVIII. Mammalian bombesin receptors: Nomenclature, distribution, pharmacology, signaling, and functions in normal and disease states. *Pharmacol. Rev.* **2008**, *60*, 1–42. [CrossRef]
8. Duan, H.; Baratto, L.; Fan, R.E.; Soerensen, S.J.C.; Liang, T.; Chung, B.I.; Thong, A.E.C.; Gill, H.; Kunder, C.; Stoyanova, T.; et al. Correlation of (68)Ga-RM2 PET with Postsurgery Histopathology Findings in Patients with Newly Diagnosed Intermediate- or High-Risk Prostate Cancer. *J. Nucl. Med.* **2022**, *63*, 1829–1835. [CrossRef]
9. Baratto, L.; Jadvar, H.; Iagaru, A. Prostate Cancer Theranostics Targeting Gastrin-Releasing Peptide Receptors. *Mol. Imaging Biol.* **2018**, *20*, 501–509. [CrossRef]
10. Maina, T.; Bergsma, H.; Kulkarni, H.R.; Mueller, D.; Charalambidis, D.; Krenning, E.P.; Nock, B.A.; de Jong, M.; Baum, R.P. Preclinical and first clinical experience with the gastrin-releasing peptide receptor-antagonist [(6)(8)Ga]SB3 and PET/CT. *Eur. J. Nucl. Med. Mol. Imaging* **2016**, *43*, 964–973. [CrossRef]
11. Ananias, H.J.; van den Heuvel, M.C.; Helfrich, W.; de Jong, I.J. Expression of the gastrin-releasing peptide receptor, the prostate stem cell antigen and the prostate-specific membrane antigen in lymph node and bone metastases of prostate cancer. *Prostate* **2009**, *69*, 1101–1108. [CrossRef]
12. Duan, H.; Ghanouni, P.; Daniel, B.; Rosenberg, J.; Thong, A.; Kunder, C.; Mari Aparici, C.; Davidzon, G.A.; Moradi, F.; Sonn, G.A.; et al. A Pilot Study of (68)Ga-PSMA11 and (68)Ga-RM2 PET/MRI for Biopsy Guidance in Patients with Suspected Prostate Cancer. *J. Nucl. Med.* **2022**, *64*, 744–750. [CrossRef] [PubMed]
13. Mapelli, P.; Ghezzo, S.; Samanes Gajate, A.M.; Preza, E.; Brembilla, G.; Cucchiara, V.; Ahmed, N.; Bezzi, C.; Presotto, L.; Bettinardi, V.; et al. Preliminary Results of an Ongoing Prospective Clinical Trial on the Use of (68)Ga-PSMA and (68)Ga-DOTA-RM2 PET/MRI in Staging of High-Risk Prostate Cancer Patients. *Diagnostics* **2021**, *11*, 2068. [CrossRef] [PubMed]
14. Minamimoto, R.; Hancock, S.; Schneider, B.; Chin, F.T.; Jamali, M.; Loening, A.; Vasanawala, S.; Gambhir, S.S.; Iagaru, A. Pilot Comparison of (6)(8)Ga-RM2 PET and (6)(8)Ga-PSMA-11 PET in Patients with Biochemically Recurrent Prostate Cancer. *J. Nucl. Med.* **2016**, *57*, 557–562. [CrossRef] [PubMed]
15. Minamimoto, R.; Sonni, I.; Hancock, S.; Vasanawala, S.; Loening, A.; Gambhir, S.S.; Iagaru, A. Prospective Evaluation of (68)Ga-RM2 PET/MRI in Patients with Biochemical Recurrence of Prostate Cancer and Negative Findings on Conventional Imaging. *J. Nucl. Med.* **2018**, *59*, 803–808. [CrossRef] [PubMed]
16. Duan, H.; Ghanouni, P.; Daniel, B.; Rosenberg, J.; Davidzon, G.A.; Aparici, C.M.; Kunder, C.; Sonn, G.A.; Iagaru, A. A Pilot Study of (68)Ga-PSMA11 and (68)Ga-RM2 PET/MRI for Evaluation of Prostate Cancer Response to High-Intensity Focused Ultrasound Therapy. *J. Nucl. Med.* **2023**, *64*, 592–597. [CrossRef]

17. Fendler, W.P.; Eiber, M.; Beheshti, M.; Bomanji, J.; Ceci, F.; Cho, S.; Giesel, F.; Haberkorn, U.; Hope, T.A.; Kopka, K.; et al. (68)Ga-PSMA PET/CT: Joint EANM and SNMMI procedure guideline for prostate cancer imaging: Version 1.0. *Eur. J. Nucl. Med. Mol. Imaging* **2017**, *44*, 1014–1024. [CrossRef]
18. Hofman, M.S.; Violet, J.; Hicks, R.J.; Ferdinandus, J.; Thang, S.P.; Akhurst, T.; Iravani, A.; Kong, G.; Ravi Kumar, A.; Murphy, D.G.; et al. [(177)Lu]-PSMA-617 radionuclide treatment in patients with metastatic castration-resistant prostate cancer (LuPSMA trial): A single-centre, single-arm, phase 2 study. *Lancet Oncol.* **2018**, *19*, 825–833. [CrossRef]
19. Fassbender, T.F.; Schiller, F.; Zamboglou, C.; Drendel, V.; Kiefer, S.; Jilg, C.A.; Grosu, A.L.; Mix, M. Voxel-based comparison of [(68)Ga]Ga-RM2-PET/CT and [(68)Ga]Ga-PSMA-11-PET/CT with histopathology for diagnosis of primary prostate cancer. *EJNMMI Res.* **2020**, *10*, 62. [CrossRef]
20. Iagaru, A. Will GRPR Compete with PSMA as a Target in Prostate Cancer? *J. Nucl. Med.* **2017**, *58*, 1883–1884. [CrossRef]
21. Eiber, M.; Maurer, T.; Souvatzoglou, M.; Beer, A.J.; Ruffani, A.; Haller, B.; Graner, F.P.; Kubler, H.; Haberkorn, U.; Eisenhut, M.; et al. Evaluation of Hybrid (6)(8)Ga-PSMA Ligand PET/CT in 248 Patients with Biochemical Recurrence After Radical Prostatectomy. *J. Nucl. Med.* **2015**, *56*, 668–674. [CrossRef]
22. Rowe, S.P.; Gage, K.L.; Faraj, S.F.; Macura, K.J.; Cornish, T.C.; Gonzalez-Roibon, N.; Guner, G.; Munari, E.; Partin, A.W.; Pavlovich, C.P.; et al. (1)(8)F-DCFBC PET/CT for PSMA-Based Detection and Characterization of Primary Prostate Cancer. *J. Nucl. Med.* **2015**, *56*, 1003–1010. [CrossRef] [PubMed]
23. Hermann, R.M.; Djannatian, M.; Czech, N.; Nitsche, M. Prostate-Specific Membrane Antigen PET/CT: False-Positive Results due to Sarcoidosis? *Case Rep. Oncol.* **2016**, *9*, 457–463. [CrossRef] [PubMed]
24. Baratto, L.; Song, H.; Duan, H.; Hatami, N.; Bagshaw, H.P.; Buyyounouski, M.; Hancock, S.; Shah, S.; Srinivas, S.; Swift, P.; et al. PSMA- and GRPR-Targeted PET: Results from 50 Patients with Biochemically Recurrent Prostate Cancer. *J. Nucl. Med.* **2021**, *62*, 1545–1549. [CrossRef] [PubMed]
25. Koller, L.; Joksch, M.; Schwarzenbock, S.; Kurth, J.; Heuschkel, M.; Holzleitner, N.; Beck, R.; von Amsberg, G.; Wester, H.J.; Krause, B.J.; et al. Preclinical Comparison of the (64)Cu- and (68)Ga-Labeled GRPR-Targeted Compounds RM2 and AMTG, as Well as First-in-Humans [(68)Ga]Ga-AMTG PET/CT. *J. Nucl. Med.* **2023**, *64*, 1654–1659. [CrossRef] [PubMed]
26. Kurth, J.; Krause, B.J.; Schwarzenbock, S.M.; Bergner, C.; Hakenberg, O.W.; Heuschkel, M. First-in-human dosimetry of gastrin-releasing peptide receptor antagonist [(177)Lu]Lu-RM2: A radiopharmaceutical for the treatment of metastatic castration-resistant prostate cancer. *Eur. J. Nucl. Med. Mol. Imaging* **2020**, *47*, 123–135. [CrossRef] [PubMed]
27. Dalm, S.U.; Bakker, I.L.; de Blois, E.; Doeswijk, G.N.; Konijnenberg, M.W.; Orlandi, F.; Barbato, D.; Tedesco, M.; Maina, T.; Nock, B.A.; et al. 68Ga/177Lu-NeoBOMB1, a Novel Radiolabeled GRPR Antagonist for Theranostic Use in Oncology. *J. Nucl. Med.* **2017**, *58*, 293–299. [CrossRef]
28. Nock, B.A.; Kaloudi, A.; Lymperis, E.; Giarika, A.; Kulkarni, H.R.; Klette, I.; Singh, A.; Krenning, E.P.; de Jong, M.; Maina, T.; et al. Theranostic Perspectives in Prostate Cancer with the Gastrin-Releasing Peptide Receptor Antagonist NeoBOMB1: Preclinical and First Clinical Results. *J. Nucl. Med.* **2017**, *58*, 75–80. [CrossRef]
29. Mansi, R.; Fleischmann, A.; Macke, H.R.; Reubi, J.C. Targeting GRPR in urological cancers--from basic research to clinical application. *Nat. Rev. Urol.* **2013**, *10*, 235–244. [CrossRef]
30. Gruber, L.; Jimenez-Franco, L.D.; Decristoforo, C.; Uprimny, C.; Glatting, G.; Hohenberger, P.; Schoenberg, S.O.; Reindl, W.; Orlandi, F.; Mariani, M.; et al. MITIGATE-NeoBOMB1, a Phase I/IIa Study to Evaluate Safety, Pharmacokinetics, and Preliminary Imaging of (68)Ga-NeoBOMB1, a Gastrin-Releasing Peptide Receptor Antagonist, in GIST Patients. *J. Nucl. Med.* **2020**, *61*, 1749–1755. [CrossRef]
31. Michalski, K.; Kemna, L.; Asberger, J.; Grosu, A.L.; Meyer, P.T.; Ruf, J.; Sprave, T. Gastrin-Releasing Peptide Receptor Antagonist [(68)Ga]RM2 PET/CT for Staging of Pre-Treated, Metastasized Breast Cancer. *Cancers* **2021**, *13*, 6106. [CrossRef]
32. Colbert, L.E.; Rebueno, N.; Moningi, S.; Beddar, S.; Sawakuchi, G.O.; Herman, J.M.; Koong, A.C.; Das, P.; Holliday, E.B.; Koay, E.J.; et al. Dose escalation for locally advanced pancreatic cancer: How high can we go? *Adv. Radiat. Oncol.* **2018**, *3*, 693–700. [CrossRef] [PubMed]
33. Nagasaki, S.; Nakamura, Y.; Maekawa, T.; Akahira, J.; Miki, Y.; Suzuki, T.; Ishidoya, S.; Arai, Y.; Sasano, H. Immunohistochemical analysis of gastrin-releasing peptide receptor (GRPR) and possible regulation by estrogen receptor betacx in human prostate carcinoma. *Neoplasma* **2012**, *59*, 224–232. [CrossRef] [PubMed]
34. Beer, M.; Montani, M.; Gerhardt, J.; Wild, P.J.; Hany, T.F.; Hermanns, T.; Muntener, M.; Kristiansen, G. Profiling gastrin-releasing peptide receptor in prostate tissues: Clinical implications and molecular correlates. *Prostate* **2012**, *72*, 318–325. [CrossRef] [PubMed]
35. Duan, H.; Davidzon, G.A.; Moradi, F.; Liang, T.; Song, H.; Iagaru, A. Modified PROMISE Criteria for Standardized Interpretation of Gastrin Realising Peptide Receptor (GRPR)-targeted PET. *Eur. J. Nucl. Med. Mol. Imaging* **2023**, *50*, 4087–4095. [CrossRef] [PubMed]
36. R Core Team. R: A Language and Environment for Statistical Computing. 2013. Available online: http://www.R-project.org/ (accessed on 31 March 2022).
37. Faul, F.; Erdfelder, E.; Lang, A.G.; Buchner, A. G*Power 3: A flexible statistical power analysis program for the social, behavioral, and biomedical sciences. *Behav. Res. Methods* **2007**, *39*, 175–191. [CrossRef]

38. Perner, S.; Hofer, M.D.; Kim, R.; Shah, R.B.; Li, H.; Moller, P.; Hautmann, R.E.; Gschwend, J.E.; Kuefer, R.; Rubin, M.A. Prostate-specific membrane antigen expression as a predictor of prostate cancer progression. *Hum. Pathol.* **2007**, *38*, 696–701. [CrossRef]
39. Silver, D.A.; Pellicer, I.; Fair, W.R.; Heston, W.D.; Cordon-Cardo, C. Prostate-specific membrane antigen expression in normal and malignant human tissues. *Clin. Cancer Res.* **1997**, *3*, 81–85.
40. Eder, M.; Schafer, M.; Bauder-Wust, U.; Haberkorn, U.; Eisenhut, M.; Kopka, K. Preclinical evaluation of a bispecific low-molecular heterodimer targeting both PSMA and GRPR for improved PET imaging and therapy of prostate cancer. *Prostate* **2014**, *74*, 659–668. [CrossRef]
41. Hofman, M.S.; Emmett, L.; Sandhu, S.; Iravani, A.; Joshua, A.M.; Goh, J.C.; Pattison, D.A.; Tan, T.H.; Kirkwood, I.D.; Francis, R.J.; et al. TheraP: ^{177}Lu-PSMA-617 (LuPSMA) versus cabazitaxel in metastatic castration-resistant prostate cancer (mCRPC) progressing after docetaxel—Overall survival after median follow-up of 3 years (ANZUP 1603). *J. Clin. Oncol.* **2022**, *40*, 5000. [CrossRef]
42. Merkens, L.; Sailer, V.; Lessel, D.; Janzen, E.; Greimeier, S.; Kirfel, J.; Perner, S.; Pantel, K.; Werner, S.; von Amsberg, G. Aggressive variants of prostate cancer: Underlying mechanisms of neuroendocrine transdifferentiation. *J. Exp. Clin. Cancer Res.* **2022**, *41*, 46. [CrossRef]
43. Mannweiler, S.; Amersdorfer, P.; Trajanoski, S.; Terrett, J.A.; King, D.; Mehes, G. Heterogeneity of prostate-specific membrane antigen (PSMA) expression in prostate carcinoma with distant metastasis. *Pathol. Oncol. Res.* **2009**, *15*, 167–172. [CrossRef] [PubMed]
44. Staal, J.; Beyaert, R. Inflammation and NF-kappaB Signaling in Prostate Cancer: Mechanisms and Clinical Implications. *Cells* **2018**, *7*, 122. [CrossRef] [PubMed]
45. Matouk, I.; Raveh, E.; Ohana, P.; Lail, R.A.; Gershtain, E.; Gilon, M.; De Groot, N.; Czerniak, A.; Hochberg, A. The increasing complexity of the oncofetal h19 gene locus: Functional dissection and therapeutic intervention. *Int. J. Mol. Sci.* **2013**, *14*, 4298–4316. [CrossRef] [PubMed]
46. Liang, W.C.; Fu, W.M.; Wong, C.W.; Wang, Y.; Wang, W.M.; Hu, G.X.; Zhang, L.; Xiao, L.J.; Wan, D.C.; Zhang, J.F.; et al. The lncRNA H19 promotes epithelial to mesenchymal transition by functioning as miRNA sponges in colorectal cancer. *Oncotarget* **2015**, *6*, 22513–22525. [CrossRef]
47. Zhang, Z.; Yao, L.; Yang, J.; Wang, Z.; Du, G. PI3K/Akt and HIF-1 signaling pathway in hypoxia-ischemia (Review). *Mol. Med. Rep.* **2018**, *18*, 3547–3554. [CrossRef]
48. Danza, G.; Di Serio, C.; Rosati, F.; Lonetto, G.; Sturli, N.; Kacer, D.; Pennella, A.; Ventimiglia, G.; Barucci, R.; Piscazzi, A.; et al. Notch signaling modulates hypoxia-induced neuroendocrine differentiation of human prostate cancer cells. *Mol. Cancer Res.* **2012**, *10*, 230–238. [CrossRef]
49. Markwalder, R.; Reubi, J.C. Gastrin-releasing peptide receptors in the human prostate: Relation to neoplastic transformation. *Cancer Res.* **1999**, *59*, 1152–1159.
50. de Visser, M.; van Weerden, W.M.; de Ridder, C.M.; Reneman, S.; Melis, M.; Krenning, E.P.; de Jong, M. Androgen-dependent expression of the gastrin-releasing peptide receptor in human prostate tumor xenografts. *J. Nucl. Med.* **2007**, *48*, 88–93.
51. Yu, Z.; Ananias, H.J.; Carlucci, G.; Hoving, H.D.; Helfrich, W.; Dierckx, R.A.; Wang, F.; de Jong, I.J.; Elsinga, P.H. An update of radiolabeled bombesin analogs for gastrin-releasing peptide receptor targeting. *Curr. Pharm. Des.* **2013**, *19*, 3329–3341. [CrossRef]
52. Constantinides, C.; Lazaris, A.C.; Haritopoulos, K.N.; Pantazopoulos, D.; Chrisofos, M.; Giannopoulos, A. Immunohistochemical detection of gastrin releasing peptide in patients with prostate cancer. *World J. Urol.* **2003**, *21*, 183–187. [CrossRef]
53. Giesel, F.L.; Knorr, K.; Spohn, F.; Will, L.; Maurer, T.; Flechsig, P.; Neels, O.; Schiller, K.; Amaral, H.; Weber, W.A.; et al. Detection Efficacy of (18)F-PSMA-1007 PET/CT in 251 Patients with Biochemical Recurrence of Prostate Cancer After Radical Prostatectomy. *J. Nucl. Med.* **2019**, *60*, 362–368. [CrossRef]
54. Verhoeven, M.; Ruigrok, E.A.M.; van Leenders, G.; van den Brink, L.; Balcioglu, H.E.; van Weerden, W.M.; Dalm, S.U. GRPR versus PSMA: Expression profiles during prostate cancer progression demonstrate the added value of GRPR-targeting theranostic approaches. *Front. Oncol.* **2023**, *13*, 1199432. [CrossRef]
55. Annunziata, S.; Cuccaro, A.; Calcagni, M.L.; Hohaus, S.; Giordano, A.; Rufini, V. Interim FDG-PET/CT in Hodgkin lymphoma: The prognostic role of the ratio between target lesion and liver SUVmax (rPET). *Ann. Nucl. Med.* **2016**, *30*, 588–592. [CrossRef]
56. Wang, C.; Zhao, K.; Hu, S.; Huang, Y.; Ma, L.; Li, M.; Song, Y. The PET-Derived Tumor-to-Liver Standard Uptake Ratio (SUV (TLR)) Is Superior to Tumor SUVmax in Predicting Tumor Response and Survival After Chemoradiotherapy in Patients With Locally Advanced Esophageal Cancer. *Front. Oncol.* **2020**, *10*, 1630. [CrossRef]
57. Mansi, R.; Wang, X.; Forrer, F.; Waser, B.; Cescato, R.; Graham, K.; Borkowski, S.; Reubi, J.C.; Maecke, H.R. Development of a potent DOTA-conjugated bombesin antagonist for targeting GRPr-positive tumours. *Eur. J. Nucl. Med. Mol. Imaging* **2011**, *38*, 97–107. [CrossRef]
58. Eder, M.; Schafer, M.; Bauder-Wust, U.; Hull, W.E.; Wangler, C.; Mier, W.; Haberkorn, U.; Eisenhut, M. 68Ga-complex lipophilicity and the targeting property of a urea-based PSMA inhibitor for PET imaging. *Bioconjug. Chem.* **2012**, *23*, 688–697. [CrossRef]
59. Reile, H.; Armatis, P.E.; Schally, A.V. Characterization of high-affinity receptors for bombesin/gastrin releasing peptide on the human prostate cancer cell lines PC-3 and DU-145: Internalization of receptor bound 125I-(Tyr4) bombesin by tumor cells. *Prostate* **1994**, *25*, 29–38. [CrossRef]

60. Yadav, M.P.; Ballal, S.; Sahoo, R.K.; Tripathi, M.; Damle, N.A.; Shamim, S.A.; Kumar, R.; Seth, A.; Bal, C. Long-term outcome of 177Lu-PSMA-617 radioligand therapy in heavily pre-treated metastatic castration-resistant prostate cancer patients. *PLoS ONE* **2021**, *16*, e0251375. [CrossRef]
61. Beheshti, M.; Taimen, P.; Kemppainen, J.; Jambor, I.; Muller, A.; Loidl, W.; Kahkonen, E.; Kakela, M.; Berndt, M.; Stephens, A.W.; et al. Value of (68)Ga-labeled bombesin antagonist (RM2) in the detection of primary prostate cancer comparing with [(18)F]fluoromethylcholine PET-CT and multiparametric MRI-a phase I/II study. *Eur. Radiol.* **2023**, *33*, 472–482. [CrossRef]
62. Fernández, R.; Kramer, V.; Hurtado de Mendoza, A.; Flores, J.; Amaral, H. Preliminary Evaluation of Tumor Uptake and Laboratory parameters After a Single Dose of 177Lu-RM2 Radioligand therapy in Metastatic Castrate-Resistant Prostate Cancer. *Eur. J. Nucl. Med. Mol. Imaging* **2019**, *46*, 952. [CrossRef]
63. Eapen, R.S.; Buteau, J.P.; Jackson, P.; Mitchell, C.; Oon, S.F.; Alghazo, O.; McIntosh, L.; Dhiantravan, N.; Scalzo, M.J.; O'Brien, J.; et al. Administering [(177)Lu]Lu-PSMA-617 Prior to Radical Prostatectomy in Men with High-risk Localised Prostate Cancer (LuTectomy): A Single-centre, Single-arm, Phase 1/2 Study. *Eur. Urol.* **2023**. [CrossRef] [PubMed]

Disclaimer/Publisher's Note: The statements, opinions and data contained in all publications are solely those of the individual author(s) and contributor(s) and not of MDPI and/or the editor(s). MDPI and/or the editor(s) disclaim responsibility for any injury to people or property resulting from any ideas, methods, instructions or products referred to in the content.

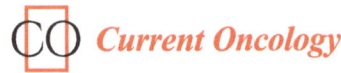 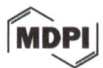

Case Report

Mixed Adenosquamous Cell Carcinoma of the Prostate with Paired Sequencing on the Primary and Liver Metastasis

Emmanuella Oyogoa [1,*], Maya Sonpatki [2], Brian T. Brinkerhoff [3], Nicole Andeen [3], Haley Meyer [4], Christopher Ryan [3] and Alexandra O. Sokolova [5]

1. Department of Medicine, Oregon Health and Science University, Portland, OR 97239, USA
2. Department of Microbiology, Oregon State University, Corvallis, OR 97331, USA
3. Department of Pathology and Laboratory Medicine, Oregon Health and Science University, Portland, OR 97239, USA
4. Department of Internal Medicine, Mayo Clinic, Rochester, MN 55902, USA
5. Division of Hematology and Medical Oncology, Knight Cancer Institute, Oregon Health and Sciences University, Portland, OR 97239, USA
* Correspondence: oyogoa@ohsu.edu

Abstract: This report aims to shed light on the intricate challenges encountered during the diagnosis and treatment of an uncommon variant of prostate cancer—mixed adenosquamous cell carcinoma of the prostate. Prostate cancers of this nature pose distinctive diagnostic and therapeutic dilemmas due to their rarity and complex histological composition. We present a case of a 63-year-old man with metastatic prostate cancer, featuring adenocarcinoma with squamous cell differentiation, who underwent a multimodal treatment approach. The patient responded to first-line carboplatin, docetaxel, and androgen deprivation therapy, followed by androgen receptor pathway inhibitor (ARPI) maintenance. However, disease progression led to radiation therapy and a subsequent switch to Lutetium (177Lu) vipivotide tetraxetan after chemotherapy challenges. Comprehensive genetic profiling revealed shared mutations in the prostate and liver lesions, emphasizing the role of targeted therapies. Prostate-specific membrane antigen (PSMA)-targeted therapy resulted in a notable PSA decline. This case highlights the evolving treatment landscape for rare prostate cancers, integrating genetic insights for tailored interventions. In conclusion, squamous cell carcinoma (SCC) of the prostate is rare, emphasizing the imperative for enhanced comprehension in diagnosis and management. Our case suggests the potential efficacy of ARPI and PSMA-targeted therapies. Our findings advocate for a more nuanced approach to the management of this rare prostate cancer variant, leveraging genomic insights for personalized treatment strategies. This exploration serves as a foundation for further research and clinical considerations in addressing the challenges posed by mixed adenosquamous cell carcinoma of the prostate.

Keywords: squamous cell carcinoma of the prostate; mixed adenosquamous cell carcinoma of the prostate; prostate cancer; prostate-specific membrane antigen positron emission tomography (PSMA PET)

1. Introduction

Prostate cancer stands as the most prevalent non-cutaneous malignancy among American men [1], with an estimated 288,300 new cases in 2023 [2]. Adenocarcinoma constitutes 95% of prostate cancer cases, representing the predominant histology. Conversely, squamous cell carcinoma (SCC) of the prostate is a rare manifestation accounting for less than 1% of cases [3,4]. Typically, mixed adenosquamous cell carcinoma of the prostate emerges as a transformation of adenocarcinoma, while in certain cases, it is thought to be primary, although the origin of primary prostate SCC is still debated [5]. The genetic and molecular intricacies of prostate SCC remain inadequately explored [5]. This case report presents a case of mixed adenosquamous cell carcinoma of the prostate, providing paired sequencing data from both the primary prostate tumor and liver metastasis.

2. Case Report

A 63-year-old man with past medical history of diabetes type 2, a family history of prostate cancer in his father and no smoking history was diagnosed with metastatic prostate cancer at the age of 61 after presenting with urinary retention. At the time of presentation, the PSA was 14.8 ng/mL. A prostate biopsy revealed prostate adenocarcinoma with squamous cell differentiation and a Gleason score of 5 + 4 (Figure 1A,B). A bone scan showed osseous lesions in the ribs and pelvic bones, and CT of the chest, abdomen and pelvis revealed visceral metastasis to the liver. The stage at diagnosis was T3AN1M1c. A CT-guided liver biopsy revealed poorly differentiated carcinoma, positive for NKX3.1 via immunohistochemistry (Figure 1C).

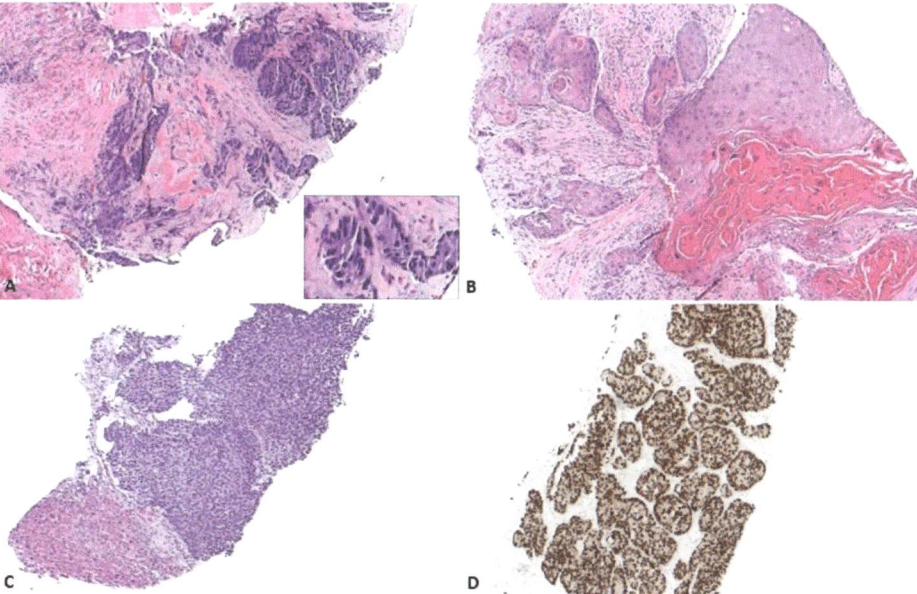

Figure 1. Biopsies of the (**A**) prostate showed high-grade adenocarcinoma (inset showing high power view of glandular component (400×)) with areas of (**B**) keratinizing squamous differentiation. Liver biopsies showed a (**C**) poorly differentiated adenocarcinoma with (**D**) immunoreactivity for the prostate marker NKX3.1 (all images at 100×).

Comprehensive genetic profiling, using institutional tumor next-generation sequencing panel Genetrails, of the pretreatment prostate biopsy showed genomic alterations in *PIK3CA* p.E542K, *MUTYH* p.G393D and androgen receptor (AR) amplification (11 copies). Other potential clinically significant mutations include the following: *ATRX* loss, *MLH1* loss, *PTEN* loss, *SUFU* loss, *TP53* K123R and loss, *SMAD4* loss and *CDKN1B* splice site. Genomic studies from the liver lesion biopsy obtained before the initiation of therapy showed the same mutations as those from the prostate, including *AR* amplification (17 copies), *PIK3CA* p.E542K and *MUTYH* p.G393D. Germline testing revealed monoallelic *MUTYH* p.G396D alteration and was negative for *TP53* and DNA damage repair gene alterations.

The initiation of carboplatin and docetaxel, in conjunction with androgen deprivation therapy (ADT), was prompted by the SCC component identified in the patient's prostate biopsy. He responded well to therapy with PSA decline from 14 ng/mL to 2 ng/mL and radiographic response (decrease in size and extent of hepatic metastases and lymphadenopathy and stable osseous lesions with no new sites of metastases). After completing six cycles of carboplatin and docetaxel, he continued ADT and started AR pathway inhibitor (ARPI) therapy due to his adenocarcinoma component. He started two ARPIs, apalutamide and abiraterone, on a clinical trial (Figure 2) [6]. PSA further declined during ARPI therapy, with a PSA nadir of 0.9 ng/mL. After 25 weeks of therapy, his PSA started rising to 4 ng/mL. His restaging imaging showed interval development of a single new lytic destruction and soft tissue component of the right posterior acetabular metastasis, no other new disease, decreased hepatic metastases and no change in the enlarged abdominal/pelvic lymph nodes. Lutetium-177 therapy was discussed and PSMA PET imaging was performed, which showed PSMA uptake in all known metastases: liver, lymph nodes and bone metastasis (Figure 3A). The patient opted for radiation therapy (XRT) to the single lesion's progression, the acetabulum, and a continuation of ARPI and ADT therapy. PSA declined reaching a nadir of 1.78 ng/mL. Four months after XRT, PSA started rising again during ARPI therapy, and imaging showed a new liver metastasis and increases in the size of the soft tissue component of osseous metastasis. The patient had a repeat PSMA PET scan (Figure 3B) and opted to undergo Lutetium (177Lu) vipivotide tetraxetan therapy. Unfortunately, this therapy became unavailable due to supply issues, and the patient received one cycle of cabazitaxel and carboplatin chemotherapy before initiating PSMA-targeted therapy. Initially, the patent showed a response to Lutetium (177Lu) vipivotide tetraxetan therapy with a PSA decline from 33 ng/mL to 15 ng/mL after the first cycle. Unfortunately, PSA started rising after cycle 3, and he had radiographic progression after cycle 3 with new and enlarging pulmonary, hepatic and bone metastasis. The patient was hospitalized for altered mental status, raising concerns about leptomeningeal metastasis despite the absence of clear radiographic evidence. Although the altered mental status resolved, the patient later developed pneumonia. Opting for a transition to comfort care, he passed away.

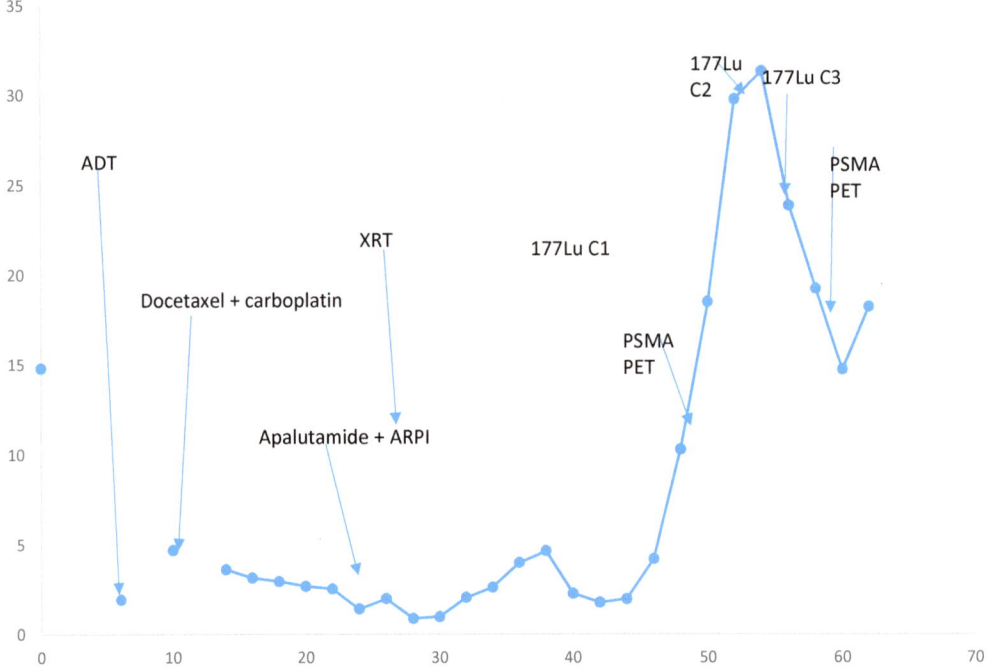

Figure 2. PSA levels and corresponding treatment course with time on the X axis and PSA (ng/mL) on the Y axis.

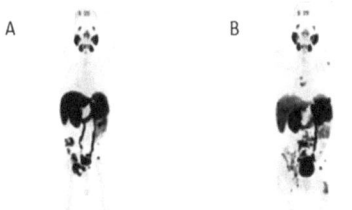

Figure 3. PSMA PET imaging. (**A**) PSMA imaging obtained after completion of chemotherapy treatment with hepatic, pelvic bone and pelvic lymph node uptake. (**B**) PSMA imaging obtained 6 months after (**A**) while on ADT and ARPI. Compared to 3A, increased osseous lesion, hepatic lesions and lymph nodes. New uptake present in spinal bone. Decreased uptake in pelvic bone.

3. Discussion

Outcome data for SCC of the prostate are limited but suggest a more aggressive phenotype and worse treatment outcomes compared to adenocarcinoma [7]. For localized SCC cases, several reports have suggested the efficacy of multimodal therapy [8]: a combination of radiation and/or radical prostatectomy with androgen deprivation therapy (ADT) and chemotherapy [9]. There is no standard of care for metastatic SCC, and chemotherapy is typically offered as the first-line therapy along with ADT [10]. Generally, the same treatment options are available for both SCC and adenocarcinoma. However, chemotherapy doublets are preferred in SCC of the prostate. The treatment response to systemic therapies for squamous cell carcinoma is less than what is observed for adenocarcinoma [11].

SCC of the prostate is associated with a more aggressive disease phenotype compared to adenocarcinoma, and is more likely to have metastasized to bone, liver or lungs at the time of diagnosis [12], to have lower prostate-specific antigen (PSA) with advanced disease [13] and has worse survival [14]. In 11 case reports of primary squamous cell carcinoma of the prostate, the median overall survival was 11 months with survival ranging between 3 months and 6 years [3,15–24]. At the time of diagnosis, PSA is often low, even in the setting of metastases. It is often challenging to identify the origin of SCC, and some experts propose that SCC originates from the urothelium and then migrates to the prostate [5,11,13,25]. The presence of prostate-specific alterations, such as *TMPRSS2-ERG* or *SPOP*, can help determine the prostate primary origin of the SCC [25]. The data on the somatic mutation profile of the SCC of prostate cancer is limited.

In this case, we present matching pretreatment biopsies of prostate and liver metastasis. Overall genomic fundings were very similar in these two biopsies and showed activation of the PI3K/AKT pathway, *AR* amplification and *T53* mutation.

In the presented case, PI3K/AKT pathway activation was evident with *PIK3CA* p.E542K alteration and *PTEN* loss. PI3K/AKT pathway activation is common in many cancer types, including SCC of different origins (cervix, oral cavity, head and neck and skin) [26]. It is present in about 40% of early prostate cancer cases and up to 70–100% of advanced cases [27–30]. It is unclear if PI3K/AKT activation in the presented case is associated with the SCC or adenocarcinoma component. Two other prostate SCC case reports reported *PTEN* alterations; one case reported *PTEN* alteration in both primary and metastatic biopsies [25], suggesting it might be an early alteration in the tumorigenesis of SCC of the prostate. PI3K/AKT pathway activation is associated with resistance to androgen deprivation therapy and poor outcomes in conventional adenocarcinoma of the prostate. Several therapeutic strategies are being evaluated to target the PIK/AKT pathway, with AKT inhibitors being the most promising. Phase III trial, IPATential150, demonstrated improved radiographic progression-free survival with the AKT inhibitor Ipatasertib in combination with abiraterone compared to placebo plus abiraterone among patients with mCRPC with PTEN-loss [31]. Another phase III trial evaluating the role of capivasertib, an AKT inhibitor, is ongoing [32]. Clinical trial participation with an AKT inhibitor was a potential therapeutic option for our patient but was not available when Lu-117 therapy started.

AR amplification is a common alteration in castration-resistant adenocarcinoma of the prostate and is present in up to 50% of cases [33–36]. However, it is rarely present in untreated prostate tumors [37]. In this case, of SCC of the prostate, *AR* amplification was present in both the liver biopsy and the prostate tissue that were obtained prior to the initiation of treatment, suggesting an early event. *AR* amplification is associated with resistance to the *AR* pathway inhibitors [38,39]. The presented case had *AR* amplification and SCC component of the tumor—both predictive of poor response to ARPI. However, the patient had a longer-than-expected response to ARPI and completed 10 months of ARPI therapy with a stable disease, except single oligometastatic progression treated with XRT. This case suggests that there could be a role for ARPI therapy in mixed adenosquamous cell carcinoma prostate tumors.

As is found in many cancers, we detected a somatic mutation of *TP53* in the primary tumor and liver metastases, and there was no evidence of a germline alteration on genetic testing. Somatic *TP53* mutations are common in many tumors, including prostate tumors. Sweeney et al. found that about 46% (n = 37/76) of patients who had no prior treatment with abiraterone or enzalutamide had a somatic *TP53* mutation. In comparison, 41% (n = 108/262) of patients treated with abiraterone and/or enzalutamide had a somatic *TP53* mutation [40]. Although somatic *TP53* mutation did not appear to play a major role in the characterization of SCC of the prostate in this case, germline *TP53* mutations were recently shown to have an association with increased risk of developing prostate cancer [41].

PSMA is a mostly prostate-specific transmembrane protein with 100- to 1000-fold higher expression in prostatic adenocarcinoma compared to benign prostate [42]. Up to 87% of patients with mCRPC have PSMA-avid tumors [43]. PSMA uptake among the SCC of the prostate has not been characterized. In the presented case, all known metastases had PSMA uptake, and the patient pursued PSMA-directed therapy with the initial response, which unfortunately was not durable. This case highlights the potential role of PSMA PET and PSMA-directed therapy (e.g., Lutetium (177Lu) vipivotide tetraxetan) in the SCC of the prostate.

Overall, SCC of the prostate is a rare disease. This case highlights the need for a better understanding of the diagnosis, treatment and management of pure and mixed adenosquamous cell carcinoma of the prostate. Tumor sequencing can help to identify the origin of SCC and suggest therapeutic approaches. Our case suggests a role for ARPI and PSMA-targeted therapies in mixed adenosquamous cell carcinoma of the prostate. Future directives should include the role of targeted therapy and screening for certain somatic and germline mutations present in prostate cancer. In particular, more research and clinical trials are needed for targeted treatment in pure and mixed adenosquamous cell carcinoma of the prostate.

Author Contributions: Conceptualization, A.O.S.; writing—original draft preparation, E.O.; writing—review and editing, E.O., M.S., B.T.B., N.A., H.M., C.R. and A.O.S.; supervision, A.O.S. All authors have read and agreed to the published version of the manuscript.

Funding: Prostate Cancer Foundation Young Investigator Award, NCI CA097186 (PNW SPORE) and P30 CA015704; DOD PCRP W81XWH2220021; PNW SPORE PILOT P50 CA097186-16A1.

Institutional Review Board Statement: Ethical review and approval were waived for this study as this is a case report.

Informed Consent Statement: Informed consent was obtained from all subjects involved in the study.

Data Availability Statement: No new data were created or analyzed in this study. Data sharing is not applicable to this article.

Conflicts of Interest: The authors declare no conflicts of interest.

References

1. Hsing, A.W.; Chokkalingam, A.P. Prostate Cancer Epidemiology. *Front. Biosci. J. Virtual Libr.* **2006**, *11*, 1388–1413. [CrossRef] [PubMed]
2. Cancer of the Prostate—Cancer Stat Facts. Available online: https://seer.cancer.gov/statfacts/html/prost.html (accessed on 22 July 2023).
3. Little, N.A.; Wiener, J.S.; Walther, P.J.; Paulson, D.F.; Anderson, E.E. Squamous Cell Carcinoma of the Prostate: 2 Cases of a Rare Malignancy and Review of the Literature. *J. Urol.* **1993**, *149*, 137–139. [CrossRef] [PubMed]
4. Autio, K.; McBride, S. Oligometastatic Squamous Cell Transformation from Metastatic Prostate Adenocarcinoma Treated with Systemic and Focal Therapy: A Case Report. *J. Immunother. Precis. Oncol.* **2022**, *5*, 79–83. [CrossRef] [PubMed]
5. Braslis, K.G.; David, R.C.; Nelson, E.; Civantos, F.; Soloway, M.S. Squamous Cell Carcinoma of the Prostate: A Transformation from Adenocarcinoma after the Use of a Luteinizing Hormone-Releasing Hormone Agonist and Flutamide. *Urology* **1995**, *45*, 329–331. [CrossRef] [PubMed]
6. Graff, J. *Advanced ChemoHormonal Therapy for Treatment Naïve Metastatic Prostate Cancer: Apalutamide and Abiraterone Acetate with Prednisone and Androgen Deprivation Therapy after Treatment with Docetaxel and Androgen Deprivation Therapy*; clinicaltrials.gov; NIH: Bethesda, MD, USA, 2023.
7. He, X.; Yang, K.; Chen, G.; Zheng, J. Squamous Cell Carcinoma of the Prostate with Lower Urinary Tract Symptoms: A Case Report. *Urol. Case Rep.* **2021**, *39*, 101796. [CrossRef]
8. John, T.T.; Bashir, J.; Burrow, C.T.; Machin, D.G. Squamous Cell Carcinoma of the Prostate—A Case Report. *Int. Urol. Nephrol.* **2005**, *37*, 311–313. [CrossRef] [PubMed]
9. Hutten, R.J.; Weil, C.R.; Tward, J.D.; Lloyd, S.; Johnson, S.B. Patterns of Care and Treatment Outcomes in Locoregional Squamous Cell Carcinoma of the Prostate. *Eur. Urol. Open Sci.* **2021**, *23*, 30–33. [CrossRef]
10. Atagi, K.; Fukuhara, H.; Ishiguro, M.; Osakabe, H.; Satoshi, F.; Tamura, K.; Karashima, T.; Inoue, K. Successful Treatment with DCF Chemotherapy and Radiotherapy for Primary Squamous Cell Carcinoma of the Prostate. *IJU Case Rep.* **2021**, *4*, 421–424. [CrossRef]
11. Li, J.; Wang, Z. The Pathology of Unusual Subtypes of Prostate Cancer. *Chin. J. Cancer Res. Chung-Kuo Yen Cheng Yen Chiu* **2016**, *28*, 130–143. [CrossRef]
12. Malik, R.D.; Dakwar, G.; Hardee, M.E.; Sanfilippo, N.J.; Rosenkrantz, A.B.; Taneja, S.S. Squamous Cell Carcinoma of the Prostate. *Rev. Urol.* **2011**, *13*, 56–60.
13. Arva, N.C.; Das, K. Diagnostic Dilemmas of Squamous Differentiation in Prostate Carcinoma Case Report and Review of the Literature. *Diagn. Pathol.* **2011**, *6*, 46. [CrossRef] [PubMed]
14. Biswas, T.; Podder, T.; Lepera, P.A.; Walker, P. Primary Squamous Carcinoma of the Prostate: A Case Report of a Rare Clinical Entity. *Future Sci. OA* **2015**, *1*, FSO18. [CrossRef] [PubMed]
15. Thompson, G.J.; Albers, D.D.; Broders, A.C. Unusual Carcinomas Involving the Prostate Gland. *J. Urol.* **1953**, *69*, 416–425. [CrossRef] [PubMed]
16. Corder, M.P.; Cicmil, G.A. Effective Treatment of Metastatic Squamous Cell Carcinoma of the Prostate with Adriamycin. *J. Urol.* **1976**, *115*, 222. [CrossRef]
17. Horan, A.H. Sequential Cryotherapy for Prostatic Carcinoma: Does It Palliate the Bone Pain? *Conn. Med.* **1975**, *39*, 81–83.
18. Berbis, P.; Andrac, L.; Daou, N.; Privat, Y. Single Nodule on the Glans Penis: Metastatic Lesion from an Unusual Carcinoma of the Prostate. *Dermatologica* **1987**, *175*, 152–155. [CrossRef] [PubMed]
19. Gray, G.F.; Marshall, V.F. Squamous Carcinoma of the Prostate. *J. Urol.* **1975**, *113*, 736–738. [CrossRef] [PubMed]
20. Moskovitz, B.; Munichor, M.; Bolkier, M.; Livne, P.M. Squamous Cell Carcinoma of the Prostate. *Urol. Int.* **1993**, *51*, 181–183. [CrossRef] [PubMed]
21. Pérez García, F.J.; Veiga González, M.; Rodríguez Martínez, J.J.; Rabade Rey, C.J.; Fernández Gómez, J.M.; Escaf, S.; Martín Benito, J.L. Squamous cell carcinoma of the prostate. Presentation of a case and review of the literature. *Actas Urol. Esp.* **1997**, *21*, 931–935.
22. Sarma, D.P.; Weilbaecher, T.G.; Moon, T.D. Squamous Cell Carcinoma of Prostate. *Urology* **1991**, *37*, 260–262. [CrossRef]
23. Sharma, S.K.; Malik, A.K.; Bapna, B.C. Squamous Cell Carcinoma of Prostate. *Indian J. Cancer* **1980**, *17*, 134–135. [PubMed]
24. Uchibayashi, T.; Hisazumi, H.; Hasegawa, M.; Shiba, N.; Muraishi, Y.; Tanaka, T.; Nonomura, A. Squamous Cell Carcinoma of the Prostate. *Scand. J. Urol. Nephrol.* **1997**, *31*, 223–224. [CrossRef] [PubMed]
25. Dizman, N.; Salgia, M.; Ali, S.M.; Wu, H.; Arvanitis, L.; Chung, J.H.; Pal, S.K. Squamous Transformation of Prostate Adenocarcinoma: A Report of Two Cases with Genomic Profiling. *Clin. Genitourin. Cancer* **2020**, *18*, e289–e292. [CrossRef] [PubMed]
26. Ghafouri-Fard, S.; Noie Alamdari, A.; Noee Alamdari, Y.; Abak, A.; Hussen, B.M.; Taheri, M.; Jamali, E. Role of PI3K/AKT Pathway in Squamous Cell Carcinoma with an Especial Focus on Head and Neck Cancers. *Cancer Cell Int.* **2022**, *22*, 254. [CrossRef] [PubMed]
27. Carver, B.S.; Chapinski, C.; Wongvipat, J.; Hieronymus, H.; Chen, Y.; Chandarlapaty, S.; Arora, V.K.; Le, C.; Koutcher, J.; Scher, H.; et al. Reciprocal Feedback Regulation of PI3K and Androgen Receptor Signaling in PTEN-Deficient Prostate Cancer. *Cancer Cell* **2011**, *19*, 575–586. [CrossRef] [PubMed]
28. Taylor, B.S.; Schultz, N.; Hieronymus, H.; Gopalan, A.; Xiao, Y.; Carver, B.S.; Arora, V.K.; Kaushik, P.; Cerami, E.; Reva, B.; et al. Integrative Genomic Profiling of Human Prostate Cancer. *Cancer Cell* **2010**, *18*, 11–22. [CrossRef] [PubMed]

29. Crumbaker, M.; Khoja, L.; Joshua, A.M. AR Signaling and the PI3K Pathway in Prostate Cancer. *Cancers* **2017**, *9*, 34. [CrossRef] [PubMed]
30. Pearson, H.B.; Li, J.; Meniel, V.S.; Fennell, C.M.; Waring, P.; Montgomery, K.G.; Rebello, R.J.; Macpherson, A.A.; Koushyar, S.; Furic, L.; et al. Identification of Pik3ca Mutation as a Genetic Driver of Prostate Cancer That Cooperates with Pten Loss to Accelerate Progression and Castration-Resistant Growth. *Cancer Discov.* **2018**, *8*, 764–779. [CrossRef] [PubMed]
31. Sweeney, C.; Bracarda, S.; Sternberg, C.N.; Chi, K.N.; Olmos, D.; Sandhu, S.; Massard, C.; Matsubara, N.; Alekseev, B.; Parnis, F.; et al. Ipatasertib plus Abiraterone and Prednisolone in Metastatic Castration-Resistant Prostate Cancer (IPATential150): A Multicentre, Randomised, Double-Blind, Phase 3 Trial. *Lancet Lond. Engl.* **2021**, *398*, 131–142. [CrossRef]
32. AstraZeneca. *A Phase III Double-Blind, Randomised, Placebo-Controlled Study Assessing the Efficacy and Safety of Capivasertib + Abiraterone versus Placebo+Abiraterone as Treatment for Patients with DeNovo Metastatic Hormone-Sensitive Prostate Cancer Characterised by PTEN Deficiency*; clinicaltrials.gov; NIH: Bethesda, MD, USA, 2023.
33. Visakorpi, T.; Hyytinen, E.; Koivisto, P.; Tanner, M.; Keinänen, R.; Palmberg, C.; Palotie, A.; Tammela, T.; Isola, J.; Kallioniemi, O.P. In Vivo Amplification of the Androgen Receptor Gene and Progression of Human Prostate Cancer. *Nat. Genet.* **1995**, *9*, 401–406. [CrossRef]
34. Grasso, C.S.; Wu, Y.-M.; Robinson, D.R.; Cao, X.; Dhanasekaran, S.M.; Khan, A.P.; Quist, M.J.; Jing, X.; Lonigro, R.J.; Brenner, J.C.; et al. The Mutational Landscape of Lethal Castration-Resistant Prostate Cancer. *Nature* **2012**, *487*, 239–243. [CrossRef]
35. Robinson, D.; Van Allen, E.M.; Wu, Y.-M.; Schultz, N.; Lonigro, R.J.; Mosquera, J.-M.; Montgomery, B.; Taplin, M.-E.; Pritchard, C.C.; Attard, G.; et al. Integrative Clinical Genomics of Advanced Prostate Cancer. *Cell* **2015**, *161*, 1215–1228. [CrossRef]
36. Djusberg, E.; Jernberg, E.; Thysell, E.; Golovleva, I.; Lundberg, P.; Crnalic, S.; Widmark, A.; Bergh, A.; Brattsand, M.; Wikström, P. High Levels of the AR-V7 Splice Variant and Co-Amplification of the Golgi Protein Coding YIPF6 in AR Amplified Prostate Cancer Bone Metastases. *Prostate* **2017**, *77*, 625–638. [CrossRef]
37. Cancer Genome Atlas Research Network. The Molecular Taxonomy of Primary Prostate Cancer. *Cell* **2015**, *163*, 1011–1025. [CrossRef]
38. Azad, A.A.; Volik, S.V.; Wyatt, A.W.; Haegert, A.; Le Bihan, S.; Bell, R.H.; Anderson, S.A.; McConeghy, B.; Shukin, R.; Bazov, J.; et al. Androgen Receptor Gene Aberrations in Circulating Cell-Free DNA: Biomarkers of Therapeutic Resistance in Castration-Resistant Prostate Cancer. *Clin. Cancer Res. Off. J. Am. Assoc. Cancer Res.* **2015**, *21*, 2315–2324. [CrossRef]
39. Romanel, A.; Gasi Tandefelt, D.; Conteduca, V.; Jayaram, A.; Casiraghi, N.; Wetterskog, D.; Salvi, S.; Amadori, D.; Zafeiriou, Z.; Rescigno, P.; et al. Plasma AR and Abiraterone-Resistant Prostate Cancer. *Sci. Transl. Med.* **2015**, *7*, 312re10. [CrossRef]
40. Sweeney, P.L.; Lanka, S.M.; Jang, A.; Gupta, K.; Caputo, S.; Casado, C.; Huang, M.; Pocha, O.; Hawkins, M.; Lieberman, A.; et al. Analysis of TP53 Gain of Function Mutations in Metastatic Castration-Resistant Prostate Cancer. *J. Clin. Oncol.* **2023**, *41*, 246. [CrossRef]
41. Maxwell, K.N.; Cheng, H.H.; Powers, J.; Gulati, R.; Ledet, E.M.; Morrison, C.; Le, A.; Hausler, R.; Stopfer, J.; Hyman, S.; et al. Inherited TP53 Variants and Risk of Prostate Cancer. *Eur. Urol.* **2022**, *81*, 243–250. [CrossRef]
42. Evans, M.J.; Smith-Jones, P.M.; Wongvipat, J.; Navarro, V.; Kim, S.; Bander, N.H.; Larson, S.M.; Sawyers, C.L. Noninvasive Measurement of Androgen Receptor Signaling with a Positron-Emitting Radiopharmaceutical That Targets Prostate-Specific Membrane Antigen. *Proc. Natl. Acad. Sci. USA* **2011**, *108*, 9578–9582. [CrossRef]
43. Sartor, O.; de Bono, J.; Chi, K.N.; Fizazi, K.; Herrmann, K.; Rahbar, K.; Tagawa, S.T.; Nordquist, L.T.; Vaishampayan, N.; El-Haddad, G.; et al. Lutetium-177-PSMA-617 for Metastatic Castration-Resistant Prostate Cancer. *N. Engl. J. Med.* **2021**, *385*, 1091–1103. [CrossRef]

Disclaimer/Publisher's Note: The statements, opinions and data contained in all publications are solely those of the individual author(s) and contributor(s) and not of MDPI and/or the editor(s). MDPI and/or the editor(s) disclaim responsibility for any injury to people or property resulting from any ideas, methods, instructions or products referred to in the content.

MDPI AG
Grosspeteranlage 5
4052 Basel
Switzerland
Tel.: +41 61 683 77 34

MDPI Books Editorial Office
E-mail: books@mdpi.com
www.mdpi.com/books

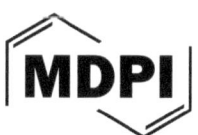

Disclaimer/Publisher's Note: The title and front matter of this reprint are at the discretion of the Topic Editors. The publisher is not responsible for their content or any associated concerns. The statements, opinions and data contained in all individual articles are solely those of the individual Editors and contributors and not of MDPI. MDPI disclaims responsibility for any injury to people or property resulting from any ideas, methods, instructions or products referred to in the content.

www.ingramcontent.com/pod-product-compliance
Lightning Source LLC
LaVergne TN
LVHW072344090526
838202LV00019B/2479